Gynecologic Cancer

Guest Editor

ROSS S. BERKOWITZ, MD

HEMATOLOGY/ONCOLOGY CLINICS OF NORTH AMERICA

www.hemonc.theclinics.com

Consulting Editors
GEORGE P. CANELLOS, MD
NANCY BERLINER, MD

February 2012 • Volume 26 • Number 1

SAUNDERS an imprint of ELSEVIER, Inc.

W.B. SAUNDERS COMPANY
A Division of Elsevier Inc.

1600 John F. Kennedy Blvd. • Suite 1800 • Philadelphia, PA 19103-2899

http://www.theclinics.com

HEMATOLOGY/ONCOLOGY CLINICS OF NORTH AMERICA Volume 26, Number 1
February 2012 ISSN 0889-8588, ISBN 13: 978-1-4557-3874-8

Editor: Patrick Manley
Developmental Editor: Donald Mumford

Hematology/Oncology Clinics (ISSN 0889-8588) is published bimonthly by Elsevier Inc., 360 Park Avenue South, New York, NY 10010-1710. Months of issue are February, April, June, August, October, and December. Business and Editorial Offices: 1600 John F. Kennedy Blvd., Ste. 1800, Philadelphia, PA 19103-2899. Customer Service Office: 3251 Riverport Lane, Maryland Heights, MO 63043. Periodicals postage paid at New York, NY and at additional mailing offices. Subscription prices are $353.00 per year (domestic individuals), $576.00 per year (domestic institutions), $173.00 per year (domestic students/residents), $401.00 per year (Canadian individuals), $705.00 per year (Canadian institutions) $477.00 per year (international individuals), $705.00 per year (international institutions), and $233.00 per year (international and Canadian students/residents). International air speed delivery is included in all *Clinics* subscription prices. All prices are subject to change without notice. **POSTMASTER:** Send address changes to *Hematology/Oncology Clinics of North America*, Elsevier Health Sciences Division, Subscription Customer Service, 3251 Riverport Lane, Maryland Heights, MO 63043. Customer Service (orders, claims, online, change of address): Elsevier Health Sciences Division, Subscription Customer Service, 3251 Riverport Lane, Maryland Heights, MO 63043. Tel: 1-800-654-2452 (U.S. and Canada); 314-447-8871 (outside U.S. and Canada). Fax: 314-447-8029. E-mail: journalscustomerservice-usa@elsevier.com (for print support); journalsonlinesupport-usa@elsevier.com (for online support).

Reprints. For copies of 100 or more, of articles in this publication, please contact the Commercial Reprints Department, Elsevier Inc., 360 Park Avenue South, New York, New York 10010-1710; Tel.: 212-633-3813, Fax: 212-462-1935, E-mail: reprints@elsevier.com.

Hematology/Oncology Clinics of North America is covered in *MEDLINE/PubMed (Index Medicus), EMBASE/ Excerpta Medica, and BIOSIS.*

Printed in the United States of America.

Contributors

CONSULTING EDITORS

GEORGE P. CANELLOS, MD
William Rosenberg Professor of Medicine, Department of Medical Oncology, Dana-Farber Cancer Institute, Boston, Massachusetts

NANCY BERLINER, MD
Chief, Division of Hematology, Brigham and Women's Hospital; Professor of Medicine, Harvard Medical School, Boston, Massachusetts

GUEST EDITOR

ROSS S. BERKOWITZ, MD
William H. Baker Professor of Gynecology, Harvard Medical School, Director of Gynecology and Gynecologic Oncology, Brigham and Women's Hospital and Dana Farber Cancer Institute, Boston, Massachusetts

AUTHORS

RICHARD R. BARAKAT, MD
Chief, Gynecology Service, Vice Chairman Clinical Affairs, Department of Surgery, Memorial Sloan-Kettering Cancer Center, New York, New York

JONATHAN S. BEREK, MD, MMS
Professor and Director, Stanford Women's Cancer Center, Stanford Cancer Institute; Chair, Department of Obstetrics & Gynecology, Stanford University School of Medicine, Stanford, California

JESSICA L. BERGER, MD
Chief Resident, Department of Obstetrics and Gynecology, Banner Good Samaritan Medical Center, Phoenix, Arizona

ROSS S. BERKOWITZ, MD
William H. Baker Professor of Gynecology, Harvard Medical School, Director of Gynecology and Gynecologic Oncology, Brigham and Women's Hospital and Dana Farber Cancer Institute, Boston, Massachusetts

JEANNE CARTER, PhD
Assistant Attending, Gynecology Service, Departments of Surgery, and Psychiatry and Behavioral Sciences, Memorial Sloan-Kettering Cancer Center, New York, New York

DENNIS S. CHI, MD
Deputy Chief, Gynecology Service, Memorial Sloan-Kettering Cancer Center, New York, New York

DANIEL W. CRAMER, MD, ScD
Professor of Obstetrics, Gynecology and Reproductive Medicine, Department of Obstetrics and Gynecology, Brigham and Women's Hospital, Obstetrics and Gynecology Epidemiology Center, Boston, Massachusetts

DANIEL ECHELMAN, AB
Women's Cancer Program, Dana Farber Cancer Institute, Boston, Massachusetts

M. HEATHER EINSTEIN, MD, MS
Assistant Professor, Division of Gynecologic Oncology, Hartford Hospital, University of Connecticut, Hartford, Connecticut

ERIC E. EISENHAUER, MD
Assistant Professor, The Ohio State University, Columbus, Ohio

SARAH FELDMAN, MD, MPH
Division of Gynecologic Oncology, Brigham and Women's Hospital, Dana Farber Cancer Institute, Harvard Medical School, Boston, Massachusetts

KATHERINE C. FUH, MD
Fellow and Clinical Instructor, Division of Gynecologic Oncology, Department of Obstetrics and Gynecology, Stanford University School of Medicine, Stanford, California

DONALD PETER GOLDSTEIN, MD
Professor of Obstetrics, Gynecology and Reproductive Biology, Harvard Medical School; Division of Gynecologic Oncology, New England Trophoblastic Disease Center, Dana Farber/Brigham and Women's Cancer Center, Boston, Massachusetts

LAURA L. HOLMAN, MD
Fellow, Department of Gynecologic Oncology and Reproductive Medicine, The University of Texas MD Anderson Cancer Center, Houston, Texas

NEIL HOROWITZ, MD
Assistant Professor of Obstetrics and Gynecology, Harvard Medical School; Director of Clinical Research, Division of Gynecologic Oncology, Department of Obstetrics and Gynecology, Brigham and Women's Hospital, Boston, Massachusetts

KAREN H. LU, MD
Professor, Department of Gynecologic Oncology and Reproductive Medicine, The University of Texas MD Anderson Cancer Center, Houston, Texas

URSULA A. MATULONIS, MD
Director and Program Leader, Medical Gynecologic Oncology, Department of Medical Oncology; Associate Professor of Medicine, Harvard Medical School, Boston, Massachusetts

RICHARD PENSON, MD, MRCP
Clinical Director, Medical Gynecologic Oncology; Associate Professor, Harvard Medical School, Massachusetts General Hospital, Boston, Massachusetts

PEDRO T. RAMIREZ, MD
Professor, Director of Minimally Invasive Surgical Research and Education, Department of Gynecologic Oncology, University of Texas MD Anderson Cancer Center, Houston, Texas

LAUREL W. RICE, MD
Professor and Chair, Division of Gynecologic Oncology, Department of Obstetrics and Gynecology, Paul B. Carbone Cancer Center, University of Wisconsin, Madison, Wisconsin

JOHN O. SCHORGE, MD
Chief, Gynecologic Oncology, Massachusetts General Hospital, Harvard Medical School, Boston, Massachusetts

AKILA N. VISWANATHAN, MD, MPH
Associate Professor of Radiation Oncology, Department of Radiation Oncology, Brigham and Women's Hospital, Boston, Massachusetts

LARI WENZEL, PhD
Professor, Department of Medicine and Public Health, University of California, Irvine, Irvine, California

Contents

Late menarche, giving birth, breastfeeding, oral contraceptive use, IUD use, and tubal ligation decrease risk for both endometrial and ovarian cancer, while more ovulatory cycles, obesity, use of talc in genital hygiene, and late menopause increase risk. Despite these similarities, different explanations are proposed: estrogen excess for endometrial and incessant ovulation for ovarian cancer. Common pathways could include reproductive tissue turnover with accumulation of *PTEN* or p53 mutations or an immune-based explanation involving mucin proteins. Seeking unified explanations for risk factors common to both cancers could lead to new perspectives on how to prevent these common and lethal gynecologic cancers.

Hereditary cancer syndromes are responsible for 5% of endometrial cancers and 10% of ovarian cancers. Hereditary breast and ovarian cancer syndrome and Lynch syndrome account for most of these inherited cases. Significant advances have been made in the identification and management of women with these syndromes. In addition, recent advances have highlighted the prognostic and therapeutic implications for women with gynecologic cancers and inherited cancer syndromes.

The incidence and mortality of cervical cancer have decreased dramatically over the past 70 years in well-developed countries through successful screening programs using cytologic examination, followed by evaluation and treatment of high-grade precancers of the cervix. In less-well-developed countries, cervical cancer incidence and mortality remain high. However, moving forward, a combination of the human papillomavirus (HPV) vaccine, new HPV screening capability, and simple see-and-treat techniques may help to decrease the cervical cancer burden in these countries.

Vulvar cancer is surgically staged and is categorized by the pathologic evaluation of the vulvar tumor and the inguinofemoral lymph nodes. All tumors more invasive than 1 mm and larger than 2 cm require pathologic assessment of inguinofemoral lymph nodes. Sentinel node biopsy is an alternative to inguinofemoral lymphadenectomy in many cases that require a lymphadenectomy. Radical local excision with inguinofemoral lymph node assessment is the preferred procedure for early-stage disease. Primary neoadjuvant chemoradiation is used for most advanced-stage tumors.

Cervical cancer is the second most common cancer in women worldwide. In developed countries screening programs have decreased the incidence of this disease and improved the detection of early-stage disease amenable to surgical intervention. This article discusses the scope of surgical treatment of cervical carcinoma, including conization for the earliest-stage and lowest-risk patients, radical hysterectomy with lymphadenectomy, radical trachelectomy for appropriately selected patients who desire future fertility, and pelvic exenteration for recurrent disease. In addition, current surgical advances such as surgical staging methods and minimally invasive approaches are discussed.

Despite being the most common gynecologic cancer in developed countries, there are many unanswered questions regarding optimal surgical management of endometrial cancer, including who should undergo surgical staging. There is evidence supporting the lower complication rate achieved with laparoscopic surgery compared with traditional open staging and building evidence to support laparoscopic-assisted robotic surgery for early endometrial cancer. Surgery plays an important role in the treatment of advanced stage disease, with retrospective studies showing some benefit to optimal cytoreduction. This review discusses the role of surgery in the management of endometrial cancer, with an emphasis on current controversies.

Surgical management of ovarian cancer requires excellent judgment and mastery of a wide array of procedures. Involvement of a gynecologic oncologist improves outcomes. Staging of apparent stage I disease is important. Minimally invasive techniques provide advantages. Primary debulking surgery provides the best long-term survival of any strategy in advanced ovarian cancer. Aggressive surgical paradigms have the greatest success. Further cytoreductive surgery may be appropriate. Most relapsed patients require management of bowel obstruction at some point. Palliative intervention can enhance quality of life. Surgical correction may extend survival. For end-stage patients with progressive disease, the treating gynecologic oncologist must manage expectations.

Gestational trophoblastic neoplasms are malignant lesions that arise from placental villous and extravillous trophoblast. Four clinicopathologic conditions make up this entity: invasive mole (IM), choriocarcinoma (CCA), placental-site trophoblastic tumor (PSTT), and epithelioid trophoblastic tumor (ETT). IM and CCA, which make up the majority of these tumors, are highly responsive to chemotherapy with an overall cure rate exceeding 90%, making it usually possible to achieve cure while preserving reproductive function. PSTT and ETT, which rarely occur, are relatively resistant to chemotherapy, making surgery the primary treatment modality, chemotherapy being used only when the disease has metastasized.

THE CLINICS ARE NOW AVAILABLE ONLINE!

Access your subscription at:
www.theclinics.com

Preface

Gynecologic Cancer

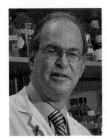

Ross S. Berkowitz, MD
Guest Editor

Like many areas in oncology, gynecologic oncology has made several important recent advances in both the prevention and the treatment of reproductive malignancies. New knowledge related to risk factors for endometrial and ovarian cancer has led to novel strategies to reduce risks through diet, contraception choices, and other factors. Important advances have also occurred in the understanding of genetic risks for gynecologic cancers and genetic testing can now identify individuals at substantial risk. Patients at genetic risk can reduce their risk through the use of oral contraception and other choices if they have not completed their families or undergo definitive prophylactic surgery when they no longer desire future pregnancies. Cervical cancer is an area of particular advancement in prevention due to cytologic screening, human papillomavirus (HPV) testing, and HPV vaccination. Globally, cervical cancer can be dramatically reduced with currently available technology. An important area in the innovative treatment of gynecologic malignancy is the application of new findings concerning the molecular biology of these cancers and utilizing new biologic therapies. Both surgical and radiation therapy have made important progress in using new technologies such as minimally invasive surgery and radiologic imaging to guide radiation treatment to maintain high cure rates while minimizing morbidity. The desire to assure that the quality of the life of patients is importantly considered in all treatment decisions has been strengthened by the increased interest and valuation of quality-of-life research in gynecologic cancer. Gynecologic oncology is strongly committed to maintaining and improving cure rates while limiting the morbidity of therapy and considering all aspects of patients' well-being including emotional and sexual health in treatment decisions.

This issue of the *Hematology/Oncology Clinics of North America* provides both a broad and an in-depth review of the many important advances that have occurred in gynecologic cancer in recent years. I would like to thank all of the contributors due to their scholarly and thoughtful contributions. While much progress has been made,

Hematol Oncol Clin N Am 26 (2012) xi–xii
doi:10.1016/j.hoc.2011.12.001
0889-8588/12/$ – see front matter © 2012 Elsevier Inc. All rights reserved.

much more progress needs to be achieved. The enclosed articles not only insightfully review current progress but also point to a better future where less women suffer from reproductive malignancy.

Ross S. Berkowitz, MD
Harvard Medical School
Brigham and Women's Hospital and
Dana Farber Cancer Institute
75 Francis Street
Boston, MA 02115, USA

E-mail address:
Ross_Berkowitz@dfci.harvard.edu

The Epidemiology of Endometrial and Ovarian Cancer

Daniel W. Cramer, MD, ScD

KEYWORDS

- Ovarian cancer • Endometrial cancer • Tumor heterogeneity
- Risk factors

The epidemiology of ovarian cancer and endometrial cancer is closely entwined. Age-specific incidence curves and the international rates for both sites parallel each other, and histologic subtypes of cancer arising from the endometrium mirror types found in the ovary. Most of the personal factors that increase or decrease risk for one of these cancers act in the same direction for the other. For these reasons, this article considers the epidemiology of ovarian and endometrial cancer together, with the goal of providing a more unified perspective. The author does not address the epidemiology of cervical cancer in this article, though this is not for lack of importance. Worldwide cervical cancer is a greater source of morbidity and mortality than endometrial and ovarian cancer combined (**Table 1**). However, there are far fewer epidemiologic uncertainties related to cervical cancer, and the means of its prevention and early detection are in hand, if not yet fully implemented where they are most needed.

TUMOR HETEROGENEITY AS IT MAY AFFECT EPIDEMIOLOGIC ASSOCIATIONS

Before discussing the epidemiology of endometrial and ovarian cancer, it must be pointed out that neither of these cancers is homogeneous from a histopathologic standpoint. Cancer registries often include endometrial cancer under the broader category "cancers of the uterine corpus," which includes sarcomas that arise from the endometrial stroma or from the smooth muscle of the uterus. Adenocarcinomas comprise the vast majority of cancers of the uterine corpus, and most epidemiologic studies are restricted to these. In turn, endometrial adenocarcinomas may be further subdivided, with endometrioid (or Type I) cancers accounting for majority, about 85%, and the remainder designated Type II and including adenosquamous, serous papillary, clear cell, and undifferentiated types, similar to those found in the ovary.[1,2]

This work was supported by NIH Grant U01CA086381, and P50CA105009.
Department of Obstetrics and Gynecology, Obstetrics and Gynecology Epidemiology Center, Brigham and Women's Hospital, 221 Longwood Avenue RFB 365, Boston, MA 02115, USA
E-mail address: DCRAMER@PARTNERS.ORG

Hematol Oncol Clin N Am 26 (2012) 1–12
doi:10.1016/j.hoc.2011.10.009
0889-8588/12/$ – see front matter © 2012 Elsevier Inc. All rights reserved.

Table 1
Age-adjusted incidence rates[a] for endometrial and ovarian cancers in different regions of the world

Region	Incidence			Mortality		
	Cervix	Endometrium	Ovary	Cervix	Endometrium	Ovary
World	15.3	8.2	6.3	7.8	2.0	3.8
More developed regions	9.1	13.0	9.3	3.1	2.3	5.1
Less developed regions	17.8	5.9	5.0	9.8	1.7	3.1
Eastern Africa	34.5	2.4	4.0	25.3	0.8	3.3
Middle Africa	23.0	1.9	4.3	17.0	0.7	3.6
Northern Africa	6.6	2.2	4.8	4.0	0.7	3.7
Southern Africa	26.8	6.9	3.8	14.8	2.1	2.8
Western Africa	33.7	1.9	3.8	24.0	0.7	3.1
Caribbean	20.8	9.0	4.3	9.4	3.3	2.7
Central America	22.2	6.1	5.2	11.1	2.5	3.4
South America	24.1	4.4	6.2	10.8	1.7	3.4
Northern America	5.7	16.4	8.7	1.7	2.4	5.4
Eastern Asia	9.6	10.3	4.3	3.9	2.2	1.8
South-Eastern Asia	15.8	5.7	6.6	8.3	2.0	4.4
South-Central Asia	24.6	2.1	5.5	14.1	1.1	4.1
Western Asia	4.5	5.6	4.8	2.1	1.5	3.6
Central and Eastern Europe	14.7	14.6	11.0	6.2	3.4	5.9
Northern Europe	8.4	13.8	11.8	2.5	2.2	6.5
Southern Europe	8.1	10.4	8.4	2.5	1.9	4.2
Western Europe	6.9	11.2	8.9	2.0	1.8	4.9
Oceania	8.0	10.8	7.6	3.6	1.7	4.7
Australia/New Zealand	5.0	11.5	7.8	1.4	1.6	4.6
Melanesia	23.7	5.2	5.1	16.6	2.0	4.2
Micronesia	9.5	8.0	6.1	3.4	5.3	5.2
Polynesia	16.7	11.5	5.0	6.0	2.6	3.8

[a] Age-adjusted incidence rates are per 100,000 and are adjusted to the World Standard.
Data from Ferley J, Shin HR, Bray F, et al. GLOBOCAN 2008 v1.2, cancer incidence and mortality worldwide: IARC cancer base no. 10. Lyon (France): International Agency for Research on Cancer; 2010. Available at: http://globocan.iarc.fr. Accessed October 5, 2011.

There is an even greater degree of heterogeneity for ovarian cancer. Ovarian malignancies may arise from germ cell, stromal, or epithelial compartments. Counting benign neoplasms, about 25% of all ovarian tumors are of germ cell origin. Most common is the mature teratoma (dermoid), which accounts for nearly one-third of all benign ovarian neoplasms, but only 2% to 3% of germ cell tumors are malignant.[3] Ovarian stromal tumors account for 6% of all benign and malignant ovarian tumors with the most common being the granulosa cell tumor, which accounts for approximately 10% of malignant ovarian cancers. The most common types of malignant ovarian cancers are epithelial and parallel the same types arising in the endometrium. Four major histologic subtypes of epithelial ovarian cancer have been described, each resembling different types of epithelia found in the female reproductive tract.[4] Features associated with fallopian tube, endocervical epithelium, or endometrial epithelium are observed in serous, mucinous, and endometrioid forms of ovarian cancer, respectively. Clear cell tumors are the fourth major histologic subtype and are identified by clear, peglike cells that resemble the lining of the endometrial glands during pregnancy. The majority of malignant ovarian tumors fall into the invasive serous category followed by endometrioid, clear cell, and mucinous types.

A distinction made for ovarian cancer that does not have an exact parallel in endometrial cancer is the designation of borderline or low malignant potential (LMP) ovarian tumor types that may spread beyond the ovary, yet generally have an indolent course and account for about 17% to 18% of ovarian cancers. The Surveillance, Epidemiology, and End Result (SEER) agency at the National Cancer Institute decided to no longer count LMP ovarian tumors as cancers after January 1, 2004. As a consequence, about a 20% "decrease" in the incidence of ovarian cancer and a 5% decrease in mortality occurred between 2004 and 2006.

In conclusion, then, epidemiologic patterns observed for endometrial cancer are most likely to pertain to the Type I cancers whereas those for ovarian cancer tend toward invasive serous. However, because of the greater heterogeneity of ovarian cancer, the mix of cases from study to study may influence epidemiologic associations reported for ovarian cancer, especially if LMP tumors are included.

AGE AND GEOGRAPHIC DISTRIBUTION

In the United States endometrial cancer is the most common gynecologic cancer, accounting for 40,100 new cases and 7470 deaths.[5] Ovarian cancer accounts for fewer cases (21,650) but more deaths (15,520).[5] Ovarian cancer is the leading cause of death from a gynecologic cancer and the fifth leading cause of cancer deaths overall in the United States. Endometrial and ovarian cancer share similar patterns of distribution by age and geography. The incidence of both cancers increases sharply during the perimenopausal years and reaches a peak well after the menopause (**Fig. 1**). Endometrial cancer rates drop after age 70 years, but ovarian cancer rates continue

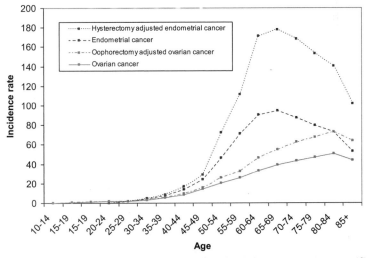

Fig. 1. Age-specific incidence rates of endometrial and ovarian cancers. Age-specific cancer incidence rates are per 100,000 and are age-adjusted. Rates include all races and pertain to invasive cancers only. (*Data from* Ries L, Melbert D, Krapcho M, et al. SEER cancer statistics review, 1975–2005. 2008. Available at: http://seer.cancer.gov/csr/1975_2005.)

to increase into a woman's eighties. It should be appreciated that the age-specific rates for ovarian cancer calculated by SEER are based on the entire United States population of females, including those who have had hysterectomy or hysterectomy and oophorectomy.[6] Except when the surgery was done for endometrial or ovarian cancer, women who have had such operations are virtually at no future risk for these cancers. For this reason it is estimated that rates overall are about 33% higher for endometrial cancer and about 15% higher for ovarian cancer, although the exact percentages differ somewhat by age.[7] The corresponding dashed lines in **Fig. 1** illustrate the predicted higher incidence rates for women who still have their uterus or ovaries. Using these corrected incidence rates, the lifetime risk for endometrial cancer is about 5.7% if women with hysterectomy for benign conditions are excluded and about 2.5% for ovarian cancer if women with hysterectomy and oophorectomy are excluded.

Worldwide, higher rates of endometrial and ovarian cancer are observed in industrialized and northern European populations, and lower rates in Third World countries (**Table 1**).[8] There is a positive correlation between the occurrence of endometrial cancer and ovarian cancer that is significant (Pearson correlation = 0.76, $P<.001$). For comparison, the rates of cervical cancer are also shown, and are inversely correlated with both endometrial cancer (Pearson correlation = -0.64, $P<.001$) and ovarian cancer (Pearson correlation = -0.57, $P = .003$).

RISK FACTORS

This section considers personal risk factors for endometrial and ovarian cancers organized under the following headings: menstrual and reproductive events, medical history, and habits and environment (**Table 2**). Genetic risk for these cancers is treated in a separate article by Karen Lu elsewhere in this issue.

Menstrual and Reproductive Events

Personal risk factors for endometrial and ovarian cancer often operate in the same direction, and many of these relate to menstrual and reproductive events. Factors that decrease risk for both endometrial and ovarian cancer include a late age at menarche,[9,10] early age at first birth[9–12] as well as last pregnancy at a later age,[12–14] a greater number of children,[9–14] and longer period of breastfeeding children.[15–19] With the exception of estrogen-dominant sequential oral contraceptives, which have been linked to endometrial cancer, in case reports[20] longer use of combination oral contraceptives reduces the risk for both endometrial and ovarian cancer.[21–24] Short or irregular cycles[9,10] and a late age at menopause are associated with increased risk for both endometrial cancer and ovarian cancers.[13,25] These events can be fit into a composite variable that estimates years of ovulation or, when average cycle length is included, number of ovulatory cycles. An increasing number of ovulatory cycles clearly correlates with increased risk for ovarian cancer.[26,27] Though less well studied, ovulatory cycles also appear to correlate directly with endometrial cancer risk.[28]

Despite the appeal of an ovulatory cycles model for consolidating many of the reproductive factors, it is also true that other contraceptive methods not associated with cessation of ovulation may also affect endometrial and ovarian cancer. Intrauterine device (IUD) use, even hormonally inert types, decreases the risk for endometrial cancer,[29,30] and studies suggest that IUD use (at least short term) may also decrease the risk for ovarian cancer.[31,32] Similarly, tubal ligation is a strong protective risk factor for ovarian cancer that may also decrease the risk for endometrial

Table 2
Risk factors for endometrial, breast, and ovarian cancers[a]

Factor	Endometrium	Ovary	References
Menstrual and Reproductive Events			
Late age at menarche	↓	↓	9,10
Short or irregular cycle lengths	↑	↑	9,10
Late age at menopause	↑	↑	13,25
Early age at first birth or late age at last birth	↓	↓	9–14
More children	↓	↓	9–14
Breastfeeding	↓	↓	15–19
Oral contraceptive use	↓	↓	21–24
Greater number of ovulatory cycles	↑	↑	26–28
Intrauterine device use	↓	↓	29,32
Tubal ligation	↓	↓	33–36
Menopausal hormones, especially estrogen only	↑	↑	37–42
Medical Events			
High body mass index	↑	↑	43,45–48
Polycystic ovarian syndrome	↑	↑	49–51
History of bone fracture	↓	↓	32,52,53
Systemic lupus erythematosus	↓	↓	54
Habits and Environment			
Smoking	↓	↑[b]	55,56
Talc use	↑	↑	57,58
Physical activity/exercise	↓	↓	59–62

[a] Increased risk is indicated by ↑, decreased risk by ↓.
[b] Only for mucinous types of ovarian cancer.
 Data from Bokhman JV. Two pathogenetic types of endometrial carcinoma. Gynecol Oncol 1983;15(1):10–7.

cancer.[33–36] Another risk factor for endometrial and ovarian cancer is menopausal hormone use, with higher risk largely confined to users of estrogen-only forms unopposed by a progestin.[37–42]

Medical History

High body mass index (BMI) is a well-established risk factor for Type I endometrial cancer and has been linked to elevated levels of estrogen, particularly in postmenopausal women for whom adipose tissue is the main site of estrogen production from androgen precursors.[43–45] High BMI also appears to be associated with increased ovarian cancer risk, possibly through similar hormonal mechanisms, although the risk is not as strong as that for endometrial cancer.[46–48] Polycystic ovarian syndrome, a condition characterized by ovarian hyperandrogenism, chronic anovulation, and progesterone deficiency, has also been associated with increased risk for both ovarian and endometrial cancer.[49–51] A history of bone fracture may decrease the risk for endometrial and possibly ovarian cancer[32,52,53] and may reflect long-term hypoestrogenic status. For reasons not entirely clear, systemic lupus erythematosus may decrease the risk for endometrial and ovarian cancer.[54]

Habits and Environmental Factors

Current smoking is associated with a reduced risk for endometrial cancer, particularly in postmenopausal women, possibly due to the antiestrogenic effects of smoking such as reduced body weight, lower age at menopause, and differences in estrogen metabolism.[55] Current smoking has also been associated with a decreased risk for clear cell ovarian tumors; however, no association was observed with serous and endometrioid tumors, and smoking doubled the risk of mucinous ovarian cancers.[56] Talc use is another factor found to consistently increase the risk for ovarian cancer[57] and has been recently reported to increase the risk for endometrial cancer as well,[58] raising intriguing questions related to the pathogenic mechanism underlying these associations. Increased exercise and physical activity decreases the risk for endometrial[59–61] and possibly ovarian cancer.[62]

In summary, this brief review of epidemiologic risk factors for endometrial and ovarian cancers reveals a surprising number of similarities, which suggests that there are also shared mechanisms in their pathogenesis.

MECHANISMS

An ultimate goal of epidemiology is to clarify the biological basis for observations made about a disease, leading to a better understanding of its pathogenesis and strategies for its control. For endometrial cancer, it has been accepted for many years that its epidemiology is largely explained by conditions that lead to an excess of estrogen relative to progesterone. A natural experiment that tested this explanation was the increase in endometrial cancer incidence that followed the increased use of unopposed estrogen to treat menopausal symptoms during the 1970s.[63] The strong link between obesity and endometrial cancer is likely explained by the fact that fat possesses aromatase capable of converting androstenedione into estrone, a biologically active estrogen.[43] That endometrial cancer increases dramatically during the perimenopause when anovulatory cycles become more common provides further physiologic support. The protective effect of smoking on endometrial cancer risk may relate to the possible antiestrogenic effects of smoking. However, it is more difficult to explain how estrogen excess fits with the association between endometrial cancer and ovulatory cycles, and even less clear how IUD use, tubal ligation, or talc use fits with estrogen excess.

The most popular explanation for ovarian cancer risk factors is the "incessant ovulation" theory,[64] and this may be relevant to the connection between ovulatory cycles and endometrial cancer. For ovarian cancer, it has been proposed that the monthly disruption and repair of the surface epithelium of the ovary may lead to genetic damage due to the accumulation of mutations of the tumor suppressor, p53, in the ovarian and, possibly, fallopian tube epithelium[65,66]; however, this mechanism would not explain the association with endometrial cancer. One possibility is that incessant ovulation largely equates with incessant menstruation, involving repeated disruption and regrowth of the uterine lining. A greater number of cycles of endometrial regeneration may increase the likelihood of random genetic mutations because DNA replication errors occur during cell division, and thus are more likely to occur in tissues undergoing many cell divisions. Estimates of the rate of sporadic mutagenesis in human cells, on the order of 10^{-7} mutations per gene per cell division,[67] suggest that the number of cells with "first hits" on a multistep carcinogenesis pathway[68] may number in the hundreds for every gram (10^9 cells/g) of proliferative tissue. It is no surprise, then, to find that sporadic mutations of another tumor suppressor gene, *PTEN*, are observed in almost half (43%) of histologically normal endometria of naturally cycling premenopausal women.[69] Thus, accumulation of mutations in p53 or PTEN associated with reproductive tissue turnover could be the common explanation that links ovulatory cycles with risk for both endometrial and ovarian cancer.

Another popular theory offered to explain ovarian cancer risk factors is inflammation associated with ovulation, talc use, or endometriosis.[70] This theory could explain why tubal ligation would be protective by blocking talc or menstrual debris from reaching the ovaries. However, this theory would not explain why tubal ligation may also protect against endometrial cancer or why IUD use protects against endometrial and possibly ovarian cancer as well. No existing theory readily explains an inverse association between mumps (parotitis) and ovarian cancer reported in early studies.[71,72]

Recently, the author's group proposed a new paradigm[32] for ovarian cancer that may also explain aspects of endometrial cancer risk. Risk factors for ovarian cancer may be determined by factors affecting the immune system: acute events in younger life that primed the immune system to recognize and eliminate ovarian cancer precursors, and/or chronic events that led to persistent antigen challenge and immune tolerance of an emerging cancer.[32] The acute events include mumps, mastitis, tubal ligation, and others that affect tissues which express surface glycoproteins known as mucins (MUC), especially MUC1, including salivary glands, breast ducts, fallopian tubes, and others. Normally MUC1 is expressed at low levels in a highly glycosylated form, whereas in cancer, MUC1 is expressed at high levels in a less glycosylated form whereby backbone peptides are exposed to the immune system and evoke anti-MUC1 antibodies described in a variety of cancers[73] as well as certain inflammatory conditions such as ulcerative colitis.[74] The "inflammatory" form of MUC1 is similar to the tumorlike form of MUC1, and hence might prime the immune system to recognize nascent cancer cells or precursor lesions that express this form of MUC1.[73] The number and diversity of these acute events, their age at occurrence, and whether their benefits are negated by chronic inflammatory events determine whether effective, long-term immune surveillance is created. The chronic events, such as incessant ovulation, talc use, and endometriosis, also affect tissues that express MUC1 and may also lead to expression of an inflammatory form of mucins. However, because the events are chronic, the author hypothesizes that they lead to immune tolerance of an emerging cancer.

Supporting this theory are findings that events such as tubal ligation and mastitis, which raised anti-MUC1 antibody levels in controls from the New England Case Control study, are associated with lower risk for ovarian cancer; and, conversely, factors that decreased anti-MUC1 antibody levels (eg, talc use and estimated ovulatory cycles) increased the risk for ovarian cancer.[32,75] Prospective data from the Nurses Health Studies (NHS) confirmed the importance of tubal ligation raising antibodies and ovulatory cycles lowering them.[76] Of importance, the NHS study found that the presence of anti-MUC1 antibodies in blood drawn at least 3 years before a clinical diagnosis of ovarian cancer predicted lower risk for ovarian cancer in women younger than 64 years at blood draw. In women older than 64 at blood draw, a protective association was not apparent for two reasons. First, anti-MUC1 antibody levels in controls declined after age 64, likely due to aging of the immune system (immunosenescence), a well-described phenomenon in vaccine literature.[77] Second, it would appear that women with the lowest anti-MUC1 antibody levels may develop ovarian cancer soonest, leaving older women destined to develop ovarian cancer with relatively higher (but ineffective) levels of antibodies. As a final piece of evidence, the author and colleagues[78] found that individuals going through a mumps infection have significantly higher anti-MUC1 antibody levels than blood-bank or community controls, providing evidence that mumps may have exerted its protective effect through MUC1 immunity.

In summary, reproductive tissue turnover and mucin-related immunity both offer more comprehensive explanations for endometrial and ovarian cancer risk factors than the separate models currently proposed. As Cramer and Finn[79] recently argued in an article addressing immune surveillance in cancer, an appeal of an immune-based model is that it is capable of explaining risk factors for many types of cancer based on possible deleterious effects of aging, obesity, smoking, lack of childhood illness, and even talc use on the immune system.

STRATEGIES FOR PREVENTION

Epidemiologists are primarily concerned with ways to prevent disease from occurring in the first place or detecting the disease at an earlier stage so that it can be more successfully treated. Because many of the risk factors for endometrial and ovarian cancer are similar, suggestions for preventing endometrial cancer may pertain to ovarian cancer as well. Maintenance of a healthy weight and a lifetime commitment to exercise would be beneficial in the prevention of both ovarian and endometrial cancer. Breastfeeding after pregnancy and use of birth-control pills are two equally important recommendations to reduce risk. Avoiding talc in pelvic hygiene is good advice to women to lower ovarian cancer risk, which may also help lower endometrial cancer risk. Many women come to hysterectomy for benign conditions and are obviously no longer at risk for endometrial cancer. Careful selection of women for incidental oophorectomy would prevent them from developing ovarian cancer as well. The author's group have recently described a risk-scoring scheme to help physicians and patients decide who might be advised to have an oophorectomy.[80]

There are currently no recommendations regarding general population screening for either endometrial or ovarian cancer, although screening may be warranted in groups at high risk for ovarian or endometrial cancer. Should more sensitive and specific screening tests become available, the sharply rising incidence of these cancers in the 50- to 65-year age range suggests this would be a good age group to target screening efforts.

SUMMARY

This review highlights similarities in the epidemiology of endometrial and ovarian cancer, including highly correlated incidence rates and similar risk factor profiles. Factors that decrease risk for both cancers include a late menarche, early age at first birth, giving birth and breastfeeding, and use of oral contraceptives. Short or irregular cycles and late menopause are associated with increased risk for both. Other risk factors that appear to operate in a similar direction include decreased risk associated with IUD use or a tubal ligation, and increased risk associated with obesity, lack of exercise, and use of talc powders in genital hygiene. Estrogen excess is proposed as the underlying mechanism for most endometrial cancers, whereas incessant ovulation has been suggested as the explanation for ovarian cancer. However, an increased number of estimated ovulatory cycles correlates directly with risk for both endometrial and ovarian cancer, suggesting that reproductive tissue turnover with an accumulation of *PTEN* or p53 mutations represents a possible common mechanism. An immune-based explanation involving mucin proteins represents another common mechanism that could explain additional risk factors. Maintenance of ideal weight, breastfeeding children, use of oral contraceptives, and avoidance of talc powders in genital hygiene are measures that could lower the risk for both types of cancer. Careful selection of patients for prophylactic oophorectomy for those women who are coming to hysterectomy for benign disease is an additional measure to consider for ovarian cancer.

REFERENCES

1. Bokhman JV. Two pathogenetic types of endometrial carcinoma. Gynecol Oncol 1983;15(1):10–7.
2. Deligdisch L, Holinka CF. Endometrial carcinoma: two diseases? Cancer Detect Prev 1987;10(3–4):237–46.
3. Scully R. Tumors of the ovary and maldeveloped gonads. Vol Second Series. Washington, DC: Armed Forces Institute of Pathology; 1979.
4. Russell P. Surface epithelial-stromal tumors of the ovary. In: Kurman RJ, editor. Blaustein's pathology of the female genital tract. 4th edition. New York: Springer-Verlag; 1994. p. 705–82.
5. American Cancer Society. Cancer Facts & Figures, 2008, Atlanta: American Cancer Society; 2008.
6. Ries L, Melbert D, Krapcho M, et al. SEER Cancer statistics review, 1975-2005. 2008. Available at: http://seer.cancer.gov/csr/1975_2005. Accessed May 10, 2011.
7. Merrill RM. Impact of hysterectomy and bilateral oophorectomy on race-specific rates of corpus, cervical, and ovarian cancers in the United States. Ann Epidemiol 2006;16(12):880–7.
8. Ferley J, Shin HR, Bray F, et al. GLOBOCAN 2008 v1.2, cancer incidence and mortality worldwide: IARC cancer base no. 10. Lyon (France): International Agency for Research on Cancer; 2010. Available at: http://globocan.iarc.fr. Accessed October 5, 2011.
9. Brinton LA, Berman ML, Mortel R, et al. Reproductive, menstrual, and medical risk factors for endometrial cancer: results from a case-control study. Am J Obstet Gynecol 1992;167(5):1317–25.
10. Titus-Ernstoff L, Perez K, Cramer DW, et al. Menstrual and reproductive factors in relation to ovarian cancer risk. Br J Cancer 2001;84(5):714–21.
11. Henderson BE, Casagrande JT, Pike MC, et al. The epidemiology of endometrial cancer in young women. Br J Cancer 1983;47(6):749–56, 2011352.
12. Whittemore AS, Harris R, Itnyre J. Characteristics relating to ovarian cancer risk: collaborative analysis of 12 US case-control studies. II. Invasive epithelial ovarian cancers in white women. Collaborative Ovarian Cancer Group. Am J Epidemiol 1992;136(10):1184–203.
13. Dossus L, Allen N, Kaaks R, et al. Reproductive risk factors and endometrial cancer: the European Prospective Investigation into Cancer and Nutrition. Int J Cancer 2010;127(2):442–51.
14. Lambe M, Wuu J, Weiderpass E, et al. Childbearing at older age and endometrial cancer risk (Sweden). Cancer Causes Control 1999;10(1):43–9.
15. Newcomb PA, Trentham-Dietz A. Breast feeding practices in relation to endometrial cancer risk, USA. Cancer Causes Control 2000;11(7):663–7.
16. Okamura C, Tsubono Y, Ito K, et al. Lactation and risk of endometrial cancer in Japan: a case-control study. Tohoku J Exp Med 2006;208(2):109–15.
17. Rosenblatt KA, Thomas DB. Prolonged lactation and endometrial cancer. WHO Collaborative Study of Neoplasia and Steroid Contraceptives. Int J Epidemiol 1995;24(3):499–503.

18. Salazar-Martinez E, Lazcano-Ponce EC, Gonzalez Lira-Lira G, et al. Reproductive factors of ovarian and endometrial cancer risk in a high fertility population in Mexico. Cancer Res 1999;59(15):3658–62.
19. Siskind V, Green A, Bain C, et al. Breastfeeding, menopause, and epithelial ovarian cancer. Epidemiology 1997;8(2):188–91.
20. Silverberg SG, Makowski EL. Endometrial carcinoma in young women taking oral contraceptive agents. Obstet Gynecol 1975;46(5):503–6.
21. La Vecchia C. Oral contraceptives and ovarian cancer: an update, 1998-2004. Eur J Cancer Prev 2006;15(2):117–24.
22. Maxwell GL, Schildkraut JM, Calingaert B, et al. Progestin and estrogen potency of combination oral contraceptives and endometrial cancer risk. Gynecol Oncol 2006;103(2):535–40.
23. Schlesselman JJ. Risk of endometrial cancer in relation to use of combined oral contraceptives. A practitioner's guide to meta-analysis. Hum Reprod 1997;12(9): 1851–63.
24. Weiderpass E, Adami HO, Baron JA, et al. Use of oral contraceptives and endometrial cancer risk (Sweden). Cancer Causes Control 1999;10(4):277–84.
25. Chiaffarino F, Pelucchi C, Parazzini F, et al. Reproductive and hormonal factors and ovarian cancer. Ann Oncol 2001;12(3):337–41.
26. Casagrande JT, Louie EW, Pike MC, et al. "Incessant ovulation" and ovarian cancer. Lancet 1979;2(8135):170–3.
27. Purdie DM, Bain CJ, Siskind V, et al. Ovulation and risk of epithelial ovarian cancer. Int J Cancer 2003;104(2):228–32.
28. McPherson CP, Sellers TA, Potter JD, et al. Reproductive factors and risk of endometrial cancer. The Iowa Women's Health Study. Am J Epidemiol 1996;143(12): 1195–202.
29. Beining RM, Dennis LK, Smith EM, et al. Meta-analysis of intrauterine device use and risk of endometrial cancer. Ann Epidemiol 2008;18(6):492–9.
30. Hubacher D, Grimes DA. Noncontraceptive health benefits of intrauterine devices: a systematic review. Obstet Gynecol Surv 2002;57(2):120–8.
31. Ness RB, Dodge RC, Edwards RP, et al. Contraception methods, beyond oral contraceptives and tubal ligation, and risk of ovarian cancer. Ann Epidemiol 2011;21(3):188–96.
32. Cramer DW, Titus-Ernstoff L, McKolanis JR, et al. Conditions associated with antibodies against the tumor-associated antigen MUC1 and their relationship to risk for ovarian cancer. Cancer Epidemiol Biomarkers Prev 2005;14(5):1125–31.
33. Castellsague X, Thompson WD, Dubrow R. Tubal sterilization and the risk of endometrial cancer. Int J Cancer 1996;65(5):607–12.
34. Green A, Purdie D, Bain C, et al. Tubal sterilisation, hysterectomy and decreased risk of ovarian cancer. Int J Cancer 1997;71:948–51.
35. Lacey JV Jr, Brinton LA, Mortel R, et al. Tubal sterilization and risk of cancer of the endometrium. Gynecol Oncol 2000;79(3):482–4.
36. Rosenblatt K, Thomas D. Association between tubal ligation and endometrial cancer. Int J Cancer 1997;71(1):129–30.
37. Beral V, Bull D, Reeves G. Endometrial cancer and hormone-replacement therapy in the Million Women Study. Lancet 2005;365(9470):1543–51.
38. Garg PP, Kerlikowske K, Subak L, et al. Hormone replacement therapy and the risk of epithelial ovarian carcinoma: a meta-analysis. Obstet Gynecol 1998; 92(3):472–9.
39. Grady D, Gebretsadik T, Kerlikowske K, et al. Hormone replacement therapy and endometrial cancer risk: a meta-analysis. Obstet Gynecol 1995;85(2):304–13.

40. Pearce CL, Chung K, Pike MC, et al. Increased ovarian cancer risk associated with menopausal estrogen therapy is reduced by adding a progestin. Cancer 2009;115(3):531–9.
41. Rodriguez C, Patel AV, Calle EE, et al. Estrogen replacement therapy and ovarian cancer mortality in a large prospective study of US women. JAMA 2001;285(11): 1460–5.
42. Rossouw JE, Anderson GL, Prentice RL, et al. Risks and benefits of estrogen plus progestin in healthy postmenopausal women: principal results From the Women's Health Initiative randomized controlled trial. JAMA 2002;288(3):321–33.
43. Calle EE, Kaaks R. Overweight, obesity and cancer: epidemiological evidence and proposed mechanisms. Nat Rev Cancer 2004;4(8):579–91.
44. Swanson CA, Potischman N, Wilbanks GD, et al. Relation of endometrial cancer risk to past and contemporary body size and body fat distribution. Cancer Epidemiol Biomarkers Prev 1993;2(4):321–7.
45. Weiderpass E, Persson I, Adami HO, et al. Body size in different periods of life, diabetes mellitus, hypertension, and risk of postmenopausal endometrial cancer (Sweden). Cancer Causes Control 2000;11(2):185–92.
46. Leitzmann MF, Koebnick C, Danforth KN, et al. Body mass index and risk of ovarian cancer. Cancer 2009;115(4):812–22.
47. Schouten LJ, Rivera C, Hunter DJ, et al. Height, body mass index, and ovarian cancer: a pooled analysis of 12 cohort studies. Cancer Epidemiol Biomarkers Prev 2008;17(4):902–12.
48. Kuper H, Cramer DW, Titus-Ernstoff L. Risk of ovarian cancer in the United States in relation to anthropometric measures: does the association depend on menopausal status? Cancer Causes Control 2002;13(5):455–63.
49. Escobedo LG, Lee NC, Peterson HB, et al. Infertility-associated endometrial cancer risk may be limited to specific subgroups of infertile women. Obstet Gynecol 1991;77(1):124–8.
50. Schildkraut JM, Schwingl PJ, Bastos E, et al. Epithelial ovarian cancer risk among women with polycystic ovary syndrome. Obstet Gynecol 1996;88(4 Pt 1):554–9.
51. Wild S, Pierpoint T, Jacobs H, et al. Long-term consequences of polycystic ovary syndrome: results of a 31 year follow-up study. Hum Fertil (Camb) 2000;3(2): 101–5.
52. Persson I, Adami HO, McLaughlin JK, et al. Reduced risk of breast and endometrial cancer among women with hip fractures (Sweden). Cancer Causes Control 1994;5(6):523–8.
53. Newcomb PA, Trentham-Dietz A, Egan KM, et al. Fracture history and risk of breast and endometrial cancer. Am J Epidemiol 2001;153(11):1071–8.
54. Bernatsky S, Ramsey-Goldman R, Foulkes WD, et al. Breast, ovarian, and endometrial malignancies in systemic lupus erythematosus: a meta-analysis. Br J Cancer 2011;104(9):1478–81.
55. Terry PD, Rohan TE, Franceschi S, et al. Cigarette smoking and the risk of endometrial cancer. Lancet Oncol 2002;3(8):470–80.
56. Jordan SJ, Whiteman DC, Purdie DM, et al. Does smoking increase risk of ovarian cancer? A systematic review. Gynecol Oncol 2006;103(3):1122–9.
57. Cramer DW, Liberman RF, Titus-Ernstoff L, et al. Genital talc exposure and risk of ovarian cancer. Int J Cancer 1999;81(3):351–6.
58. Karageorgi S, Gates MA, Hankinson SE, et al. Perineal use of talcum powder and endometrial cancer risk. Cancer Epidemiol Biomarkers Prev 2010;19(5):1269–75.
59. John EM, Koo J, Horn-Ross PL. Lifetime physical activity and risk of endometrial cancer. Cancer Epidemiol Biomarkers Prev 2010;19(5):1276–83.

60. Friedenreich CM, Cook LS, Magliocco AM, et al. Case-control study of lifetime total physical activity and endometrial cancer risk. Cancer Causes Control 2010;21(7):1105–16.

61. Arem H, Irwin ML, Zhou Y, et al. Physical activity and endometrial cancer in a population-based case-control study. Cancer Causes Control 2011;22(2):219–26.

62. Olsen CM, Bain CJ, Jordan SJ, et al. Recreational physical activity and epithelial ovarian cancer: a case-control study, systematic review, and meta-analysis. Cancer Epidemiol Biomarkers Prev 2007;16(11):2321–30.

63. Weiss NS, Szekely DR, Austin DF. Increasing incidence of endometrial cancer in the United States. N Engl J Med 1976;294(23):1259–62.

64. Fathalla MF. Incessant ovulation—a factor in ovarian neoplasia? Lancet 1971; 2(7716):163.

65. Schildkraut JM, Bastos E, Berchuck A. Relationship between lifetime ovulatory cycles and overexpression of mutant p53 in epithelial ovarian cancer. J Natl Cancer Inst 1997;89(13):932–8.

66. Saleemuddin A, Folkins AK, Garrett L, et al. Risk factors for a serous cancer precursor ("p53 signature") in women with inherited BRCA mutations. Gynecol Oncol 2008;111(2):226–32.

67. Cairns J. Mutation and cancer: the antecedents to our studies of adaptive mutation. Genetics 1998;148(4):1433–40.

68. Moolgavkar SH, Knudson AG Jr. Mutation and cancer: a model for human carcinogenesis. J Natl Cancer Inst 1981;66(6):1037–52.

69. Mutter GL, Ince TA, Baak JP, et al. Molecular identification of latent precancers in histologically normal endometrium. Cancer Res 2001;61(11):4311–4.

70. Ness RB, Cottreau C. Possible role of ovarian epithelial inflammation in ovarian cancer. J Natl Cancer Inst 1999;91(17):1459–67.

71. Newhouse ML, Pearson RM, Fullerton JM, et al. A case control study of carcinoma of the ovary. Br J Prev Soc Med 1977;31(3):148–53.

72. West RO. Epidemiologic study of malignancies of the ovaries. Cancer 1966; 19(7):1001–7.

73. Ho SB, Niehans GA, Lyftogt C, et al. Heterogeneity of mucin gene expression in normal and neoplastic tissues. Cancer Res 1993;53(3):641–51.

74. Hinoda Y, Nakagawa N, Nakamura H, et al. Detection of a circulating antibody against a peptide epitope on a mucin core protein, MUC1, in ulcerative colitis. Immunol Lett 1993;35(2):163–8.

75. Terry KL, Titus-Ernstoff L, McKolanis JR, et al. Incessant ovulation, mucin 1 immunity, and risk for ovarian cancer. Cancer Epidemiol Biomarkers Prev 2007;16(1): 30–5.

76. Pinheiro SP, Hankinson SE, Tworoger SS, et al. Anti-MUC1 antibodies and ovarian cancer risk: prospective data from the Nurses' Health Studies. Cancer Epidemiol Biomarkers Prev 2010;19(6):1595–601.

77. Kumar R, Burns EA. Age-related decline in immunity: implications for vaccine responsiveness. Expert Rev Vaccines 2008;7(4):467–79.

78. Cramer DW, Vitonis AF, Pinheiro SP, et al. Mumps and ovarian cancer: modern interpretation of an historic association. Cancer Causes Control 2010;21(8): 1193–201.

79. Cramer DW, Finn OJ. Epidemiologic perspective on immune-surveillance in cancer. Curr Opin Immunol 2011;23(2):265–71.

80. Vitonis AF, Titus-Ernstoff L, Cramer DW. Assessing ovarian cancer risk when considering elective oophorectomy at the time of hysterectomy. Obstet Gynecol 2011;117(5):1042–50.

Genetic Risk and Gynecologic Cancers

Laura L. Holman, MD, Karen H. Lu, MD*

KEYWORDS

- Gynecologic cancer • Genetic • BRCA • Lynch syndrome

Approximately 5% of endometrial cancers and 10% of ovarian cancers can be attributed to an inherited predisposition.[1,2] Given the current incidence of these diseases in the United States, hereditary cancer syndromes will lead to approximately 2200 new cases of ovarian cancer and 2300 new cases of endometrial cancer in 2011.[3] Hereditary breast and ovarian cancer (HBOC) syndrome and Lynch syndrome account for most inherited gynecologic cancers. Other syndromes associated with gynecologic malignancies, such as Cowden syndrome, Li-Fraumeni syndrome, and Peutz-Jeghers syndrome, are rare.

Since the identification of the *BRCA1* and *BRCA2* genes and Lynch syndrome genes almost 20 years ago, significant advances have been made in the management of individuals who carry these gene mutations. In addition, important discoveries related to prognosis and treatment of the patient who has ovarian cancer with a *BRCA1* or *BRCA2* gene mutation have highlighted the role of genetic testing in the care of gynecologic oncology patients. This article reviews the 2 main inherited cancer syndromes relevant to gynecologic cancers, HBOC syndrome and Lynch syndrome.

HBOC SYNDROME

HBOC syndrome is caused by mutations in the *BRCA1* or *BRCA2* genes, which were first identified and cloned in the early 1990s.[4,5] The prevalence of mutations in *BRCA1* and *BRCA2* among the general population has been estimated to be as high as 1 in 400.[6] However, this varies among different populations. In certain populations that have undergone a period of relative isolation, founder mutations in *BRCA1* and *BRCA2* have been identified. For example, Ashkenazi Jews have a prevalence of approximately 1 in 40.[7]

BRCA1 is localized to chromosome 17q, whereas *BRCA2* is localized to chromosome 13q. As tumor suppressor genes, the proteins coded for by *BRCA1* and *BRCA2* are involved in recognition and repair of DNA damage, specifically

Department of Gynecologic Oncology and Reproductive Medicine, The University of Texas MD Anderson Cancer Center, Unit 1362, 1155 Pressler, CPB6.3244, Houston, TX 77030-3721, USA
* Corresponding author.
E-mail address: khlu@mdanderson.org

Hematol Oncol Clin N Am 26 (2012) 13–29
doi:10.1016/j.hoc.2011.11.003
0889-8588/12/$ – see front matter © 2012 Published by Elsevier Inc.

hemonc.theclinics.com

double-stranded DNA breaks.[8] They are large genes, with *BRCA1* having 24 exons and *BRCA2* having 27 exons.[9] More than 1200 inherited mutations have been found to occur throughout each gene.[8,10] Approximately 80% of these mutations are either nonsense or frameshift mutations resulting in truncated, nonfunctioning protein.[8]

Women with a *BRCA1* mutation have a risk of ovarian cancer by age 70 years of 39% to 46% and a lifetime risk of breast cancer by age 70 years of 65% to 85%. Reported risks of ovarian and breast cancers in women by age 70 years among *BRCA2* carriers are 10% to 27% and 45% to 85%, respectively.[9,11] Germline *BRCA1* and *BRCA2* mutations express incomplete penetrance. Furthermore, penetrance can be highly variable within families with the same BRCA mutation.[12]

BRCA mutation carriers are also at risk for several other cancers. Those rarer cancers reported to be associated with BRCA mutations are male breast, pancreatic, and prostate cancers, although lifetime risk of these cancers is low compared with female breast and ovarian cancer. Other malignancies, such as melanoma and biliary cancers, have also been reported to occur in BRCA carriers.[12–16] Aside from malignancies, there are no known physical abnormalities or other conditions associated with BRCA mutations.

Pathology of BRCA-associated Ovarian Cancers

Multiple studies have noted that BRCA-associated ovarian cancers are more likely to be high-grade serous adenocarcinoma than sporadic ovarian cancers. Although only 44% to 59% of sporadic ovarian cancers are serous, up to 86% of BRCA-associated ovarian cancers have serous histology.[12,17,18] In addition, endometrioid, mucinous, and low malignant potential tumors are rarely diagnosed in BRCA-positive women.[19–21] Low-grade serous cancers are also unlikely to be part of the BRCA cancer spectrum.[22] When comparing the histology of *BRCA1* and *BRCA2* patients, no difference has been found.[17,21,23]

Theory of the Fallopian Tube as a Potential Origin of BRCA-associated Serous Cancers

Most pelvic serous carcinomas are classified as ovarian. These cancers have been presumed to arise from the ovarian surface epithelium.[18] However, there has recently been increasing interest in the fallopian tube as the potential site of origin of many BRCA-associated serous malignancies, including cancers that are typically diagnosed as ovarian.

This hypothesis developed as BRCA carriers and other high-risk women began to undergo risk-reducing salpingo-oophorectomy (RRSO) in the 1990s. The pathologic examination of these patients revealed early-stage, asymptomatic malignancies, with many located in the distal tube or fimbria. Most of these tumors were microscopic.[24–31] However, not all of the tumors diagnosed in these studies were found in the tube. According to a recent summary of the published cases of malignancies found in RRSO specimens in BRCA carriers, approximately 21% of occult cancers involved the ovary alone, bringing into question whether the fallopian tube is the sole site of origin for serous carcinomas.[31] Nevertheless, that most of the tumors found on RRSO are tubal is in contrast with the fact that fallopian tube cancer is rarely diagnosed in patients who present with late-stage serous carcinomas, with an incidence rate of only 0.41 per 100,000 women.[32]

To explain why fallopian tube carcinomas are diagnosed more frequently in early occult malignancies than in patients with large tumors or metastatic disease, it has been proposed that many BRCA-associated pelvic serous carcinomas originate in the fallopian tube and subsequently spread to the ovary and other peritoneal surfaces. A lesion called serous tubal intraepithelial carcinoma (STIC) has been hypothesized to be the origin of most pelvic serous carcinomas. STICs are distinguishable from the normal fallopian tube and seem to have the ability to shed malignant cells without invading the tube.[18] Several investigators have reported the presence of STICs in patients with positive peritoneal cytology.[25,31,33,34] This finding explains how patients may have a large volume of tumor on the ovary and peritoneum (and therefore diagnosed as ovarian or primary peritoneal carcinoma) but little tubal disease, although their cancer originated in the tube.

Prognosis and Novel Therapies for BRCA-associated Ovarian Cancer

Multiple studies have found a significant progression-free and overall survival advantage for patients who have ovarian cancer with a BRCA mutation compared with women who are BRCA mutation-negative. Earlier studies evaluated only patients with Ashkenazi Jewish BRCA founder mutations.[35–37] However, more recent studies comparing survival in non-Jewish BRCA-positive patients who have ovarian cancer with BRCA-negative patients have also identified a survival advantage in BRCA mutation carriers. In the largest evaluation of non-Ashkenazi Jewish BRCA carriers to date, Lacour and colleagues[38] found significantly longer progression-free (27.9 vs 17.9 months) and overall (101.7 vs 54.3 months) survival when compared with patients with sporadic ovarian cancer. In addition, these investigators noted that BRCA status was an independent predictor of progression-free and overall survival.

The cause of the survival advantage for BRCA carriers with ovarian cancer is unknown. Although several hypotheses exist, the theory that BRCA mutations improve chemotherapy sensitivity has garnered the most evidence.[39,40] BRCA1 plays an important role in the repair of double-stranded DNA breaks, a process called homologous recombination. Because mutated BRCA is unable to recognize and repair double-stranded DNA breaks, BRCA mutation carriers may be incapable of repairing chemotherapy-induced DNA damage, thus leading to improved treatment response. Ongoing research into the function of these 2 genes may help to elucidate the underlying improved prognosis seen in clinical studies.

A novel class of therapeutics, PARP (poly[ADP-ribose] polymerase pathway) inhibitors, exploit the inability of BRCA mutated cancers to adequately repair double-stranded DNA breaks. PARP is involved in the repair of single-stranded DNA breaks. Therefore, the combination of PARP inhibition with defective BRCA function in ovarian tumors leads to enhanced cell death, a concept termed synthetic lethality. Phase I and II studies of olaparib (an oral PARP inhibitor) have reported it to be efficacious with minimal side effects in BRCA-associated ovarian and breast cancers. In the phase II study, olaparib at a dose of 400 mg twice daily showed a 33% response rate. In addition, it seems to be most effective in platinum-sensitive patients.[41,42]

Identifying Women at Risk for HBOC

Given their propensity for developing other malignancies, and the risk of having family members with the same mutation, it is important to identify patients with a BRCA mutation. The Society of Gynecologic Oncologists (SGO) has developed guidelines to aid in identifying patients at risk for HBOC.[11] These same guidelines were also endorsed by the American College of Obstetricians and Gynecologists (ACOG).[10] **Table 1** details the SGO criteria.

There may be patients who do not meet these criteria but warrant genetic risk assessment. For example, families in which there are few female relatives or those in which multiple family members have undergone oophorectomy or hysterectomy at a young age may lead one to falsely assume a low risk of HBOC. In addition, women who are adopted may have little or no knowledge of their family history. Women with

Table 1	
SGO guidelines for genetic risk assessment for HBOC	
Risk Assessment Helpful	**Risk Assessment Recommended**
Women with breast cancer ≤40 years	Women with a personal history of breast
Women with bilateral breast cancer,	and ovarian cancer
especially if the first cancer was	Women with ovarian cancer and a first-
at ≤50 years	degree, second-degree, or third-degree
Women with breast cancer at ≤50 years and	relative with breast cancer at ≤50 years
a first-degree, second-degree, or third-	or ovarian cancer at any age
degree relative with breast cancer	Ashkenazi Jewish women with
at ≤50 years	ovarian cancer
Ashkenazi Jewish women with breast cancer	Women with breast cancer at ≤50 years and
at ≤50 years	a first-degree, second-degree, or third-
Women with breast or ovarian cancer at any	degree relative with ovarian cancer
age and ≥2 first-degree, second-degree, or	or male breast cancer
third-degree relatives with breast cancer at	Ashkenazi Jewish women with breast
any age, especially if ≥1 breast cancer was	cancer at ≤40 years
at ≤50 years	Women with a first-degree or second-degree
Unaffected women with a first-degree or	relative with a BRCA mutation
second-degree relative meeting one of the	
above criteria	
Patients with one of the above criteria have	Patients with one of the above criteria have
a 5%–10% chance of a BRCA mutation	a 20%–25% chance of a BRCA mutation

Data from Lancaster JM, Powell CB, Kauff ND, et al. SGO Committee Statement. Society of Gynecologic Oncologists Education Committee statement on risk assessment for inherited gynecologic cancer predispositions. Gynecol Oncol 2007;107(2):159–62.

breast or ovarian cancer who present with one of these family histories should be considered for BRCA testing.[10–12]

As expected, women diagnosed with a BRCA-associated cancer have a greater risk of having a *BRCA1* or *BRCA2* mutation than the general population. For example, women with high-grade ovarian cancer (excluding Ashkenazi Jewish women, who have a substantially increased risk) have an estimated 1 in 8 to 1 in 10 risk of one of these mutations.[23,43,44] Based on this increased prevalence, it has been suggested that it is reasonable to offer BRCA testing to all women diagnosed with high-grade ovarian cancer.[23] In general, women less than 21 years old should not be tested.[10]

Kwon and colleagues[45] recently performed an analysis highlighting the importance of genetic testing of patients with ovarian cancer. This study found that applying the SGO criteria to determine which patients with ovarian cancer to test for BRCA1 and BRCA2 mutations resulted in a cost-effective strategy for the prevention of future cancers in first-degree relatives of women who were tested. Many women who are high risk for HBOC are never referred for genetic assessment. In their retrospective study, Meyer and colleagues[46] found that 48% of patients with ovarian cancer who in 2007 fulfilled the criteria outlined earlier were referred to genetic counseling. Although it seems that most providers are aware of referral criteria, a substantial portion are still not referring their high-risk patients for genetic testing.[47] Reasons for this discrepancy are unclear, although a contributing factor may be that clinicians are not consistently able to identify patients at high risk for HBOC.[48] A recent study noted that only 19% of primary care physicians were able to delineate low-risk from high-risk patients in a survey of clinical scenarios.[49]

There is currently no consensus on the timing of referral for genetic testing for patients at high risk for HBOC. In the breast literature, many providers report a preference to refer their patients after they complete adjuvant treatment.[47] However, most patients wish their physicians had broached the subject of genetic counseling earlier in their treatment course.[50] In a study of patients with ovarian cancer who underwent BRCA testing, one-third had not been referred for genetic counseling until they had recurrent disease. Given the poor prognosis of recurrent ovarian cancer, the investigators argue for genetic counseling referral at initial diagnosis.[51]

Surveillance

It is generally agreed that women diagnosed with a BRCA mutation should be routinely screened for cancers of which they are at risk.[12] To date, there is limited evidence that ovarian cancer screening leads to improved survival. An evaluation of 13 ovarian cancer screening studies in high-risk women noted that of the 70 tumors discovered, only 24% were early stage.[52] This finding is similar to the incidence of early-stage disease in the general population of unscreened patients, arguing that there may be no difference in mortality between screened and unscreened populations.[53] However, survival outcome was unavailable for all but one of the studies included in the analysis. Large, prospective trials are under way in the United States and the United Kingdom to better determine the best way to screen women at high risk of ovarian cancer.[53,54]

Expert consensus groups agree that BRCA-carriers with intact ovaries should be offered periodic screening given their high risk for developing ovarian cancer. Screening consisting of twice-yearly CA125 and transvaginal ultrasonography beginning at age 30 to 35 years, or 5 years earlier than the earliest age of ovarian cancer in the family, has been recommended by ACOG and the National Comprehensive Cancer Network (NCCN).[10,55,56] Patients should be made aware that these recommendations are based on presumptive benefit only. The benefit of surveillance to women who have undergone salpingo-oophorectomy is unknown, and there are currently no recommendations for screening these patients for peritoneal cancer.[10]

Chemoprevention

The protective effect of oral contraceptives against ovarian cancer in high-risk women has been shown in multiple studies. One of the largest studies to date, a case-control study of more than 3000 BRCA-positive women with and without ovarian cancer, noted an increasingly reduced risk of ovarian cancer with each year of use for up to 3 to 5 years. The decreased risk existed for both *BRCA1* and *BRCA2* carriers.[57] Several other studies have also reported a protective effect of oral contraceptive use against ovarian cancer in BRCA-positive women, with longer use associated with decreased risk.[58–60] Together, these studies suggest it may be reasonable for BRCA carriers with intact ovaries to use oral contraceptives to decrease their risk of ovarian cancer. However, there is conflicting evidence on the effect of oral contraceptive use on the risk of breast cancer in BRCA-positive women.[61–63] Therefore, as with any intervention, women and physicians should have a balanced discussion of potential risks and benefits before initiating oral contraceptives.

RRSO

RRSO is the practice of removing the bilateral ovaries and fallopian tubes in BRCA carriers, and is the most efficacious method of ovarian cancer risk reduction. Oophorectomy has been recognized as a method of decreasing ovarian cancer risk since the 1950s.[64] More recently, there have been multiple prospective and retrospective studies evaluating RRSO in BRCA-positive women. The most recent was a multicenter cohort study of almost 2500 BRCA-positive women who underwent either RRSO or surveillance. This study found an 86% decrease in ovarian cancer risk in patients who had a previous history of breast cancer and a 72% decrease in risk in women without breast cancer history.[65] Other studies have reported a 75% to 96% decrease in ovarian cancer risk in BRCA carriers who underwent RRSO.[66–69] A risk of 1% to 6% of primary peritoneal cancer remains after RRSO. Although small, this risk seems to persist for up to 20 years after oophorectomy.[64,69,70] In addition, there is evidence that RRSO provides a survival advantage. Grann and colleagues[71] reported that women who had undergone RRSO prolonged their survival by 2.6 years. Other studies have noted a 60% to 72% decrease in overall mortality in BRCA carriers who have undergone RRSO compared with those who have not.[65,72]

RRSO should be recommended to all BRCA carriers at the age of 40 years or after conclusion of childbearing.[10] This guideline was developed because less than 2% to 3% of women with BRCA mutations develop ovarian cancer before the age of 40 years. In addition, BRCA1 mutation carriers' chance of developing ovarian cancer increases exponentially during their 40s. Although BRCA2 mutation carriers' risk of ovarian cancer does not increase until a later age, they have a greater decrease in their risk of breast cancer the earlier their ovaries are removed.[10,73]

During RRSO, it is important to ensure that all ovarian and fallopian tube tissue is excised. In addition, pelvic washings should be performed at the beginning of the case because there are reports of positive cytology with no tumor found in the tissue specimen.[74] There is currently insufficient evidence to recommend routine hysterectomy at the time of RRSO in the absence of other uterine or cervical pathologic results. Proponents of the procedure argue that it removes the intramural fallopian tube tissue and eliminates the possible increased risk of endometrial cancer in BRCA carriers. However, there have been no reports of patients developing cancer from the small amount of intramural fallopian tube tissue, and it remains unclear if BRCA-positive women truly have an increased risk of endometrial cancer.[15,75]

Studies of pathologic specimens from RRSO have noted that up to 12% have an occult malignancy that is not grossly visible.[28,29,66,67] Therefore, it is important that the entire pathologic specimen is carefully evaluated. It has been recommended that the entire tube and ovary be serially cut into 2-mm to 3-mm sections.[64] In addition, clear communication with the pathologist is important to ensure that the specimen is assessed appropriately.

Although RRSO has definite benefits, concerns remain regarding the adverse effects for these young women undergoing surgical menopause, including osteoporosis and cardiovascular disease risks.[64,76] Based on these concerns and emerging evidence of the fimbria as the site of origin for serous carcinomas, Leblanc and colleagues[77] recently reported their experience on radical fimbriectomy in a cohort of BRCA mutation carriers undergoing risk-reducing surgery. With this procedure, the patients had most of their ovarian tissue left in situ, with plans to undergo a bilateral oophorectomy at a later date. Although the investigators found the procedure to be safe, they caution that the risks of an incomplete risk-reducing surgery are unknown and further studies are warranted.

LYNCH SYNDROME

Lynch syndrome, also known as hereditary nonpolyposis colorectal cancer (HNPCC) syndrome, accounts for most inherited endometrial cancer cases. The original family was described in 1913 by Aldred Warthin, although the syndrome was not characterized until the 1960s and 1970s.[78–80] Since that time, Lynch syndrome has been recognized as an inherited mutation in one of the DNA mismatch repair genes (*MLH1*, *MSH2*, *MSH6*, or *PMS2*). The prevalence of these mutations in the general population is approximately 1 in 500 to 1 in 1000.[81]

Inheritance and Penetrance

MLH1, *MSH2*, *MSH6*, and *PMS2* are all inherited in an autosomal-dominant pattern. These genes function to repair base-base mismatches and eliminate insertion or deletion loops of repetitive sequences that occur during DNA replication. Mutations in the mismatch repair genes are typically point mutations that lead to nonsense or missense mutations. Genomic deletions have also been observed. More than 1200 mutations have been described in these genes.[82]

Most patients with Lynch syndrome are found to have a mutation in either *MLH1* (50%) or *MSH2* (40%). Approximately 10% of cases are attributable to an *MSH6* mutation.[83] Only a few patients have a mutation in *PMS2*. Mutations in other mismatch repair genes have been described as associated with Lynch syndrome, including *MLH3* and *MSH3*. However, they have been only in isolated families.[84]

Mutations in the mismatch repair genes associated with Lynch syndrome all express incomplete penetrance. In addition, the amount of penetrance seems to vary based on factors such as gene mutation. For example, *MSH2* mutation carriers have been noted to have a significantly more increased risk of developing cancers than *MSH1* mutation carriers.[85] In addition, *MSH6* mutations have been found to be responsible for a lower incidence of colorectal cancer, but a higher incidence of endometrial cancer.[86,87] The reasons for these differences in penetrance are unknown.

Lynch-associated Malignancies

In women, Lynch syndrome is most commonly associated with colorectal and endometrial cancers, with a 40% to 60% lifetime risk of each. These patients typically develop endometrial cancer at an earlier age than the general population, with the mean age at diagnosis being 50 years.[88] Approximately 10% of women diagnosed with endometrial cancer less than the age of 50 years have Lynch syndrome.[89] Multiple other malignancies are associated with Lynch syndrome, which are listed in **Table 2**.

Pathology of Lynch-associated Endometrial and Ovarian Cancers

Compared with sporadic endometrial cancers, the histology of Lynch syndrome-associated tumors is heterogeneous. A study comparing Lynch-associated endometrial cancers with sporadic cancers in women less than the age of 50 years and sporadic microsatellite instability-high cancers noted that although most of the tumors were of endometrioid histology, women with Lynch syndrome frequently had nonendometrioid histology and more stage II, III, and IV disease. The nonendometrioid tumors included clear cell carcinomas, carcinosarcomas, and mixed papillary serous and clear cell carcinomas, with most of these malignancies arising in *MSH2* mutation carriers.[90] In addition, studies have noted an important association between lower uterine segment tumors and Lynch syndrome.[91] Westin and colleagues[92] found that 29% of these uncommon tumors were in patients with Lynch syndrome.

Although limited data exist regarding Lynch-associated ovarian cancers, it seems that they are also heterogeneous. In the largest study of these malignancies to date, Watson and colleagues[93] found that most were epithelial cancers with a wide variety of histologies. However, 85% were well or moderately differentiated. Ten percent to 22% of Lynch-associated ovarian cancers arise in the setting of a synchronous

Table 2 HNPCC-associated malignancies	
Malignancy	**Lifetime Risk (%)**
Endometrial	40–60
Colorectal (women)	40–60
Gastric	13
Ovary	6–12
Renal pelvis/ureter	4–8
Small bowel	<5
Brain	4
Biliary tract	2

Data from Refs.[81,112–114]

endometrial cancer, whereas approximately 5% of endometrial cancers are associated with a synchronous ovarian cancer.[93,94]

Prognosis of Lynch Syndrome-associated Endometrial Cancer

In general, patients with Lynch syndrome-associated colorectal cancer have a better prognosis than those with sporadic tumors. However, there are limited data regarding endometrial and ovarian cancer prognosis for these women. Boks and colleagues[95] found no statistical difference in survival rates between women with sporadic endometrial cancers and those with Lynch syndrome-associated tumors. An additional study of patients with ovarian cancer found a significant survival advantage for women with Lynch syndrome.[96] However, both of these studies were small and have not been validated.

Identifying Women at Risk for Lynch Syndrome

Given their propensity for developing more than 1 primary malignancy, and the risk of having family members with the same mutation, it is important to identify patients with Lynch syndrome. Initial guidelines to assist physicians in identifying patients with Lynch syndrome were focused on colorectal cancer.[97] However, women with HNPCC have an equal risk of colorectal and endometrial cancers. In addition, there is evidence that approximately 50% of patients with Lynch syndrome diagnosed with both endometrial and colon cancer were diagnosed with endometrial cancer first.[98] For these reasons, screening guidelines that incorporate the risk of endometrial cancer are necessary. The SGO has published guidelines to aid with determining which patients should be screened for Lynch syndrome (**Table 3**).

Surveillance

Although there are compelling data to recommend colonoscopy every 1 to 2 years for individuals with Lynch syndrome, there is currently no strong evidence on how to screen these women for gynecologic malignancies.[99] A study based on families diagnosed with Amsterdam II criteria found that only approximately 3% to 7% of gynecologic malignancies would develop before 30 to 35 years if screening were begun at this age.[100] Studies have attempted to evaluate transvaginal ultrasonography alone, transvaginal ultrasonography with CA125, and endometrial biopsy with hysteroscopy as screening methods for endometrial cancer in patients with Lynch syndrome.[101–103] Other studies have examined the use of transvaginal ultrasonography with endometrial biopsy and the combination of transvaginal ultrasonography, endometrial biopsy,

Table 3 SGO guidelines for genetic risk assessment for Lynch syndrome	
Risk Assessment Helpful	**Risk Assessment Recommended**
Patients with endometrial or colorectal cancer diagnosed before 50 years Patients with endometrial or ovarian cancer with synchronous or metachronous Lynch-associated malignancies Patients with colorectal or endometrial cancer and more than 2 first-degree relatives with a Lynch-associated malignancy Patient with a first-degree or second-degree relative meeting the above criteria	Patients meeting revised Amsterdam criteria[a] Patients with synchronous or metachronous colorectal and ovarian or endometrial cancers Patients with a first-degree or second-degree relative with a known MMR mutation
Patients with one of the above criteria have a 5%–10% chance of Lynch syndrome	Patients with one of the above criteria have a 20%–25% chance of Lynch syndrome

[a] Revised Amsterdam criteria are as follows: (1) at least 3 relatives with a Lynch-associated cancer in 1 lineage; (2) one affected individual is a first-degree relative of the other two; (3) at least 2 successive affected generations; (4) at least 1 Lynch-associated cancer is diagnosed before age 50 years.[115]

Data from Lancaster JM, Powell CB, Kauff ND, et al. SGO Committee Statement: Society of Gynecologic Oncologists Education Committee Statement on Risk Assessment for Inherited Gynecologic Cancer Predispositions. Gynecol Oncol 2007;107(2):159–62.

and CA125.[104,105] In general, it has been noted that these tests have low sensitivity for detecting disease, although studies that include endometrial biopsy seem to be the most effective. Although endometrial cancer is typically characterized by abnormal vaginal bleeding, women with Lynch syndrome are often premenopausal, and abnormal bleeding may not be recognized promptly. Based on these limited data, expert opinion has generally recommended that women with Lynch syndrome should receive annual endometrial biopsies and transvaginal ultrasonography once they reach the age of 30 to 35 years.[99]

Risk-reducing Surgery

In 1997, the Cancer Genetics Studies Consortium stated "evidence of benefit is lacking" in regards to the risk-reducing surgery for women with Lynch syndrome.[55] However, since that time there have been additional studies addressing the ability of prophylactic hysterectomy and bilateral salpingo-oophorectomy to decrease the risk of gynecologic malignancies for these women. Schmeler and colleagues[106] reported their experience with 315 women with Lynch syndrome who underwent surveillance or prophylactic hysterectomy with or without salpingo-oophorectomy. These investigators found that they prevented 100% of endometrial and ovarian cancers by performing surgery, although the difference in ovarian cancer between the surgery and surveillance group was not statistically significant. A recent analytical model of 10,000 theoretic women with Lynch syndrome found it would take 28 surgeries to prevent 1 case of ovarian cancer, but only 6 surgeries to prevent 1 case of endometrial cancer.[107] These and other studies have led experts to recommend that prophylactic hysterectomy and bilateral salpingo-oophorectomy be offered to all women with Lynch syndrome at the age of 35 years or once childbearing is complete.[99,106] Women undergoing risk-reducing surgery may still be at risk for primary peritoneal cancer, and should be counseled accordingly. However, the amount of risk is unknown because only case reports are available.[108]

As with BRCA mutation carriers, it is important that patients with Lynch syndrome undergoing prophylactic surgery have all pathologic specimens carefully examined. Schmeler and colleagues[106] noted that 5% of women undergoing prophylactic surgery had an occult endometrial cancer. In addition, it has been suggested that patients undergo preoperative endometrial biopsy, transvaginal ultrasonography, and CA125 to aid with diagnosis of these occult malignancies before surgery.

OTHER SYNDROMES

Several other rare hereditary cancer syndromes have gynecologic manifestations, including Peutz-Jeghers syndrome (PJS), Cowden syndrome (CS), and Li-Fraumeni syndrome (LFS). Given their rarity, there are few data regarding screening, prognosis, and treatment.

Pigmented lesions on the lips and buccal mucosa, as well as increased risk for tumors and malignancies at multiple sites, including the breast, gastrointestinal system, and the gynecologic organs, characterize PJS. PJS results from germline mutations in the LKB1 gene. Uniquely, patients with PJS are at risk for sex cord-stromal tumors with annular tubules of the ovary and adenoma malignum of the cervix.[109] Expert opinion currently recommends annual pelvic examination and pap smear starting at age 18 years and transvaginal ultrasonography and CA125 testing starting at age 25 years for women with PJS.[110]

CS, also known as multiple hamartoma syndrome, is distinguished by hamartomas, distinct dermatologic changes, and various malignancies. CS is caused by germline mutations in the PTEN gene.[109] Endometrial cancer is one of the major diagnostic criteria for CS. According to the NCCN, women with CS should be offered periodic endometrial biopsies starting at age 30 to 35 years, or 5 years earlier than the earliest endometrial cancer in the family.[56] However, there are no data regarding the efficacy of these recommendations.

LFS is characterized by multiple primary tumors with the absence of any other physical abnormalities, and results from germline p53 mutations.[109] Gynecologic malignancies are not common in women with LFS, although the most frequently diagnosed gynecologic cancer is ovarian adenocarcinoma, with an average age of onset of 39.5 years.[111] There are no ovarian cancer surveillance recommendations for patients with LFS.[56]

SUMMARY

Although most gynecologic malignancies are sporadic, hereditary cancer syndromes cause a substantial portion of these cancers. Given that the diagnosis of these syndromes has prognostic and therapeutic implications for the patient, as well as preventive implications for her family members, genetic testing is now an accepted part of the management of the patient who has gynecologic cancer.

REFERENCES

1. Gruber SB, Thompson WD. A population-based study of endometrial cancer and familial risk in younger women. Cancer and hormone study group. Cancer Epidemiol Biomarkers Prev 1996;5(6):411–7.
2. Lancaster JM. Clinical relevance of hereditary ovarian cancer. In: Lu KH, editor. Hereditary gynecologic cancer: risk, prevention, and management. New York: Informa Healthcare; 2008. p. 1–13.

3. Siegel R, Ward E, Brawley O, et al. Cancer statistics, 2011. The impact of eliminating socioeconomic and racial disparities on premature cancer deaths. CA Cancer J Clin 2011;61(4):212–36.
4. Miki Y, Swensen J, Shattuck-Eidens D, et al. A strong candidate for the breast and ovarian cancer susceptibility gene BRCA1. Science 1994;266(5182): 66–71.
5. Wooster R, Bignell G, Lancaster J, et al. Identification of the breast cancer susceptibility gene BRCA2. Nature 1995;378(6559):789–92.
6. Prevalence and penetrance of BRCA1 and BRCA2 mutations in a population-based series of breast cancer cases. Anglian Breast Cancer Study Group. Br J Cancer 2000;83(10):1301–8.
7. Struewing JP, Hartge P, Wacholder S, et al. The risk of cancer associated with specific mutations of BRCA1 and BRCA2 among Ashkenazi Jews. N Engl J Med 1997;336(20):1401–8.
8. Copeland LJ. Epithelial ovarian cancer. In: DiSaia PJ, Creasman WT, editors. Clinical gynecologic oncology. 7th edition. Philadelphia: Mosby Elsevier; 2007. p. 311–67.
9. Garber JE, Offit K. Hereditary cancer predisposition syndromes. J Clin Oncol 2005;22(2):276–92.
10. American College of Obstetricians and Gynecologists, ACOG Committee on Practice Bulletins - Gynecology, ACOG Committee on Genetics, et al. ACOG Practice Bulletin No. 103: Hereditary breast and ovarian cancer syndrome. Obstet Gynecol 2009;113(4):957–66.
11. Lancaster JM, Powell CB, Kauff ND, et al. Society of Gynecologic Oncologists Education Committee statement on risk assessment for inherited gynecologic cancer predispositions. Gynecol Oncol 2007;107(2):159–62.
12. Petrucelli N, Daly MB, Feldman GL. BRCA1 and BRCA2 hereditary breast and ovarian cancer. In: Pagon RA, Bird TD, Dolan CR, editors. GeneReviews [Internet]. Seattle (WA): University of Washington; September 04, 1993–1998. [updated 2011 Jan 20].
13. Tai YC, Domcheck S, Parmigiani G, et al. Breast cancer risk among male BRCA1 and BRCA2 mutation carriers. J Natl Cancer Inst 2007;99(23):1811–4.
14. The Breast Cancer Linkage Consortium. Cancer risks in BRCA2 mutation carriers. J Natl Cancer Inst 1999;91(15):1310–6.
15. Thompson D, Easton DF, Consortium TBCL. Cancer incidence in BRCA1 mutation carriers. J Natl Cancer Inst 2002;94(18):1358–65.
16. Risch HA, McLaughlin JR, Cole DEC, et al. Population BRCA1 and BRCA2 mutation frequencies and cancer penetrances: A kin-cohort study in Ontario, Canada. J Natl Cancer Inst 2006;98(23):1694–706.
17. Shaw PA, McLaughlin JR, Zweemer RP, et al. Histopathologic features of genetically determined ovarian cancer. Int J Gynecol Pathol 2002;21(4):407–11.
18. Jarboe EA, Folkins AK, Crum CP, et al. Pathology of BRCA-associated ovarian cancers, including occult cancers. In: Lu KH, editor. Hereditary gynecologic cancer: risk, prevention, and management. New York: Informa Healthcare; 2008. p. 29–43.
19. Narod SA. Clinical genetics of gynecologic cancer. In: Barakat RR, Perelman RO, Markman M, et al, editors. Principles and practice of gynecologic oncology. 5th edition. Philadelphia: Lippincott Williams & Wilkins; 2009. p. 31–6.
20. Rubin SC, Benjamin I, Behbakht K, et al. Clinical and pathological features of ovarian cancer in women with germ-line mutations of BRCA1. N Engl J Med 1996;335(19):1413–6.

21. Werness BA, Ramus SJ, CiCioccio RA, et al. Histopathology, FIGO stage, and BRCA mutation status of ovarian cancers from the Gilda Radner Familial Ovarian Cancer Registry. Int J Gynecol Pathol 2004;23(1):29–34.

22. Vineyard MA, Daniels MS, Urbauer DL, et al. Is low-grade serous ovarian cancer part of the tumor spectrum of hereditary breast and ovarian cancer. Gynecol Oncol 2011;120(2):229–32.

23. Pal T, Permuth-Wey J, Betts JA, et al. BRCA1 and BRCA2 mutations account for a large proportion of ovarian carcinoma cases. Cancer 2005;104(12):2807–16.

24. Callahan MJ, Crum CP, Medeiros F, et al. Primary fallopian tube malignancies in BRCA-positive women undergoing surgery for ovarian cancer risk reduction. J Clin Oncol 2007;25(25):3985–90.

25. Leeper K, Garcia R, Swisher E, et al. Pathologic findings in prophylactic oophorectomy specimens in high-risk women. Gynecol Oncol 2002;87(1):52–6.

26. Medeiros F, Muto MG, Lee Y, et al. The tubal fimbria is a preferred site for early adenocarcinoma in women with familial ovarian cancer syndrome. Am J Surg Pathol 2006;30(2):230–6.

27. Finch A, Shaw P, Rosen B, et al. Clinical and pathologic findings of prophylactic salpingo-oophorectomies in 159 BRCA1 and BRCA2 carriers. Gynecol Oncol 2006;100(1):58–64.

28. Powell CB, Kenley E, Chen LM, et al. Risk-reducing salpingo-oophorectomy in BRCA mutation carriers: role of serial sectioning in the detection of occult malignancy. J Clin Oncol 2005;23(1):127–32.

29. Lu KH, Garber JE, Cramer DW, et al. Occult ovarian tumors in women with BRCA1 or BRCA2 mutations undergoing prophylactic oophorectomy. J Clin Oncol 2000;18(14):2728–32.

30. Colgan TJ, Murphy J, Cole DE, et al. Occult carcinoma in prophylactic oophorectomy specimens: prevalence and association with BRCA germline mutation status. Am J Surg Pathol 2001;25(10):1283–9.

31. Yates MS, Meyer LA, Deavers MT, et al. Microscopic and early-stage ovarian cancers in BRCA1/2 mutation carriers: building a model for early BRCA-associated tumorigenesis. Cancer Prev Res (Phila) 2011;4(3):463–70.

32. Stewart SL, Wike JM, Foster SL, et al. The incidence of primary fallopian tube cancer in the United States. Gynecol Oncol 2007;107(3):392–7.

33. Paley PJ, Swisher EM, Garcia RL, et al. Occult cancer of the fallopian tube in BRCA-1 germline mutation carriers at prophylactic oophorectomy: a case for recommending hysterectomy at surgical prophylaxis. Gynecol Oncol 2001;80(2):176–80.

34. Agoff SN, Garcia RL, Goff B, et al. Follow-up of in situ and early-stage fallopian tube carcinoma in patients undergoing prophylactic surgery for proven or suspected BRCA-1 or BRCA-2 mutations. Am J Surg Pathol 2004;28(8):1112–4.

35. Boyd J, Sonoda Y, Federici MG, et al. Clinicopathologic features of BRCA-linked and sporadic ovarian cancer. JAMA 2000;283(17):2260–5.

36. Ben David Y, Chetrit A, Hirsh-Yechezkel G, et al. Effect of BRCA mutations on the length of survival in epithelial ovarian tumors. J Clin Oncol 2002;20(2):463–6.

37. Chetrit A, Hirsh-Yechezkel G, Ben David Y, et al. Effect of BRCA1/2 mutations on long-term survival of patients with invasive ovarian cancer: the national Israeli study of ovarian cancer. J Clin Oncol 2008;26(1):20–5.

38. Lacour RA, Westin SN, Meyer LA, et al. Improved survival in non-Ashkenazi Jewish ovarian cancer patients with BRCA1 and BRCA2 gene mutations. Gynecol Oncol 2011;121(2):358–63.

39. Cass I, Baldwin RL, Varkey T, et al. Improved survival in women with BRCA-associated ovarian carcinoma. Cancer 2003;97(9):2187–95.
40. Husain A, He G, Venkatraman ES, et al. BRCA1 up-regulation is associated with repair-mediated resistance to cis-diamminedichloroplatinum(II). Cancer Res 1998;58(6):1120–3.
41. Fong PC, Boss DS, Yap TA, et al. Inhibition of poly(ADP-ribose) polymerase in tumors from BRCA mutation carriers. N Engl J Med 2009;361(2):123–34.
42. Audeh MW, Carmichael J, Penson RT, et al. Oral poly(ADP-ribose) polymerase inhibitor olaparib in patients with BRCA1 or BRCA2 mutations and recurrent ovarian cancer: a proof-of-concept trial. Lancet 2010;376(9737):245–51.
43. Risch HA, McLaughlin JR, Cole DE, et al. Prevalence and penetrance of germline BRCA1 and BRCA2 mutations in a population series of 649 women with ovarian cancer. Am J Hum Genet 2001;68(3):700–10.
44. Hirsh-Yechezkel G, Chetrit A, Lubin F, et al. Population attributes affecting the prevalence of BRCA mutation carriers in epithelial ovarian cancer cases in Israel. Gynecol Oncol 2003;89(3):494–8.
45. Kwon JS, Daniels MS, Sun CC, et al. Preventing future cancers by testing women with ovarian cancer for BRCA mutations. J Clin Oncol 2010;28(4): 675–82.
46. Meyer LA, Anderson ME, Lacour RA, et al. Evaluating women with ovarian cancer for BRCA1 and BRCA2 mutations. Obstet Gynecol 2010;115(5):945–52.
47. van Riel E, Warlam-Rodenhuis CC, Verhoef S, et al. BRCA testing of breast cancer patients: medical specialists' referral patterns, knowledge and attitudes to genetic testing. Eur J Cancer Care (Engl) 2009;19(3):369–76.
48. Trivers KF, Baldwin LM, Miller JW, et al. Reported referral for genetic counseling or BRCA 1/2 testing among United States physicians. Cancer 2011;117(23): 5334–43.
49. Bellcross CA, Kolor K, Goddard KA, et al. Awareness and utilization of BRCA1/2 testing among U.S. primary care physicians. Am J Prev Med 2011;40(1):61–6.
50. Schlich-Bakker KJ, ten Kroode HF, Warlam-Rodenhuis CC, et al. Barriers to participating in genetic counseling and BRCA testing during primary treatment for breast cancer. Genet Med 2007;9(11):766–77.
51. Daniels MS, Urbauer DL, Stanley JL, et al. Timing of BRCA1/BRCA2 genetic testing in women with ovarian cancer. Genet Med 2009;11(9):624–8.
52. Cass I. Ovarian cancer screening. In: Lu KH, editor. Hereditary gynecologic cancer: risk, prevention, and management. New York: Informa Healthcare; 2008. p. 45–64.
53. Chan JK, Urban R, Cheung MK, et al. Ovarian cancer in younger vs older women: a population-based analysis. Br J Cancer 2006;95(10):1314–20.
54. Greene MH, Piedmonte M, Alberts D, et al. A prospective study of risk-reducing salpingo-oophorectomy and longitudinal CA-125 screening among women at increased genetic risk of ovarian cancer: design and baseline characteristics: a Gynecologic Oncology Group Study. Cancer Epidemiol Biomarkers Prev 2008;17(3):594–604.
55. Burke W, Daly M, Garber J, et al. Recommendations for follow-up care of individuals with an inherited predisposition to cancer. II. BRCA1 and BRCA2. Cancer Genetics Studies Consortium. JAMA 1997;277(12):997–1003.
56. National Comprehensive Cancer Network. Genetic/familial high-risk assessment: breast and ovarian. NCNN Clinical Practice Guidelines in Oncology V12011 2011. Available at: http://www.nccn.org/professionals/physician_gls/pdf/genetics_screening.pdf. Accessed October 31, 2011.

57. McLaughlin JR, Risch HA, Lubinski J, et al. Reproductive risk factors for ovarian cancer in carriers of BRCA1 or BRCA2 mutations: a case-control study. Lancet Oncol 2007;8(1):26–34.

58. Whittemore AS, Balise RR, Pharoah PD, et al. Oral contraceptive use and ovarian cancer risk among carriers of BRCA1 or BRCA2 mutations. Br J Cancer 2004;91(11):1911–5.

59. Narod SA, Risch H, Moslehi R, et al. Oral contraceptives and the risk of hereditary ovarian cancer. Hereditary Ovarian Cancer Clinical Study Group. N Engl J Med 1998;339(7):424–8.

60. McGuire V, Felberg A, Mills M, et al. Relation of contraceptive and reproductive history to ovarian cancer risk in carriers and noncarriers of BRCA1 gene mutations. Am J Epidemiol 2004;160(7):613–8.

61. Narod SA, Dube MP, Lubinski J, et al. Oral contraceptives and the risk of breast cancer in BRCA1 and BRCA2 mutation carriers. J Natl Cancer Inst 2002;94(23): 1773–9.

62. Brohet RM, Goldgar DE, Easton DF, et al. Oral contraceptives and breast cancer risk in the international BRCA1/2 carrier cohort study: a report from EMBRACE, GENEPSO, GEO-HEBON, and the IBCCS Collaborating Group. J Clin Oncol 2007;25(25):3831–6.

63. Iodice S, Barile M, Rotmensz N, et al. Oral contraceptive use and breast or ovarian cancer risk in BRCA1/2 carriers: a meta-analysis. Eur J Cancer 2010; 46(12):2275–84.

64. Lewin SN, Kauff ND. Risk-reducing salpingo-oophorectomy for the prevention of inherited breast and ovarian cancer. In: Lu KH, editor. Hereditary gynecologic cancer: risk, prevention, and management. New York: Informa Healthcare; 2008. p. 79–91.

65. Domchek SM, Friebel TM, Singer CF, et al. Association of risk-reducing surgery in BRCA1 or BRCA2 mutation carriers with cancer risk and mortality. JAMA 2010;304(9):967–75.

66. Kauff ND, Satagopan JM, Robson ME, et al. Risk-reducing salpingo-oophorectomy in women with a BRCA1 or BRCA2 mutation. N Engl J Med 2002;346(21):1601–15.

67. Rebbeck TR, Lynch HT, Neuhausen SL, et al. Prophylactic oophorectomy in carriers of BRCA1 or BRCA2 mutations. N Engl J Med 2002;346(1):1616–22.

68. Kauff ND, Domchek SM, Friebel TM, et al. Risk-reducing salpingo-oophorectomy for the prevention of BRCA1- and BRCA2-associated breast and gynecologic cancer: a multicenter, prospective study. J Clin Oncol 2008; 26(8):1331–7.

69. Finch A, Beiner M, Lubinski J, et al. Salpingo-oophorectomy and the risk of ovarian, fallopian tube, and peritoneal cancers in women with a BRCA1 or BRCA2 mutation. JAMA 2006;296(2):185–92.

70. Casey MJ, Synder C, Bewtra C, et al. Intra-abdominal carcinomatosis after prophylactic oophorectomy in women of hereditary breast ovarian cancer syndrome kindreds associated with BRCA1 and BRCA2 mutations. Gynecol Oncol 2005;97(2):457–67.

71. Grann VR, Jacobson JS, Thomason D, et al. Effect of prevention strategies on survival and quality-adjusted survival of women with BRCA 1/2 mutations: an updated decision analysis. J Clin Oncol 2002;20(10):2520–9.

72. Domchek SM, Friebel TM, Neuhausen SL, et al. Mortality after bilateral salpingo-oophorectomy in BRCA1 and BRCA2 mutation carriers: a prospective cohort study. Lancet Oncol 2006;7(3):223–9.

73. Eisen A, Lubinski J, Klijn J, et al. Breast cancer risk following bilateral oophorectomy in BRCA1 and BRCA2 mutation carriers: an international case-control study. J Clin Oncol 2005;23(30):7491–6.

74. Colgan TJ, Boerner SL, Murphy J, et al. Peritoneal lavage cytology: an assessment of its value during prophylactic oophorectomy. Gynecol Oncol 2002;85(3):397–403.

75. Levine DA, Lin O, Barakat RR, et al. Risk of endometrial carcinoma associated with BRCA mutation. Gynecol Oncol 2001;80(3):395–8.

76. ACOG. ACOG practice bulletin no. 89. Elective and risk-reducing salpingo-oophorectomy. Obstet Gynecol 2008;111(1):231–41.

77. Leblanc E, Narducci F, Farre I, et al. Radical fimbriectomy: a reasonable temporary risk-reducing surgery for selected women with a germ-line mutation of BRCA1 or 2 genes? Rationale and preliminary development. Gynecol Oncol 2011;121(3):472–6.

78. Lynch HT, Shaw MW, Magnuson CW, et al. Hereditary factors in cancer. Study of two large midwestern kindreds. Arch Intern Med 1966;117(2):206–12.

79. Lynch HT, Krush AJ. Cancer family "G" revisited: 1895-1970. Cancer 1971;27(6):1505–11.

80. Warthin A. Heredity with reference to carcinoma as shown by the study of the cases examined in the pathological laboratory of the University of Michigan, 1895-1913. Arch Intern Med 1913;12:546–55.

81. Lu KH. Clinical relevance of hereditary endometrial cancer. In: Lu KH, editor. Hereditary gynecologic cancer: risk, prevention, and management. New York: Informa Healthcare; 2008. p. 15–28.

82. Sheridan E. Molecular genetics and cancer risks in Lynch syndrome. In: Lu KH, editor. Hereditary gynecologic cancer: risk, prevention, and management. New York: Informa Healthcare; 2008. p. 129–48.

83. Peltomaki P. Role of DNA mismatch repair defects in the pathogenesis of human cancer. J Clin Oncol 2003;21(6):1174–9.

84. Kohlmann W, Gruber SB. Lynch syndrome. In: Pagon RA, Bird TD, Dolan CR, editors. GeneReviews [Internet]. Seattle (WA): University of Washington; February 05, 1993–2004. [updated 2011 Aug 11].

85. Vasen HF, Stormorken A, Menko FH, et al. MSH2 mutation carriers are at higher risk of cancer than MLH1 mutation carriers: a study of hereditary nonpolyposis colorectal cancer families. J Clin Oncol 2001;19(20):4074–80.

86. Plaschke J, Engel C, Kruger S, et al. Lower incidence of colorectal cancer and later age of disease onset in 27 families with pathogenic MSH6 germline mutations compared with families with MLH1 or MSH2 mutations: the German Hereditary Nonpolyposis Colorectal Cancer Consortium. J Clin Oncol 2004;22(22):4486–94.

87. Lynch HT, Boland CR, Gong G, et al. Phenotypic and genotypic heterogeneity in the Lynch syndrome: diagnostic, surveillance and management implications. Eur J Hum Genet 2006;14(4):390–402.

88. Meyer LA, Broaddus RR, Lu KH. Endometrial cancer and Lynch syndrome: clinical and pathologic considerations. Cancer Control 2009;16(1):14–22.

89. McMeekin DS, Alektiar KM, Sabbatini PJ, et al. Corpus: epithelial tumors. In: Barakat RR, Perelman RO, Markman M, et al, editors. Principles and practice of gynecologic oncology. 5th edition. Baltimore (MD): Lippincott Williams & Wilkins; 2009. p. 683–6.

90. Broaddus RR, Lynch HT, Chen LM, et al. Pathologic features of endometrial carcinoma associated with HNPCC. Cancer 2006;106(1):87–94.

91. Garg K, Leiotao MM, Kauff ND, et al. Selection of endometrial carcinomas for DNA mismatch repair protein immunohistochemistry using patient age and tumor morphology enhances detection of mismatch repair abnormalities. Am J Surg Pathol 2009;33(6):925–33.

92. Westin SN, Lacour RA, Urbauer DL, et al. Carcinoma of the lower uterine segment: a newly described association with Lynch syndrome. J Clin Oncol 2008;26(36):5965–71.

93. Watson P, Butzow R, Lynch HT, et al. The clinical features of ovarian cancer in hereditary nonpolyposis colorectal cancer. Gynecol Oncol 2001;82(2):223–8.

94. Zaino R, Whitney C, Brady MF, et al. Simultaneously detected endometrial and ovarian carcinomas–a prospective clinicopathologic study of 74 cases: a gynecologic oncology group study. Gynecol Oncol 2001;83(2):355–62.

95. Boks DE, Trujillo AP, Voogd AC, et al. Survival analysis of endometrial carcinoma associated with hereditary nonpolyposis colorectal cancer. Int J Cancer 2002;102(2):198–200.

96. Crijnen TE, Janssen-Heijnen ML, Gelderblom H, et al. Survival of patients with ovarian cancer due to a mismatch repair defect. Fam Cancer 2005;4(4):301–5.

97. Umar A, Boland CR, Terdiman JP, et al. Revised Bethesda Guidelines for hereditary nonpolyposis colorectal cancer (Lynch syndrome) and microsatellite instability. J Natl Cancer Inst 2004;96(4):261–8.

98. Lu KH, Dinh M, Kohlmann W, et al. Gynecologic cancer as a "sentinel cancer" for women with hereditary nonpolyposis colorectal cancer syndrome. Obstet Gynecol 2005;105(3):569–74.

99. Lindor NM, Petersen GM, Hadley DW, et al. Recommendations for the care of individuals with an inherited predisposition to Lynch syndrome: a systematic review. JAMA 2006;296(12):1507–17.

100. Brown GJ, St John DJ, Macrae FA, et al. Cancer risk in young women at risk of hereditary nonpolyposis colorectal cancer: implications for gynecologic surveillance. Gynecol Oncol 2001;80(3):346–9.

101. Dove-Edwin I, Boks D, Goff S, et al. The outcome of endometrial carcinoma surveillance by ultrasound scan in women at risk of hereditary nonpolyposis colorectal carcinoma and familial colorectal carcinoma. Cancer 2002;94(6):1708–12.

102. Rijcken FE, Mourits MJ, Kleibeuker JH, et al. Gynecologic screening in hereditary nonpolyposis colorectal cancer. Gynecol Oncol 2003;91(1):74–80.

103. Lecuru F, Metzger U, Scarabin C, et al. Hysteroscopic findings in women at risk of HNPCC. Results of a prospective observational study. Fam Cancer 2007;6(3):295–9.

104. Renkonen-Sinisalo L, Butzow R, Leminen A, et al. Surveillance for endometrial cancer in hereditary nonpolyposis colorectal cancer syndrome. Int J Cancer 2007;120(4):821–4.

105. Gerritzen LH, Hoogerbrugge N, Oei AL, et al. Improvement of endometrial biopsy over transvaginal ultrasound alone for endometrial surveillance in women with Lynch syndrome. Fam Cancer 2009;8(4):391–7.

106. Schmeler KM, Lynch HT, Chen LM, et al. Prophylactic surgery to reduce the risk of gynecologic cancers in the Lynch syndrome. N Engl J Med 2006;354(3):261–9.

107. Chen LM, Yang KY, Little SE, et al. Gynecologic cancer prevention in Lynch syndrome/hereditary nonpolyposis colorectal cancer families. Obstet Gynecol 2007;110(1):18–25.

108. Schmeler KM, Daniels MS, Soliman PT, et al. Primary peritoneal cancer after bilateral salpingo-oophorectomy in two patients with Lynch syndrome. Obstet Gynecol 2010;115(2 Pt 2):432–4.
109. Walsh CS, Strong LC. Other syndromes. In: Lu KH, editor. Hereditary gynecologic cancer. risk, prevention, and management. New York: Informa Healthcare; 2008. p. 195–218.
110. Giardiello FM, Trimbath JD. Peutz-Jeghers syndrome and management recommendations. Clin Gastroenterol Hepatol 2006;4(4):408–15.
111. Olivier M, Goldgar DE, Sodha N, et al. Li-Fraumeni and related syndromes: correlation between tumor type, family structure, and TP53 genotype. Cancer Res 2003;63(20):6643–50.
112. Dunlop MG, Farrington SM, Carothers AD, et al. Cancer risk associated with germline DNA mismatch repair gene mutations. Hum Mol Genet 1997;6(1): 105–10.
113. Aarnio M, Sankila R, Pukkala E, et al. Cancer risk in mutation carriers of DNA-mismatch-repair genes. Int J Cancer 1999;81(2):214–8.
114. Watson P, Vansen HF, Mecklin JP, et al. The risk of extra-colonic, extra-endometrial cancer in the Lynch syndrome. Int J Cancer 2008;123(2):444–9.
115. Vasen HF, Watson P, Mecklin JP, et al. New clinical criteria for hereditary nonpolyposis colorectal cancer (HNPCC, Lynch syndrome) proposed by the International Collaborative group on HNPCC. Gastroenterology 1999;116(6):1453–6.

Management of Cervical Precancers: A Global Perspective

Daniel Echelman, AB[a], Sarah Feldman, MD, MPH[b],*

KEYWORDS

• Cervical dysplasia • Cervical cancer • Screening
• Human papilloma virus

Cervical cancer is the third most common form of cancer among women worldwide,[1] yet it is one of the few cancers that can be detected and prevented at a precancerous stage. Most cervical cancer cases (85%) occur in the developing world, where they account for 13% of all female cancers.[1] Furthermore, cervical cancer rates in developing countries are on the rise. Breast cancer and cervical cancer combined are projected to equal maternal deaths as the leading causes of mortality among reproductive-aged women by 2025.[2] In contrast, in high-resource countries, effective screening for, and management of, precancers has precipitated a decline in the incidence and mortality due to cervical cancer over the past half-century.[3]

Cervical cancer in the developing world is a challenge of education, resources, and competing priorities. Screening for cervical cancer has historically been inadequate in lower-resource settings. In recent years, several developing nations have targeted cervical cancer with renewed focus, establishing new guidelines for prevention and management and directing resources toward increasing screening coverage (**Table 1**).[4,5] Prevention of cervical cancer in these settings has been complicated by sociocultural and infrastructural variables. Moreover, the biology of cervical cancer differs for developed versus developing settings, affected by the variable prevalence of high-risk human papillomavirus (HPV) subtypes and by the AIDS pandemic. Programs for cervical cancer prevention and management in developing nations must account for these variables while weighing financial and opportunity costs. This article reviews the current status for prevention and management of cervical precancers in health systems around the world.

[a] Women's Cancer Program, Dana Farber Cancer Institute, 450 Brookline Avenue, Boston, MA 02115, USA
[b] Division of Gynecologic Oncology, Brigham and Women's Hospital, Dana Farber Cancer Institute, Harvard Medical School, 75 Francis Street, Boston, MA 02115, USA
* Corresponding author.
E-mail address: sfeldman@partners.org

Hematol Oncol Clin N Am 26 (2012) 31–44
doi:10.1016/j.hoc.2011.11.005   hemonc.theclinics.com

Table 1
International screening guidelines overview

Country/Organization	Age Range	Interval	Primary Screening Modality
American College of Obstetricians and Gynecologists[39]	≥21 y	Every 2–3 y	Cytologic examination, optional HPV cotesting at >30 y
European Guidelines for Quality Assurance in Cervical Cancer Screening[35]	Beginning between ages 20 and 30 y until 60 y	Every 3–5 y	Cytologic examination
World Health Organization (WHO) Guidelines for Developing Countries[19]	25–49 y, 3-y interval if not resource-limited >30 y, at least 1–3 times lifetime if resource limited		Cytologic examination, other modalities are also acceptable
South Africa (Department of Health)[75]	≥30 y	3 tests, lifetime	Cytologic examination
India (Government of India/WHO collaboration)[76]	30–59 y	Every 5 y	VIA
Peru[72,74]	25–59 y	Every 2 y	Cytologic examination or VIA
Thailand[72]	35–54 y	Every 5 y	Cytologic examination nationally, VIA regionally

EPIDEMIOLOGY OF CERVICAL CANCER

Cervical cancer is the third most common cancer and the fourth leading cause of cancer-related deaths among women worldwide, with an estimated 530,232 cases diagnosed and 275,008 fatalities worldwide in 2008.[1] Cancer rates, however, vary dramatically by whether or not a country has an adequate screening program. In the United States, the disease accounted for only 1.6% of cancer cases and 1.4% of cancer mortality among women in 2008.[1] The incidence rate of cervical cancer in developed nations has decreased steadily over the last half-century.[3] This decline in incidence of cervical cancer is largely the result of improved cervical cytology services and coverage over the period.

In the United States, cervical cancer disproportionately affects racial minorities and women of lower socioeconomic standing. Invasive cervical cancer is more common among black and Hispanic women than among white women. Moreover, survival of the disease is less probable for black women than for white women.[3] Cervical cancer incidence and mortality increase with decreased socioeconomic status among all racial groups.[6]

Internationally, the burden of cervical cancer falls most heavily on developing nations. About 85% of the cases and 88% of the deaths due to cervical cancer occur in developing nations.[1] Women in developing nations are at a 35% greater lifetime risk of cervical cancer than women in high-income countries.[2] Although cervical cancer is most common in women older than 50 years, in developing nations, cervical cancer is becoming increasingly prevalent among women during their reproductive years (ages,

15–49 years). Because cervical cancer has a greater cure rate when discovered at an asymptomatic early stage, in countries without screening programs, patients are disproportionately diagnosed with advanced stage and thus incurable disease.

HPV: EPIDEMIOLOGY AND MOLECULAR BIOLOGY

Infection of the cervix with HPV is necessary, although not sufficient, to cause cervical neoplasia and cervical cancer. HPV is among the most prevalent sexually transmitted viruses in the human population. It is estimated that 50% to 80% of sexually active women contract genital HPV during their lifetime. Around 80% of HPV infections clear within 2 years and do not cause cervical neoplasia and invasive cervical cancers.[7] Persistent infection with HPV is required for the development of cervical dysplasia and invasive cervical cancer.

In the United States, an approximate 6.2 million persons are infected with the virus each year.[8] HPV infection is present in 13.3% of US women with normal cervical cytology, comparable with the global prevalence of 11.4%.[9] HPV is more common in lesser-developed regions. In Eastern Africa, where age-standardized incidence and mortality are greatest, HPV is prevalent in 33.6% of women with normal cervical cytology.[10] HPV is most commonly identified on cervical testing among adolescent women (ages, 14–24 years) and is associated with sexual debut.[11]

Certain HPV subtypes increase the likelihood that an infection of the cervix with HPV will develop into cervical dysplasia and invasive cervical cancer. Fifteen HPV subtypes are classified as high risk for cervical cancer (16, 18, 31, 33, 35, 39, 45, 51, 52, 56, 58, 59, 68, 73, and 82). HPV-16 and HPV-18, the 2 highest-risk subtypes, are present in 71% of cervical carcinoma.[12] The prevalence of HPV-16 and HPV-18 is variable worldwide, ranging from 2.0% among women with normal cervical cytology in Western Europe to 9.7% among women with normal cervical cytologic in Eastern Europe.[10]

Infection with a high-risk HPV subtype is the single greatest risk factor for invasive cervical cancer. Other risk factors include tobacco smoking, high parity, long-term hormonal contraceptive use, and infection with human immunodeficiency virus (HIV).[13] The risk of HPV infection is greater in women with multiple sexual partners, and HPV is a common coinfection with other sexually transmitted infections, including HIV.

HPV INFECTION, IMMUNE SURVEILLANCE, AND DEVELOPMENT OF NEOPLASIA

HPV are DNA viruses that infect the human anogenital tract and surface epithelium. HPV are small nonenveloped viruses, consisting of a capsid shell and a 7.9-kilobase genome. The HPV genome carries 8 protein-coding genes, 6 coding for early viral function (E1, E2, E3, E4, E6, and E7) and 2 coding for late viral function (L1 and L2). More than 100 HPV subtypes have been characterized to date. HPV subtypes are distinguished by genotypic diversity in the E6, E7, and L1 coding regions, sharing no greater than 90% genetic similarity in these regions.[14] HPV-16 and HPV-18 are associated with 71% of cervical cancers; types 31, 33, 35, 45, 52, and 58 are found in association with an additional 21% of cervical cancers.[12]

The virus is typically transmitted via sexual intercourse, during which the virus is deposited on the basement membrane of the cervical epithelium.[15] Once present on the cervical epithelium, HPV infection may be transient or may persist and lead to the eventual development of cervical neoplasia and potentially cervical cancer. The course of infection depends on several stages in the natural history of cervical cancer. HPV DNA exists in cervical cells in either an episomal or an integrated state.

Integration of viral DNA into the host genome may be necessary for persistent infection and development of cervical dysplasia.

Most HPV infections resolve within a few years and do not develop into precancerous lesions. A cell-mediated immune response is responsible for clearing viral particles and infected cells. Immunologic memory may protect against future infection, although it is limited to serologic HPV subtype,[16] because women are susceptible to a subsequent infection with a different strain.

Cervical dysplasia typically begins in undifferentiated keratinocytes in the cervical transformation zone, where proliferating subcolumnar cuboidal reserve cells replace columnar cells with squamous epithelium. This site of epithelial metaplasia is at risk for dysplastic growth.[17] Most invasive cervical cancers arise from the squamous epithelium in the transformation zone. However, between 10% and 25% of cervical cancer patients, are found to have adenocarcinoma of the glandular epithelia.[18,19]

Growth at the precancerous stage is gradual and may progress to a higher level of dysplasia but may also regress and eventually clear. Levels of dysplasia diagnosed on cervical biopsy are roughly categorized into 3 levels of dysplasia: low-grade dysplasia (with minimal risk for progression to cancer) and moderate or severe levels of dysplasia (cocategorized as high-grade dysplasia). There is a fair amount of interobserver variation as to the diagnosis of the different levels of dysplasia and, to date, no reproducible way to predict which of these high-grade precancers will progress to invasive cancer.[20]

An HPV infection in general progresses more rapidly from transmission to precancerous lesions than from precancerous lesions to cancer.[21] Cervical lesions persist for years before progressing to cancer, which allows for time to intervene and prevent progression to cancer. Even in the absence of treatment, only a minority of cervical intraepithelial neoplasias (CINs), an estimated 1% of low-grade lesions and 5% to 12% of high-grade lesions, progress to invasive carcinoma.[22] The progression of an infection to precancerous lesions and to invasive cancer is more probable and more rapid in women infected with high-risk subtypes HPV-16 and HPV-18.[23] At the cellular level, HPV-16 and HPV-18 have greater transforming potential than lower-risk HPV subtypes.[24] The oncogenicity of high-risk HPV-16 may further relate to its suppression of immune responses.[25] However, 80% to 90% of women infected with HPV-16 and HPV-18 will not develop precancerous lesions.[26]

HPV infection is more likely to persist in immunocompromised patients. Most notably, HIV coinfection is a risk for HPV infection and for the development of CIN and invasive cervical cancer. HIV broadly suppresses immune system function by killing macrophages and CD4$^+$ T cells. The virus may also increase the risk of malignancy with HPV infection by altering interactions between cancer cells and lymphocytes.[27]

SCREENING AND DIAGNOSIS OF CERVICAL PRECANCERS

At the time that cervical cytologic examination was being introduced by Papanicolaou and Traut in 1943, cervical cancer was the leading cause of cancer mortality among US women.[18] As of 2008, cervical cancer was the 15th most common cause of cancer mortality among US women.[1] Organized cervical cancer prevention programs have precipitated a decline in cervical cancer rates in the developed world. When compared against historic cohorts, such programs have reduced the incidence of cervical cancer by as much as 75%.[18]

Successful cervical cancer prevention programs integrate screening with management of cervical precancers. Three screening modalities, cervical cytologic testing

(Papanicolaou test), cervical HPV testing, and visual inspection of the cervix, are commonly used for cervical screening. Women with positive test results may be referred for colposcopy, in which the transformation zone is visualized under magnification, and abnormal lesions may be biopsied. Histologically confirmed precancerous lesions may be treated by various excisional or ablational techniques. Specific recommendations for screening and management vary according to national and institutional guidelines. In developed nations, a 3-visit model for cervical precancer management is generally used in which screening, colposcopy with directed biopsy, and treatment proceed in 3 separate steps. Alternatively, either a 1-visit approach, in which a rapid screen is followed by immediate treatment, or a 2-visit approach, in which an abnormal Papanicolaou test result is triaged to evaluation and treatment in 1 visit (both known as see and treat), may also be used.

The Papanicolaou test, or Pap smear, has been the standard screening test for much of the past half-century. The test checks for morphologic abnormalities in fixed and stained cells from cervical epithelial sampling. Conventional cytologic testing has a specificity of 94% to 97% in distinguishing high-grade CIN. However, with a sensitivity of approximately 70% to 80%,[18] false-negative results are frequent with Papanicolaou testing alone. Uneven sampling of cervical epithelia and sample loss and manipulation during preparation of cytology slides limit the sensitivity of the technique. Recently, liquid-based cytologic examination has emerged as an alternative to conventional cytologic examination. Improvements in sample preparation limit the number of unsatisfactory Papanicolaou tests, although they do not appreciably raise the sensitivity of cervical cytologic examination.[28,29] The high frequency of false-negative results with cytologic testing necessitates repeated screening. Cervical cytologic examination has been effective with screening at regular intervals because of the long lead time of cervical precancers, although such screening requirements place a larger burden on patients and health systems.

Modern techniques in molecular biology allow detection of genital HPV infection with probes for HPV DNA and RNA, HPV proteins, and cellular markers. Hybrid Capture 2 (HC2; Qiagen), which is the most widely used of these tools, uses DNA hybridization probes for type-specific detection of HPV DNA and can detect 13 high-risk HPV subtypes, including HPV-16 and HPV-18. The sensitivity of detection with HPV testing for high-grade cervical lesions is approximately 95%.[30,31] However, the technology does not discriminate between transient HPV infections and HPV-associated cervical lesions. As such, interpretation of test results is complicated by the moderate specificity of the technique, reported between 61% and 96% in various studies.[32] The specificity of HPV testing is greatest among populations in which the prevalence of HPV is low and the incidence of cervical precancer is high. In a Finnish study of primary HPV testing (N = 33,100), the specificity of the test ranged from 93.4% to 95.6% in women aged 35 years and more, who have lower HPV prevalence yet higher CIN incidence than younger cohorts, as compared with 84.4% among women aged 25 to 34 years.[33]

In clinical studies involving side-by-side comparison of cervical cytologic examination and HPV testing, sensitivity is consistently higher with HPV testing and specificity is consistently higher with cytologic examination.[29,31] Because of the complementary strengths of each technique, HPV testing has been incorporated as an adjuvant test with cytologic examination. The Canadian Cervical Cancer Screening Trial, which examined conventional cytologic examination and the HC2 HPV test in a randomized controlled trial (N = 10,154), reported 100% sensitivity and 92.5% specificity for simultaneous Papanicolaou and HPV cotesting.[30] However, a large number of additional colposcopies were required for diagnosis of each additional case of high-grade dysplasia when using combined testing than when using either test alone or when using either test only as a downstream test for abnormal screens, a process known as reflex testing. Colposcopy and biopsy adds significant additional cost as well as pain and anxiety to a screening program; thus, combined testing becomes viable only if offered at a less frequent interval than either test alone.

In much of the developed world, cervical cytologic examination remains the primary screening test. Several large-scale studies have evaluated HPV screening as a cotest along with primary cervical cytologic examination or for triage after cytologic examination, reporting greater predictive values than for cytologic examination alone.[34,35] Nevertheless, as recently as 2010, the European Guidelines for Quality Assurance in Cervical Screening maintain cytologic examination as the standard, noting the risk of overdiagnosis and inconclusive evidence on adjuvant HPV testing.[35] Specifics of screening programs vary amongst European Union nations. Recent guidelines issued from several major US organizations, including US Preventive Services Task Force,[36] American Society of Colposcopy and Cervical Pathology,[37] American Cancer Society,[38] and American College of Obstetrics and Gynecology[39] recommend Papanicolaou test alone starting at age 21 years, with reflex HPV testing for Papanicolaou tests showing atypical squamous cells of undetermined significance. These organizations have different opinions about the data suggesting that all women should undergo Papanicolaou and HPV cotesting starting at age 30 years, although they do all agree that if both tests are obtained and both show negative results, they should not be repeated before 3 years. They all agree that for regular-risk women, Papanicolaou testing alone every 3 years is acceptable for women aged 30 years and older.

MANAGEMENT OF SCREENING ABNORMALITIES

Patients with abnormal cervical cytology are typically triaged to a secondary screening evaluation, although in some nations, particularly in Central and Eastern Europe, colposcopy is used in routine cervical examination.[40] Colposcopy involves the visualization of abnormal lesions of the cervix under magnification, often with direct biopsy for histologic diagnosis. Independently, colposcopy has a sensitivity reported between 44% and 77% and a specificity reported between 85% and 90% in various studies.[32] Biopsy enables histologic diagnosis of mild, moderate, or severe dysplasia or invasive cervical cancer. Colposcopy requires equipment (a working colposcope and sterile instruments), experienced trained practitioners to perform the biopsies, and easily available pathology services to read the biopsies, relay results, and then track patients to return for repeat visits for treatment or reassessment. Such a system is costly and impractical in many lower-resource settings. Thus, easier, more practical solutions for screening and diagnosis that can be applied by lesser-trained clinicians or health care workers, which do not require easily accessible pathology services and often allowing for one see-and-treat visit, have been evaluated extensively.

TREATMENT OPTIONS

There are 2 main approaches to treatment of cervical precancers: excisional and ablative. In countries with greater resources, an excisional procedure, either a loop excision or a cold knife cone biopsy, is commonly performed. The loop procedure uses a wire loop and electrocautery and local anesthesia to excise a small area of the cervix containing an abnormality that can then be sent off for pathology review. If cancer is diagnosed, a larger therapeutic surgery can be performed. This treatment can be performed both in a 3-visit approach (screen with Papanicolaou test or HPV, followed by colposcopic-directed biopsy, followed by treatment if pathologic examination shows a high-grade precancer), or it can be performed in a 2-visit approach (abnormal Papanicolaou test result followed by evaluation and treatment at next visit).

Another treatment, cryotherapy, ablates the cervix by freezing it. This technique applies a cold probe to the external cervix and is best when used for smaller less-advanced lesions. For the treatment to be successful, the lesion must be fully visible and cannot involve the endocervical canal or the vagina. Furthermore, cryotherapy does not treat cancer and has limited efficacy (70%–92%) against CIN 3.[7] Because it is low cost and rarely results in major complications, cryotherapy is an ideal treatment when resources are scarce or when a less-trained worker is performing many see-and-treat examinations.

SCREENING IN DEVELOPING SETTINGS

Simultaneous or sequential Papanicolaou and HPV screening require additional resources, making such combination testing impractical in developing settings. HPV may be preferable to Papanicolaou testing as a stand-alone primary cervical screen in resource-limited settings. Because of the high sensitivity for the detection of moderate or severe dysplasia, HPV testing is more appropriately suited for settings in which women have few lifetime examinations.[41] Moreover, HPV tests have a higher positive predictive value in these settings because of the higher incidence of cervical cancer.[42]

Visual inspection of the cervix (visual inspection with acetic acid [VIA] or Lugol iodine [VILI]) offers an alternative screening test to Papanicolaou and HPV testing. The screen involves application of acetic acid (VIA) or Lugol iodine reagent (VILI) to the cervix, followed by examination with the naked eye or with magnification to detect well-defined lesions in the vicinity of the squamocolumnar junction. The sensitivity of VIA/VILI for detection of high-grade lesions varies widely in studies in different settings (55%–96%), although it is most frequently reported in the 70% to 85% range, roughly comparable with cervical cytologic examination.[18,32,43] However, VIA/VILI is less specific than cervical cytologic examination, with reported specificities ranging from 49% to 86% for VIA and from 73% to 93% for VILI.[32]

Cervical screening programs with VIA/VILI are likely most compatible with the available infrastructure in developing countries. VIA/VILI does not require laboratory capacity, and medical personnel can be trained in the technique in less than 10 days.[44] Moreover, VIA is the most cost-effective method of cervical screening, as measured in cost per year of life saved. In representative models based in Thailand comparing primary Papanicolaou, HPV, and VIA screening, VIA screening costs approximately $200 to $300 per year of life saved and HPV and Papanicolaou screening cost approximately $1000 to $4000 per year of life saved ($2002).[42]

Loss to follow-up is a challenge with cervical cancer screening in middle- and low-income countries. The course of care is taxing on patients and health systems, requiring multiple visits for primary screening, directed biopsy, and treatment. Thus, VIA/VILI or HPV testing can been used in combination with same-day treatment, often using low-cost cryotherapy, wherein screen-positive women are immediately triaged to treatment without colposcopy or histologic examination. See-and-treat cervical cancer prevention programs using VIA/VILI or HPV testing with cryotherapy have proven efficacious in reducing the incidence of moderate or severe dysplasia and invasive cancer in a variety of developing settings.[45–47] In a large (N = 6555) randomized trial of the approach in South Africa, participants randomized to the see-and-treat cohort with VIA/VILI and HPV screening had a 46% and a 77% lower prevalence of moderate to severe dysplasia at 12 months, respectively, than those randomized to receive delayed evaluation.[47]

See-and-treat approaches using same-day screening and cryotherapy are liable to overtreat participants. However, the technique has been generally highly acceptable to study participants, and major complications with cryotherapy are infrequent.[45,46] Moreover, see-and-treat approaches are more cost-effective than multiple-visit screening designs for resource-limited settings.[48,49] Models of see-and-treat programs in Kenya, Thailand, Peru, India, and South Africa produce a cost per year of life saved that is below the respective national per capita gross domestic products (GDPs).[49]

The efficacy and cost-effectiveness of see-and-treat screening with HPV testing may be augmented by cervicovaginal sample self-collection. In various settings, sample self-collection has been acceptable to the local population, and invitation for self-collection has increased compliance and overall screening coverage versus invitation for clinician-directed sampling.[41,50] The approach is limited by poorer specimen quality and sensitivity for detection of moderate or severe dysplasia, reported between 55.0% and 82.5%.[51,52] However, self-collection is more cost effective than clinical sample collection.[53]

See-and-treat and self-collection with cervical screening are confined to pilot programs and study trials in much of the developing world. Conventional cytologic examination remains the standard in South Africa, Brazil, and Sudan, although many nations, including India and Kenya, have shifted the focus to VIA/VILI with referral to secondary screening.

LIMITATIONS OF SCREENING SERVICES WORLDWIDE

Cervical cancer is the second most common cancer among women in low-income countries, although it accounts for only 0.6% of the overall mortality in low-income countries.[54] The design of, and resource allocation to, cervical cancer programs must be made in the context of the demands of such competing health priorities as HIV, maternal mortality, and diarrheal diseases. The standard of care in developed nations for the management of cervical precancers requires laboratory capacity for cytologic and histologic examinations and time and resource available for multiple visits for screening, colposcopy with directed biopsy, and ultimately treatment. Comparatively, see-and-treat programs, 1- or 2-visit models involving VIA/VILI or HPV screening with cryotherapy, can produce a cost per year of life saved that is below the respective national per capita GDPs[49] at which point see-and-treat screening can be considered very cost effective.[55]

Effective prevention and management of cervical precancers has yet to be realized in many developing nations and resource-poor settings. In developing nations, 65.3% of women have never received a pelvic examination. Lifetime screening coverage may be as low as 10% in poorer nations, including Zambia, Ethiopia, and Bangladesh.[56] Even in developing nations that, in recent years, have committed to cervical cancer prevention programs, screening coverage is markedly depressed as compared with coverage in developed nations. Moreover, follow-up diagnosis and treatment of cervical precancers have been complicated by inefficiencies in referral networks and care provision.[57] Efforts to address cervical cancer in developing nations are further complicated by particular regional variables, including the HIV/AIDS pandemic. Nevertheless, within controlled settings in developing nations, cervical cancer screening and management can function with comparable efficacy to programs in developed nations.[58] A host of economic, logistical, and sociocultural factors may impede the accessibility and availability of preventative and treatment services for cervical precancers. Such limitations include fragmented health care systems, inadequate health infrastructure for cervical cancer care, and a lack of training of clinicians for cervical cancer prevention and management.[59–61] In an example from an Ugandan study, 87% of final-year medical students had never performed a Papanicolaou test[59]; in Lagos, Nigeria, a study found that only 11.8% of general practitioners informed their patients about Papanicolaou tests.[62] Numerous developing nations are severely lacking in capacity for colposcopy, cryotherapy, or other vital screening or treatment infrastructure.[40]

Social and cultural barriers may also limit patient access to care. Low levels of awareness about cervical cancer pose a common barrier in many developing settings to uptake of preventative services.[60,63–65] Cultural notions of modesty and attitudes about screening further impede uptake of these services.[59,66] In a survey of attitudes about Papanicolaou testing among Kenyan women, participants did not recognize the rationale for early detection, opining, "if you are not in pain, why [do] you need a test?" and adding that "even if we went for such a test, we do not want to be told that we have cancer."[57] The utility of cancer treatment is viewed with skepticism in some settings in which cancer is regarded as a disease without a cure or as the result of witchcraft or infidelity.[61] Such patient limitations to cervical cancer screening and treatment are prevalent among lower-income and immigrant populations in developed nations as well.[66,67]

Cervical cancer prevention programs have used multiple strategies in efforts to overcome patient limitations. Interventions commonly incorporate a public educational component, which may consist of posters, pamphlets, television, or radio advertising. In regions with low literacy, person-to-person and group health education may be most important to overcoming barriers of lack of awareness. Sample self-collection by patients for HPV testing may allow screening programs to circumvent specific barriers associated with pelvic examination.

Cervical cancer programs have succeeded in developing settings in which they have addressed both provider limitations and patient limitations. In a pilot project for mass cervical cancer screening in Soweto, South Africa, laboratory capacity was organized to conduct 90,000 Papanicolaou tests annually. The project, however, garnered a low level of participation among the target population because it failed to incorporate a public awareness campaign.[65] By contrast, an intervention in Sarawak, Malaysia, that addressed both infrastructural and social barriers succeeded in reducing the late-stage presentation of both breast cancer and cervical cancer cases by approximately one-half.[68] The program trained health staff in early detection and strengthened referral systems, while also engaging an active public awareness campaign.

HPV VACCINATION

As an alternative to screening and management of cervical precancers, HPV vaccination provides primary prevention against precancers and invasive cancer. At present, 2 vaccine formulations are commercially available, the quadrivalent HPV 6/11/16/18 vaccine (Gardasil) and the bivalent HPV-16/18 vaccine (Cervarix). Both vaccines protect against infection from HPV-16 and HPV-18, which are associated with approximately 70% of cervical carcinoma.[10] Both the bivalent and quadrivalent vaccines are highly effective in protecting against HPV-16/HPV-18 infection (92%–100% efficacy) and the development of HPV-16/HPV-18–related CIN 2/3 (>90% efficacy) among HPV-naive women.[69–71] However, the vaccines are not effective in women with previous HPV exposure.[70] In the United States, vaccination is recommended for girls aged 9 to 18 years. Under certain guidelines, catch-up vaccination is recommended for women aged 18 to 26 years, who are more likely to have had previous HPV infection. Cervical screening is still recommended in vaccinated women because the current HPV vaccines cover the 2 highest-risk HPV subtypes but not the remaining 13 high-risk HPV subtypes that cumulatively account for approximately 30% of cervical cancers.

Although currently affordable only in middle- and high-income nations, HPV vaccination has the potential to close the gap in cervical cancer incidence and mortality between developed and underdeveloped nations. Various models of HPV vaccination campaigns in developing countries highlight potential reductions in lifetime risk of cervical cancer ranging from 30.1% (Senegal) to 60.1% (Ethiopia) and 60.8% (Brazil).[55,73] HPV vaccination in combination with see-and-treat HPV screening provides a 1.5- to 2-fold lifetime risk reduction versus screening alone.[33,72,73] At present, however, the cost of the vaccine is prohibitively expensive for resource-poor settings.[55] Vaccination is most cost effective in nations with the greatest cervical cancer burden, including much of Eastern Africa, Haiti, and Bolivia.[55] Several global health care organizations are currently working with vaccine manufacturers to lower the cost of the vaccine to be affordable in the poorest countries.

SUMMARY

Cervical cancer incidence and mortality have decreased dramatically over the past 50 years in countries with access and resources to provide frequent screening, evaluation, and treatment of high-grade cervical cancer precursors. For countries with fewer resources and many competing health concerns, cervical cancer remains one of the most lethal and common cancers among women. With the advent of newer technology, such as low-cost HPV vaccines and self-administered HPV tests, followed by simple well-known techniques such as VIA and cryotherapy, cervical cancer rates may well start to decrease worldwide.

REFERENCES

1. Ferlay J, Shin HR, Bray F, et al. GLOBOCAN 2008 v1.2, cancer incidence and mortality worldwide: IARC CancerBase No. 10 [Internet]. Lyon (France): International Agency for Research on Cancer; 2010. Available at: http://globocan.iarc.fr. Accessed November 6, 2011.
2. Yin D, Morris C, Allen M, et al. Institute for Health Metrics and Evaluation. The Challenge Ahead: Progress and setbacks in breast and cervical cancer. Seattle, WA: IHME; 2011.
3. Howlader N, Noone AM, Krapcho M, et al, editors. SEER cancer statistics review, 1975-2008, National Cancer Institute. Bethesda (MD). Available at: http://seer.cancer.gov/csr/1975_2008/. Based on November 2010 SEER data submission, posted to the SEER web site, 2011. Accessed November 21, 2011.
4. Mellstedt H. Cancer initiatives in developing countries. Ann Oncol 2006; 17(Suppl 8):viii24–31.
5. Hamad HM. Cancer initiatives in Sudan. Ann Oncol 2006;17(Suppl 8):viii32–6.
6. Singh GK, Miller BA, Hankey BF, et al. Persistent area socioeconomic disparities in U.S. incidence of cervical cancer, mortality, stage, and survival, 1975-2000. Cancer 2004;101(5):1051–7.
7. Sankaranarayanan R, Thara S, Esmy PO, et al. Cervical cancer: screening and therapeutic perspectives. Med Princ Pract 2008;17(5):351–64.

8. Weinstock H, Berman S, Cates W Jr. Sexually transmitted diseases among American youth: incidence and prevalence estimates, 2000. Perspect Sex Reprod Health 2004;36(1):6–10.

9. WHO/ICO Information Centre on HPV and Cervical Cancer (HPV Information Centre). Human papillomavirus and related cancers in United States of America. Summary Report 2010. Available at: www.who.int/hpvcentre. Accessed November 6, 2011.

10. WHO/ICO Information Centre on HPV and Cervical Cancer (HPV Information Centre). Human papillomavirus and related cancers in world. Summary Report 2010. Available at: www.who.int/hpvcentre. Accessed November 6, 2011.

11. Dunne EF, Unger ER, Sternberg M, et al. Prevalence of HPV infection among females in the United States. JAMA 2007;297(8):813–9.

12. de Sanjose S, Quint WG, Alemany L, et al. Retrospective International Survey and HPV Time Trends Study Group. Human papillomavirus genotype attribution in invasive cervical cancer: a retrospective cross-sectional worldwide study. Lancet Oncol 2010;11(11):1048–56.

13. Muñoz N, Castellsagué X, de González AB, et al. Chapter 1: HPV in the etiology of human cancer. Vaccine 2006;24(Suppl 3):S3/1–10.

14. Wheeler CM. Natural history of human papillomavirus infections, cytologic and histologic abnormalities, and cancer. Obstet Gynecol Clin North Am 2008; 35(4):519–36, vii.

15. Carter JR, Ding Z, Rose BR. HPV infection and cervical disease: a review. Aust N Z J Obstet Gynaecol 2011;51(2):103–8.

16. González P, Hildesheim A, Rodríguez AC, et al. Behavioral/lifestyle and immunologic factors associated with HPV infection among women older than 45 years. Cancer Epidemiol Biomarkers Prev 2010;19(12):3044–54.

17. Weinstein LC, Buchanan EM, Hillson C, et al. Screening and prevention: cervical cancer. Prim Care 2009;36(3):559–74.

18. Safaeian M, Solomon D, Castle PE. Cervical cancer prevention—cervical screening: science in evolution. Obstet Gynecol Clin North Am 2007;34(4): 739–60, ix.

19. Comprehensive cervical cancer control: a guide to essential practice. Geneva (Switzerland): World Health Organization; 2006. Available at: www.rho.org/files/WHO_CC_control_2006.pdf. Accessed November 6, 2011.

20. Dalla Palma P, Giorgi Rossi P, Collina G, et al, NTCC Pathology Group. The reproducibility of CIN diagnoses among different pathologists: data from histology reviews from a multicenter randomized study. Am J Clin Pathol 2009;132:125–32.

21. Schiffman M, Rodríguez AC. Heterogeneity in CIN3 diagnosis. Lancet Oncol 2008;9(5):404–6.

22. Ostör AG. Natural history of cervical intraepithelial neoplasia: a critical review. Int J Gynecol Pathol 1993;12(2):186–92.

23. Castle PE, Schiffman M, Wheeler CM, et al. Evidence for frequent regression of cervical intraepithelial neoplasia-grade 2. Obstet Gynecol 2009;113(1): 18–25.

24. Storey A, Pim D, Murray A, et al. Comparison of the in vitro transforming activities of human papillomavirus types. EMBO J 1988;7(6):1815–20.

25. Hasan UA, Bates E, Takeshita F, et al. TLR9 expression and function is abolished by the cervical cancer-associated human papillomavirus type 16. J Immunol 2007;178(5):3186–97.

26. Stanley M. Pathology and epidemiology of HPV infection in females. Gynecol Oncol 2010;117(Suppl 2):S5–10.

27. Fernandes AP, Gonçalves MA, Duarte G, et al. HPV16, HPV18, and HIV infection may influence cervical cytokine intralesional levels. Virology 2005;334(2):294–8.

28. Ronco G, Cuzick J, Pierotti P, et al. Accuracy of liquid based versus conventional cytology: overall results of new technologies for cervical cancer screening: randomised controlled trial. BMJ 2007;335(7609):28.

29. Whitlock EP, Vesco KK, Eder M, et al. Liquid-based cytology and human papillomavirus testing to screen for cervical cancer: a systematic review for the U.S. Preventive services task force. Ann Intern Med 2011;155:687–97.

30. Mayrand MH, Duarte-Franco E, Rodrigues I, et al, Canadian Cervical Cancer Screening Trial Study Group. Human papillomavirus DNA versus Papanicolaou screening tests for cervical cancer. N Engl J Med 2007;357(16):1579–88.

31. Pimple S, Muwonge R, Amin G, et al. Cytology versus HPV testing for the detection of high-grade cervical lesions in women found positive on visual inspection in Mumbai, India. Int J Gynaecol Obstet 2010;108(3):236–9.

32. Sankaranarayanan R, Gaffikin L, Jacob M, et al. A critical assessment of screening methods for cervical neoplasia. Int J Gynaecol Obstet 2005; 89(Suppl 2):S4–12.

33. Leinonen M, Nieminen P, Kotaniemi-Talonen L, et al. Age-specific evaluation of primary human papillomavirus screening vs conventional cytology in a randomized setting. J Natl Cancer Inst 2009;101(23):1612–23.

34. Sørbye SW, Arbyn M, Fismen S, et al. Triage of women with low-grade cervical lesions—HPV mRNA testing versus repeat cytology. PLoS One 2011;6(8):e24083.

35. Arbyn M, Anttila A, Jordan J, et al. European guidelines for quality assurance in cervical cancer screening. Second edition—summary document. Ann Oncol 2010;21(3):448–58.

36. Available at: www.uspstf.org. Accessed November 9, 2011.

37. Available at: www.asccp.org. Accessed November 9, 2011.

38. Available at: www.acs.org. Accessed November 9, 2011.

39. ACOG Committee on Practice Bulletins—Gynecology. ACOG Practice Bulletin no. 109: Cervical cytology screening. Obstet Gynecol 2009;114(6):1409–20.

40. Denny L, Quinn M, Sankaranarayanan R. Chapter 8: screening for cervical cancer in developing countries. Vaccine 2006;24(Suppl 3):S3/71–77.

41. Lazcano-Ponce E, Lorincz AT, Cruz-Valdez A, et al. Self-collection of vaginal specimens for human papillomavirus testing in cervical cancer prevention (MARCH): a community-based randomised controlled trial. Lancet 2011 Nov 1. [Epub ahead of print].

42. Mandelblatt JS, Lawrence WF, Gaffikin L, et al. Costs and benefits of different strategies to screen for cervical cancer in less-developed countries. J Natl Cancer Inst 2002;94(19):1469–83.

43. Cervical cancer screening in developing countries: report of a WHO Consultation. Geneva (Switzerland): World Health Organization; 2002. Available at: whqlibdoc. who.int/publications/2002/9241545720.pdf. Accessed November 6, 2011.

44. Blumenthal PD, Lauterbach M, Sellors JW, et al. Training for cervical cancer prevention programs in low-resource settings: focus on visual inspection with acetic acid and cryotherapy. Int J Gynaecol Obstet 2005;89(Suppl 2):S30–7.

45. Gaffikin L, Blumenthal PD, Emerson M, et al, Royal Thai College of Obstetricians and Gynaecologists (RTCOG)/JHPIEGO Corporation Cervical Cancer Prevention Group [corrected]. Safety, acceptability, and feasibility of a single-visit approach to cervical-cancer prevention in rural Thailand: a demonstration project. Lancet 2003;361(9360):814–20 [Erratum appears in: Lancet 2003;361(9373):1994]; PubMed PMID: 12642047.

46. Blumenthal PD, Gaffikin L, Deganus S, et al, Ghana Cervicare Group. Cervical cancer prevention: safety, acceptability, and feasibility of a single-visit approach in Accra, Ghana. Am J Obstet Gynecol 2007;196(4):407, e1–8 [discussion: 407, e8–9].

47. Denny L, Kuhn L, De Souza M, et al. Screen-and-treat approaches for cervical cancer prevention in low-resource settings: a randomized controlled trial. JAMA 2005;294(17):2173–81.

48. Goldie SJ, Kuhn L, Denny L, et al. Policy analysis of cervical cancer screening strategies in low-resource settings: clinical benefits and cost-effectiveness. JAMA 2001;285(24):3107–15 [Erratum appears in: JAMA 2001;286(9):1026].

49. Goldie SJ, Gaffikin L, Goldhaber-Fiebert JD, et al, Alliance for Cervical Cancer Prevention Cost Working Group. Cost-effectiveness of cervical-cancer screening in five developing countries. N Engl J Med 2005;353(20):2158–68.

50. Barbee L, Kobetz E, Menard J, et al. Assessing the acceptability of self-sampling for HPV among Haitian immigrant women: CBPR in action. Cancer Causes Control 2010;21(3):421–31.

51. Taylor S, Wang C, Wright TC, et al. A comparison of human papillomavirus testing of clinician-collected and self-collected samples during follow-up after screen-and-treat. Int J Cancer 2011;129(4):879–86.

52. Bhatla N, Dar L, Patro AR, et al. Can human papillomavirus DNA testing of self-collected vaginal samples compare with physician-collected cervical samples and cytology for cervical cancer screening in developing countries? Cancer Epidemiol 2009;33(6):446–50.

53. Balasubramanian A, Kulasingam SL, Baer A, et al. Accuracy and cost-effectiveness of cervical cancer screening by high-risk human papillomavirus DNA testing of self-collected vaginal samples. J Low Genit Tract Dis 2010; 14(3):185–95.

54. World Health Organization. Causes of death 2008 summary tables. Geneva (Switzerland): World Health Organization; 2010. Available at: http://apps.who.int/ghodata/. Accessed November 6, 2011.

55. Goldie SJ, O'Shea M, Campos NG, et al. Health and economic outcomes of HPV 16,18 vaccination in 72 GAVI-eligible countries. Vaccine 2008;26(32):4080–93.

56. Gakidou E, Nordhagen S, Obermeyer Z. Coverage of cervical cancer screening in 57 countries: low average levels and large inequalities. PLoS Med 2008;5(6): e132.

57. Gatune JW, Nyamongo IK. An ethnographic study of cervical cancer among women in rural Kenya: is there a folk causal model? Int J Gynecol Cancer 2005;15(6):1049–59.

58. Muwonge R, Mbalawa CG, Keita N, et al, IARC Multicentre Study Group on Cervical Cancer Early Detection. Performance of colposcopy in five sub-Saharan African countries. BJOG 2009;116(6):829–37.

59. Mutyaba T, Mmiro FA, Weiderpass E. Knowledge, attitudes and practices on cervical cancer screening among the medical workers of Mulago Hospital, Uganda. BMC Med Educ 2006;6:13.

60. Urasa M, Darj E. Knowledge of cervical cancer and screening practices of nurses at a regional hospital in Tanzania. Afr Health Sci 2011;11(1):48–57.

61. Ekortarl A, Ndom P, Sacks A. A study of patients who appear with far advanced cancer at Yaounde General Hospital, Cameroon, Africa. Psychooncology 2007; 16(3):255–7.

62. Anorlu RI, Ribiu KA, Abudu OO, et al. Cervical cancer screening practices among general practitioners in Lagos Nigeria. J Obstet Gynaecol 2007;27(2):181–4.

63. Lee FH, Paz-Soldan VA, Carcamo C, et al. Knowledge and attitudes of adult Peruvian women vis-à-vis human papillomavirus (HPV), cervical cancer, and the HPV vaccine. J Low Genit Tract Dis 2010;14(2):113–7.

64. Ajayi IO, Adewole IF. Knowledge and attitude of general outpatient attendants in Nigeria to cervical cancer. Cent Afr J Med 1998;44(2):41–3.

65. Sankaranarayanan R, Budukh AM, Rajkumar R. Effective screening programmes for cervical cancer in low- and middle-income developing countries. Bull World Health Organ 2001;79(10):954–62.

66. Redwood-Campbell L, Fowler N, Laryea S, et al. 'Before you teach me, I cannot know': immigrant women's barriers and enablers with regard to cervical cancer screening among different ethnolinguistic groups in Canada. Can J Public Health 2011;102(3):230–4.

67. Fernandez ME, McCurdy SA, Arvey SR, et al. HPV knowledge, attitudes, and cultural beliefs among Hispanic men and women living on the Texas-Mexico border. Ethn Health 2009;14(6):607–24.

68. Devi BC, Tang TS, Corbex M. Reducing by half the percentage of late-stage presentation for breast and cervix cancer over 4 years: a pilot study of clinical downstaging in Sarawak, Malaysia. Ann Oncol 2007;18(7):1172–6.

69. Garland SM, Hernandez-Avila M, Wheeler CM, et al, Females United to Unilaterally Reduce Endo/Ectocervical Disease (FUTURE) I Investigators. Quadrivalent vaccine against human papillomavirus to prevent anogenital diseases. N Engl J Med 2007;356(19):1928–43.

70. Paavonen J, Naud P, Salmerón J, et al, HPV PATRICIA Study Group. Efficacy of human papillomavirus (HPV)-16/18 AS04-adjuvanted vaccine against cervical infection and precancer caused by oncogenic HPV types (PATRICIA): final analysis of a double-blind, randomised study in young women. Lancet 2009; 374(9686):301–14 [Erratum appears in: Lancet 2010;376(9746):1054].

71. FUTURE II Study Group. Quadrivalent vaccine against human papillomavirus to prevent high-grade cervical lesions. N Engl J Med 2007;356(19):1915–27.

72. IARC. Cervix cancer screening. IARC handbooks of cancer prevention, volume 10. Lyon (France): IARC; 2005.

73. Goldie SJ, Kim JJ, Kobus K, et al. Cost-effectiveness of HPV 16, 18 vaccination in Brazil. Vaccine 2007;25(33):6257–70.

74. Luciani S, Winkler J. Cervical cancer prevention in Peru: lessons learned from the TATI demonstration project. Washington, DC: PAHO; 2006.

75. National Guideline for Cervical Cancer Screening Programme. Department of Health, South Africa. Available at: www.kznhealth.gov.za/cervicalcancer.pdf. Accessed November 21, 2011.

76. Guidelines for Cervical Cancer Screening Programme. National Cancer Control Program; 2006. Available at: www.cytoindia.com/cytology%20eqa/CCSP%20Guidelines.pdf. Accessed November 6, 2011.

Current Management of Vulvar Cancer

Katherine C. Fuh, MD[a], Jonathan S. Berek, MD, MMS[b],*

KEYWORDS

- Vulvar cancer • Radical local excision
- Modified radical vulvectomy
- Inguinofemoral lymphadenectomy
- Sentinel lymph node biopsy

Vulvar cancer is the fourth most common gynecologic cancer and comprises 5% of the malignancies of the female genital tract.[1] Squamous cell carcinoma of the vulva is predominantly a disease of postmenopausal women, with a mean age at diagnosis of approximately 65 years. The diagnosis is often made after years of symptoms of pruritus associated with vulvar dystrophy. The lesion is usually raised and may be fleshy, ulcerated, leukoplakic, or warty in appearance. Most squamous cell carcinomas of the vulva occur on the labia majora, but the labia minora, clitoris, and the perineum may be primary sites.

Vulvar cancer is surgically staged based on pathologic evaluation of a vulvar biopsy and of the inguinofemoral lymph nodes. A complete clinical assessment helps guide the surgical and medical approach to treatment. In particular, the diameter of the primary tumor should be measured, and the inguinal, axillary, and supraclavicular lymph nodes should be palpated. Because of the multifocal nature of squamous intraepithelial lesions, cervical cytology and colposcopy of the cervix, vagina, and vulva should be performed. Imaging, such as abdominal/pelvic computed tomography (CT) may be performed for women with tumors 2 cm or larger to detect suspected metastases to lymph node or other distant sites.

Diagnosis requires a biopsy specimen, which can be taken in the office. The biopsy specimen must include underlying dermis and connective tissue so that depth and stromal invasion can be evaluated. Staging and primary surgical treatment are typically performed as a single procedure. Staging should include the evaluation for factors related to prognosis: tumor size, depth of invasion, lymph node metastases, and distant metastases.

The authors have nothing to disclose.

[a] Division of Gynecologic Oncology, Department of Obstetrics and Gynecology, Stanford University School of Medicine, 300 Pasteur Drive, HH333, Stanford, CA 94305, USA

[b] Department of Obstetrics and Gynecology, Stanford Women's Cancer Center, Stanford Cancer Institute, Stanford University School of Medicine, 300 Pasteur Drive, HH333, Stanford, CA 94305, USA

* Corresponding author.

E-mail address: jberek@stanford.edu

Hematol Oncol Clin N Am 26 (2012) 45–62

doi:10.1016/j.hoc.2011.10.006

0889-8588/12/$ – see front matter © 2012 Elsevier Inc. All rights reserved.

hemonc.theclinics.com

STAGING

Historically, staging was based on clinical factors using the tumor, node, metastasis (TNM) classification adopted by the International Federation of Gynecology and Obstetrics (FIGO) in 1969. This staging was focused on a clinical evaluation of the primary tumor, the regional lymph nodes, and a limited search for distant metastases. However, clinical evaluation of inguinofemoral lymph nodes is inaccurate in approximately 25% to 30% of cases.[2–4] The percentage of error in clinical staging compared with surgical staging increased from 18% for stage I disease to 44% for stage IV disease.[5] In 1988, surgical staging for vulvar cancer was introduced, and updated FIGO staging occurred in 2008 (**Table 1**). Surgical staging is preferable because the diagnosis of inguinofemoral lymph node metastasis is the most important predictor of overall prognosis.

Pathology

Squamous cell carcinoma

More than 90% of vulvar malignancies are squamous cell carcinomas. There are 2 subtypes, both of which usually occur on the labia or vestibule. The keratinizing, differentiated, or simplex type is most common. This type occurs in older women and is not related to human papillomavirus (HPV) infection but is associated with vulvar dystrophies such as lichen sclerosus and, in developing countries, chronic venereal

Table 1	
FIGO staging of carcinoma of the vulva (2008)	
Stage I	Tumor confined to the vulva
IA	Lesions ≤2 cm in size, confined to the vulva or perineum and with stromal invasion ≤1.0 mm[a], no nodal metastasis
IB	Lesions >2 cm in size or with stromal invasion >1.0 mm[a], confined to the vulva or perineum, with negative nodes
Stage II	Tumor of any size with extension to adjacent perineal structures (one-third lower urethra, one-third lower vagina, anus) with negative nodes
Stage III	Tumor of any size with or without extension to adjacent perineal structures (one-third lower urethra, one-third lower vagina, anus) with positive inguinofemoral lymph nodes
IIIA	(1) With 1 lymph node metastasis (≥5 mm), or (2) 1–2 lymph node metastases (<5 mm)
IIIB	(1) With 2 or more lymph node metastases (≥5 mm), or (2) 3 or more lymph node metastases (<5 mm)
IIIC	With positive nodes with extracapsular spread
Stage IV	Tumor invades other regional (two-thirds upper urethra, two-thirds upper vagina), of distant structures
IVA	Tumor invades any of the following: (1) upper urethral and/or vaginal mucosa, bladder mucosa, rectal mucosa, or fixed to pelvic bone, or (2) fixed or ulcerated inguinofemoral lymph nodes
IVB	Any distant metastasis including pelvic lymph nodes

[a] The depth of invasion is defined as the measurement of the tumor from the epithelial-stromal junction of the adjacent most superficial dermal papilla to the deepest point of invasion.

Data from FIGO Committee on Gynecologic Oncology. Revised FIGO staging for carcinoma of the vulva cervix, and endometrium. Int J Gynecol Obs 2009;105:103–4; and *Reproduced from* Berek JS, Hacker NF. Berek and Hacker's Gynecologic Oncology. 5th edition. Philadelphia: Lippincott Williams & Wilkins; 2010; with permission.

granulomatous disease. The classic, warty, or bowenoid type is predominantly associated with HPV 16, 18, and 33, and is found in younger women.[6,7] These women tend to present with early-stage disease, although several cases of stage III/IV disease in HIV-infected women have been reported. Verrucous carcinoma is a variant of squamous cell carcinoma that has distinct features. Although cauliflowerlike in appearance, it is differentiated from squamous cell carcinoma with a verrucous configuration. The lesion grows slowly and rarely metastasizes to lymph nodes, but it may be locally destructive.

Melanoma

Melanoma is the second most common vulvar cancer histology, accounting for approximately 5% of primary vulvar neoplasms. Melanoma of the vulva occurs predominantly in postmenopausal, white, non-Hispanic women at a median age of 68 years.[8] Vulvar melanoma is usually a pigmented lesion, but amelanotic lesions also occur. Most arise de novo on the clitoris or labia minora, but can also develop within preexisting junctional or compound nevi.

Basal cell carcinoma

Two percent of vulvar cancers are basal cell cancers and 2% of basal cell cancers occur on the vulva.[9] They usually affect postmenopausal white women and may be locally invasive, although they are usually nonmetastasizing. The typical appearance is that of a rodent ulcer with rolled edges and central ulceration; the lesion may be pigmented or pearly and gray. They are often asymptomatic, but pruritus, bleeding, or pain may occur. Basal cell carcinomas are associated with a high incidence of antecedent or concomitant malignancy elsewhere in the body.[10] A thorough search for primary malignancies should be performed.

Sarcoma

Soft tissue sarcomas such as leiomyosarcomas, rhabdomyosarcomas, liposarcomas, angiosarcomas, neurofibrosarcomas, fibrous histiocytomas, and epithelioid sarcomas constitute 1% to 2% of vulvar malignancies. As with soft tissue sarcomas located elsewhere on the extremities and trunk, high-grade lesions that are larger than 5 cm in diameter, with infiltrating margins and a high mitotic rate, are most likely to recur.

Adenocarcinoma

Most primary adenocarcinomas of the vulva occur in the Bartholin gland. This gland is composed of columnar epithelium; ducts are lined by stratified squamous epithelium that changes to transitional cell epithelium as the terminal ducts are reached. Cancers arising in the Bartholin gland are most often adenocarcinomas or squamous cell carcinomas, but transitional cell carcinomas, adenosquamous carcinomas, and adenoid cystic cell carcinomas may also develop.[11,12] Median age is 57 years, and enlargement of the Bartholin gland in a postmenopausal woman is a concern for malignancy because benign inflammatory disease usually does not occur in this age group. The gland should be biopsied in older (>40 years of age) women with a mass in this location, even if the lesions appear cystic or abscessed. Metastatic disease is common in cancers of the Bartholin gland because of the rich vascular and lymphatic network.

Invasive adenocarcinoma may be present within or beneath the surface intraepithelial lesion, which is known as Paget disease.[13,14] This is an uncommon malignancy. Most patients are in their 60s and 70s and white. Pruritus is the most common symptom, present in 70% of patients. The lesion has an eczematoid appearance; it is well demarcated and has slightly raised edges and a red background, often dotted with small, pale islands. It is usually multifocal and may occur anywhere on the vulva, mons, perineum/perianal area, or inner thigh. Vulvar biopsy should be performed in patients with suspicious lesions, including those with persistent pruritic eczematous lesions that fail to resolve within 6 weeks of appropriate antieczema therapy. Women with Paget disease should be evaluated for the possibility of synchronous neoplasms because approximately 4% to 5% of these patients have a noncontiguous carcinoma involving the breast, rectum, bladder, urethra, cervix, or ovary.

SURGICAL MANAGEMENT

In the 1940s, Taussig[15] in the United States and Way[2] in Great Britain pioneered the historic standard treatment of operable vulvar cancer with en bloc radical vulvectomy and bilateral removal of the inguinofemoral and pelvic lymph nodes. This resection consists of removal of the entire vulva down to the level of the deep fascia of the thigh, to the periosteum of the pubis, and to the inferior fascia of the urogenital diaphragm. Traditionally, this procedure could be performed with 2 teams of surgeons, if appropriate, through a single incision that circumscribes the labia majora and extends to the inguinofemoral regions bilaterally. This approach has largely been abandoned because most of the vulvar cancers now treated are low stage and because neoadjuvant chemoradiation is used for most of the advanced cases.

MANAGEMENT OF STAGE I TO II VULVAR CANCER

The modern approach to the management of patients with early-stage vulvar carcinoma should be individualized. In considering the appropriate operation, it is necessary to determine independently the appropriate management of the primary lesion and the inguinofemoral lymph nodes.[16,17]

Management of the Primary Tumor

Several factors have led to modifications from the en bloc radical vulvectomy and bilateral inguinofemoral and pelvic lymphadenectomy. These factors include the more frequent presentation of smaller tumors at diagnosis in younger women, the concern of postoperative morbidity and associated long-term hospitalization, the psychosexual effects from distortion of the vulva, and the problem of lymphedema. Alternative and less radical surgical approaches that remove less of the vulva and the surrounding skin are most commonly performed.

Two factors should be taken into consideration: age and condition of the remainder of the vulva. Since the 1980s, several investigators have advocated a radical local excision rather than a radical vulvectomy for the primary lesion in patients with T1a (2 cm or less) or T1b (larger than 2 cm). It is desirable to conserve as much of the vulva as possible. For stage II disease, the most conservative excision technique should be used that results in at least a 1-cm tumor-free margin. Depending on the size, location, and depth of invasion of the lesion, this may necessitate radical local excision, or modified radical vulvectomy, and the separate incision technique of an inguinofemoral lymphadenectomy (**Table 2**).[17]

Radical Local Excision

Radical local excision or modified radical vulvectomy (removal of part or all of the vulva unilaterally, also called modified radical hemivulvectomy) is most appropriate for the lesions on the lateral or posterior aspects of the vulva where preservation of the clitoris is feasible (**Figs. 1** and **2**). For anterior lesions, clitoral-sparing modified radical

Table 2
Treatment based on size of lesion, depth of invasion, and laterality

Size of Lesion	Depth of Invasion (mm)	Location	Operation	Inguinal Femoral Lymphadenectomy or Sentinel Lymph Node Evaluation[a,b]
T1a	≤1	Lateral[c] or central	Radical local excision	No
	>1	Lateral[c]	Radical local excision	Ipsilateral
T1a	>1	Central	Radical local excision	Bilateral
T1b		Lateral	Radical local excision	Ipsilateral
T2: Any size with extension to adjacent perineal structures (lower/distal one-third urethra, lower/distal one-third vagina, anal involvement)	—	—	Modified radical[d] and/or selected chemoradiation	Bilateral
Extensive T3–T4 disease (spread to the urethra, anus, bladder, rectum, or pelvic bone)	—	—	Neoadjuvant chemoradiation[e] and selected surgery	—

[a] Sentinel node biopsy can be considered as an alternative to inguinofemoral lymphadenectomy in all cases that require a lymphadenectomy.
[b] Bilateral lymphadenectomy is performed if unilateral node is positive.
[c] Further than 1 cm from midline.
[d] Modified radical vulvectomy (terminology includes radical hemivulvectomy, anterior or posterior modified radical vulvectomy).
[e] Can consider chemoradiation as primary treatment or postoperative radiation for patients with high risk of local recurrence (those with stage IVA disease, positive or close margins, and a large number of groin nodes).

vulvectomy can be an option. However, the depth of the resection, from the skin to the urogenital diaphragm, is the same as in standard radical vulvectomy.[18]

In a retrospective study including 41 patients with squamous carcinoma of the anterior vulva not involving the clitoris, 13 patients had clitoral-sparing modified radical vulvectomy and 28 had radical vulvectomy. The 13 patients who had clitoral-sparing surgery included 8 with stage I, 2 with stage II, 2 with stage III, and 1 with stage IV disease. After a median follow-up of 59 months, none of the 13 patients having conservative surgery had locoregional failure. In another study, 122 patients with lateral T1 and T2 lesions were studied: half of these patients had radical vulvectomy and the other half a radical hemivulvectomy. Disease-free survival at 5 years was 98% and 93%, respectively. Local or distant recurrence was not more common in patients treated by radical vulvectomy or radical hemivulvectomy.[19] Another published experience at the Royal Hospital for Women in Sydney described 116 patients with FIGO stages I and II vulvar cancer who underwent radical local excision. The patients who had radical vulvectomy had multifocal tumors. With a median follow-up of 84 months, the overall 5-year survival of patients with radical local excision was 96.4%.[20]

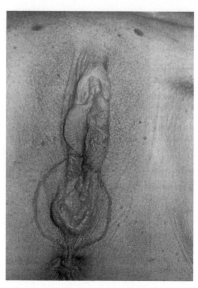

Fig. 1. Small (T1) vulvar carcinoma at the posterior fourchette. (*Reproduced from* Berek JS, Hacker NF. Berek and Hacker's Gynecologic Oncology. 5th edition. Philadelphia: Lippincott Williams & Wilkins; 2010. p. 547; with permission.)

Technique for Radical Local Excision

Radical local excision implies a deep excision of the primary tumor. The surgical margins should be at least 1 cm and should be drawn using a marking pen with the vulva in its natural state. The incision should be carried down to the inferior fascia of the urogenital diaphragm, which is coplanar with the fascia lata and the fascia over the pubic symphysis. The surgical defect is closed in 2 layers. For perineal lesions, proximity to the anus may preclude adequate surgical margins, and

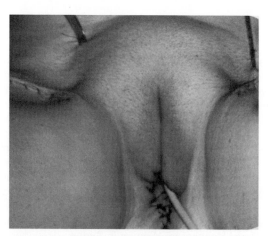

Fig. 2. Satisfactory cosmetic result after radical local excision and bilateral inguinofemoral node dissection. (*Reproduced from* Berek JS, Hacker NF. Berek and Hacker's Gynecologic Oncology. 5th edition. Philadelphia: Lippincott Williams & Wilkins; 2010. p. 548; with permission.)

consideration should be given to preoperative radiation. For periurethral lesions, the distal half of the urethra may be resected without loss of continence (**Fig. 3**).

For all types of vulvar excisions, a tumor-free margin of at least 1 cm seems to decrease the risk of local recurrence.[18,21,22] A retrospective case series (n = 135) reported a decrease in the rate of local recurrence in cases with normal tissue margins of 1 cm or greater compared with less than 8 mm (0% vs 50%).[23] Therefore, a surgical margin of at least 1 cm accounts for the 20% tissue shrinkage with formalin fixation. Care should be taken to ensure that the skin incision is made without tension.

Management of Inguinofemoral Lymph Nodes

Appropriate management of the regional lymph nodes is the single most important factor in decreasing mortality from early vulvar cancer. The only patients who are not at significant risk of lymph node metastases are those with a T1a tumor that invades the stroma to a depth of no greater than 1 mm. If a tumor is less than 2 cm in diameter, the lesion should be locally excised and analyzed histologically to determine the depth of invasion. Depth of invasion is measured from the most superficial dermal papilla adjacent to the tumor to the deepest focus of invasion.

If recurrence occurs in the undissected inguinofemoral lymph nodes, there is a high mortality. Pelvic lymphadenectomy, removal of iliac and obturator nodes, is not required for staging or therapy and has not been shown to improve survival. The choice of approach for lymphadenectomy depends on the size and location of the lesion as well as the presence of bulky positive nodes.

Tumor thickness is also measured and the average difference between tumor thickness and depth of invasion has been found to be 0.3 mm.[24–26] If the invasive focus is less than 1 mm, inguinofemoral lymphadenectomy may be omitted because the incidence of nodal metastases is essentially nil.[16,27–30] All patients with a more deeply

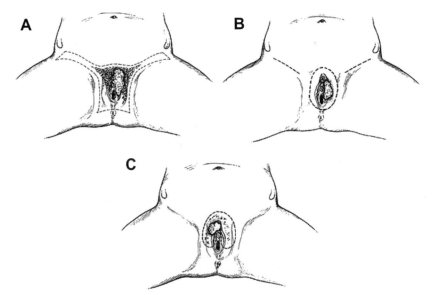

Fig. 3. Vulvar incisions for removal of primary tumor and inguinofemoral lymph nodes. (*A*) Modified butterfly incision. (*B*) Triple incision technique: a skin bridge is left between the radical vulvectomy and the groin incisions. (*C*) Anterior horseshoe incision. (*From* Elkas JC, Berek JS. Vulvar cancer: Staging, treatment and prognosis. In: UpToDate, Basow, DS (Ed), UpToDate, Waltham, MA, 2012; with permission.)

invasive T1a or T1b tumor require surgical removal of inguinofemoral lymph nodes or sentinel node evaluation (see later discussion). The Gynecologic Oncology Group (GOG) reported 6 inguinofemoral recurrences among 121 patients with T1N0 or T1N1 tumors after a superficial (inguinal) dissection, even though the inguinal nodes were reported as negative, although it is unclear whether all these recurrences were in femoral nodes.[31] Therefore, this approach has been abandoned in favor of either a complete inguinofemoral lymphadenectomy or a sentinel lymph node assessment.

Separate incision technique

The separate incision technique allows for radical excision of the primary lesion and the unilateral or bilateral pathologic analysis of the inguinofemoral lymph nodes. This operation can be performed in a modified dorsal lithotomy position using Allen stirrups. In this manner, the surgeon can modify the degree of exposure for the vulvectomy and the inguinofemoral lymphadenectomy to maximize the exposure during each portion of the operation. The radical local excision is performed to remove the primary tumor with at least a 1-cm margin.

Ipsilateral inguinofemoral lymph node assessment

The surgical evaluation of the ipsilateral inguinofemoral lymph nodes is suitable for lateralized primary lesions, when there are no metastases in the ipsilateral inguinofemoral lymph nodes. A study of 163 patients with a unilateral vulvar cancer, of whom 48 had positive inguinofemoral lymph nodes, 3 of the patients with positive contralateral nodes had negative ipsilateral nodes. In this study, the only independent risk factor for contralateral lymph node involvement was the total number of positive ipsilateral inguinofemoral lymph nodes. With each positive lymph node, the possibility of having bilateral inguinofemoral lymph node involvement increased by 84%. Central, nonlateralized lesions should have bilateral surgical assessment.[32] Ipsilateral lymphadenectomy was associated with less than a 1% risk of contralateral inguinofemoral node metastases for stage IB disease that are unifocal, lateral at least 1 cm from vulvar midline, not located in the anterior portion of the labia minora (area just posterior to the clitoris), have no palpable lymphadenopathy in either inguinofemoral region, and no lymph node metastases found at time of unilateral lymphadenectomy.[31,32]

Bilateral lymphadenectomy is performed for midline tumors or if lymph node metastases are discovered at unilateral lymphadenectomy. The rate of bilateral inguinofemoral metastases in women with lesions with unilateral lesions with stromal invasion 3 mm or deeper is 2.8% or greater.[33] If an inguinal lymphadenectomy is being performed, it should include the femoral lymph nodes because so-called superficial lymphadenectomy has been associated with a high rate of inguinofemoral recurrence.[31]

Technique for Inguinofemoral Lymphadenectomy

The patient is placed in a modified dorsal lithotomy position. Flexion at the hip is minimized. The inguinofemoral dissection routinely includes removal of the lymph nodes superficial to the inguinal ligament, nodes within the proximal femoral triangle (borders formed by the sartorius muscle and the adductor longus muscle), and the lymph nodes deep to the cribriform fascia. A linear incision is made along the aspect of a line drawn between the anterior superior iliac spine and the pubic tubercle ranging from 6 to 10 cm long. The incision is best made about 1 cm above the inguinal crease (**Fig. 4**). The incision is carried through the subcutaneous tissues to the superficial fascia.

The lateral border is the superficial circumflex iliac vessels, which have been proposed as the surgical landmark from embryologic and anatomic studies.[34] Borders

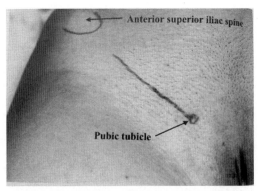

Fig. 4. Skin incision for inguinofemoral node dissection through a separate incision. (*Reproduced from* Berek JS, Hacker NF. Berek and Hacker's Gynecologic Oncology. 5th edition. Philadelphia: Lippincott Williams & Wilkins; 2010. p. 550; with permission.)

of the cephalad dissection include the pubic tubercle medially, the external oblique aponeurosis overlying the inguinal canal superiorly, the exposed sartorius muscle laterally, and the inguinal ligament inferiorly.

Borders of the caudad dissection include the borders of the femoral triangle. The index finger is used to make 1 subcutaneous tunnel over the adductor muscle and another tunnel over the sartorius muscle. The tunnels converge toward the apex of the femoral triangle on top of the fascia lata. The great saphenous vein crosses the medial border of the femoral triangle in the subcutaneous tissue (**Fig. 5**).

The cephalad dissection consists in mobilizing the fat pad overlying the inguinal ligament. The skin over the central portion of the flap is undermined parallel to the skin at a depth of 3 to 4 mm. The superficial epigastric vessels are encountered. Once the inguinal nodes lying along the inguinal ligament are encountered, the dissection gradually deepens. The dissection deepens by going through the Scarpa fascia to the external oblique aponeurosis at or superior to the skin incision. The Scarpa fascia curves downward over the inguinal ligament to insert onto the cribriform fascia, which may need to be incised before blunt development of the subcutaneous tunnels. Subcutaneous tunnels are developed with the index finger over the adductor muscle and another over the sartorius muscle. This process outlines the upper portion of the inguinofemoral fat pad, which will be removed in continuity with the nodal tissue in the femoral triangle.

Beginning the dissection superiorly, the fat pad is elevated from the external oblique aponeurosis. The fat pad will almost slide off the aponeurosis if the dissection is in the correct plane. The fat pad is mobilized to the inferior margin of the inguinal ligament. Branches of the superficial external pudendal and the superficial circumflex iliac vessels traverse the subcutaneous tissue over the inguinal ligament at the medial and lateral limits of the cephalad flap. These pedicles between the cephalad and caudad aspects of the incision are clamped, divided, and ligated. The dissection is carried 2 cm above the inguinal ligament to include all the inguinal nodes.

The caudad part of the dissection is performed superficial to the fascia lata to avoid the femoral vessels and nerve. The skin is undermined in a manner similar to the cephalad dissection using skin hooks or retractors to elevate the skin. The dissection is carried toward the apex of the femoral triangle following the medial and lateral boundaries formed by the previously created tunnels. Avoiding extensive dissection in the caudad part of the triangle minimizes paresthesias of the anterior thigh.

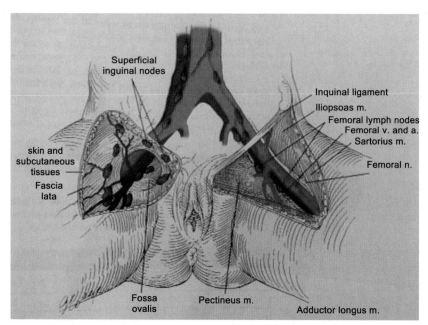

Fig. 5. Inguinofemoral lymph nodes. (*Reproduced from* Berek JS, Hacker NF. Berek and Hacker's Gynecologic Oncology. 5th edition. Philadelphia: Lippincott Williams & Wilkins; 2010. p. 541; with permission.)

Some investigators have suggested that saphenous vein sparing may decrease postoperative morbidity.[35] However, one study of 64 patients found that 31 patients who underwent saphenous sparing had no difference in postoperative fever, acute cellulitis, seroma, or lymphocyst formation.[36] All subcutaneous tissue superficial to the Scarpa fascia must be preserved to minimize skin necrosis. Once the apex of the femoral triangle is encountered, it is important to stay anterior to the fascia lata while passing an index finger or blunt instrument under the fat pad. This pedicle contains many lymphatic channels entering the femoral triangle and, by ligation, the lymphatic drainage is minimized.

The fatty tissue containing the femoral lymph nodes is removed from within the fossa ovalis. There are only 1 to 3 femoral lymph nodes, and they are always situated medial to the femoral vein in the opening of the fossa ovalis. Therefore, the fascia lata lateral to the femoral vessels does not need to be removed. The Cloquet node is not consistently present but should be checked for by retraction of the inguinal ligament cephalad over the femoral canal. A suction drain is placed in the inguinal region at the conclusion of the dissection.

SENTINEL LYMPH NODE BIOPSY

Sentinel lymph node assessment and biopsy has been used for the treatment of breast cancer and is now being used in vulvar cancer. Sentinel node evaluation has been studied as an alternative to inguinofemoral lymphadenectomy because this approach incurs less morbidity. Barton and colleagues[37] in 1992 described perilesional injections of technetium-99m-antimony trisulfide colloid followed by lymphoscintigraphy in vulvar cancer. Four of the 6 patients with central tumors or lesions that crossed the midline had bilateral inguinofemoral node uptake and 2 had unilateral uptake to the side on which the lesion was predominantly located. All patients had bilateral inguinofemoral lymphadenectomy. In 1 of the cases, metastatic spread was bilateral but isotope uptake was only unilateral. Levenback and colleagues[38] first described the use of blue dye for intraoperative lymphatic mapping in vulvar cancer. Isosulfan blue (0.5 mL) was injected into the dermis at the junction of the tumor and the normal tissue. Those with midline tumors received 2 injections at the leading border of the tumor on both sides. All 6 patients with lateral tumors had sentinel nodes identified. Of 3 patients with midline tumors, 1 had a previous wide local excision of the perineum and hence possibly altered lymphatic uptake, a second had clitoral primary blue lymphatics that were seen passing under the symphysis pubis during excision of the primary, and the third patient had the sentinel node identified on 1 side only.

The first area to receive lymphatic drainage from a lateral vulvar lesion is usually the ipsilateral superficial inguinal nodes. In theory, if the sentinel lymph node shows no evidence of metastatic involvement, then all other nodes should be negative. The best candidates for intraoperative lymphatic mapping are women with uninfected tumors limited to the lateral vulva, with no palpable enlarged inguinofemoral nodes and no history of vulvar surgery that could disrupt lymphatic drainage. Bilateral inguinofemoral node involvement is common in patients with midline vulvar cancers, even if drainage to the contralateral inguinofemoral region is not observed on lymphoscintigraphy. Sentinel lymph nodes should be detected bilaterally when the lesion is midline. If a sentinel lymph node is not found on each side, then a full inguinofemoral lymphadenectomy is required on the side without the sentinel lymph node.

In the largest observational study, 403 women with squamous cell vulvar cancer (tumor <4 cm) had sentinel node detection with a combination of radioactive tracer and blue dye.[39] The sentinel node was then removed. If a sentinel lymph node was detected and positive, or if no sentinel lymph node was detected, inguinofemoral lymphadenectomy was performed. Median follow-up was 35 months. The inguinofemoral node recurrence rate was 2.3% and 3-year survival rate was 97%. The general reported rate of inguinofemoral node recurrence after inguinofemoral lymphadenectomy ranges from 1% to 10%. Median time to inguinofemoral node recurrence was 12 months. These data suggest that sentinel lymph node evaluation and biopsy may be used for most of these patients.

There are 2 methods used for mapping: peritumoral injection of isosulfan blue dye or preoperative lymphoscintigraphy using radiolabeled colloid followed by node detection with an intraoperative γ-detecting probe. Use of a combination of blue dye and radiolabeled colloid yields more accurate results than each test alone.[38,40–44] The procedure for lymph node detection with blue dye requires a skin incision approximately the same size as that for lymphadenectomy to allow dissection down to the Camper fascia and identification of the blue afferent channel to the blue sentinel lymph node. Adding the radiolabeled colloid before surgery permits a smaller inguinofemoral lymph node dissection.

The ongoing GOG trial (GOG 173) is a validation study of sentinel biopsy comparing sentinel lymph node biopsy with inguinofemoral lymphadenectomy. The study evaluated 403 patients with squamous cell tumors between 2 cm and 6 cm. One-hundred and nine had lateralized lesions and ipsilateral inguinofemoral node dissections, whereas 294 had midline involvement and bilateral dissections. All patients had sentinel lymph node biopsy as well as complete inguinal femoral lymphadenectomy. Sentinel lymph node identification was performed with blue dye and radiolabeled colloid. The study goal was to enroll 120 patients with nodal metastases to validate the sensitivity of sentinel node detection of greater than

88%, which would lead to a false-negative predictive rate of less than 5%. Sentinel node identification was successful in 78.8% of patients using blue dye only and in 96.2% using a combination of radiolocalization and blue dye. For the 294 patients with midline lesion treated by bilateral dissection, 54% had sentinel node identified on both sides, 38.8% on 1 side, and 7.1% not identified on either side. In conclusion, the combination of blue dye and radiocolloid seems superior to blue dye alone, and further results for the cohort will be reported. These preliminary results are promising, and the long-term follow-up results will likely further validate sentinel biopsy as the technique to evaluate for inguinofemoral node disease in stage I and II disease.

MANAGEMENT OF STAGE III TO IV VULVAR CANCER

Advanced stage includes T3 tumors spread to the urethra, vagina, perineum, or anus; or T4 tumor infiltrating the bladder mucosa and/or rectal mucosa, or including the upper part of the urethral mucosa and/or fixed to the bone; or the presence of bulky, positive inguinofemoral nodes. Management should be individualized and a multidisciplinary team approach is desirable. It is advantageous to determine the most appropriate treatment of the primary tumor and inguinofemoral and pelvic lymph nodes. In most cases in which distant metastases are not found, pelvic and groin neoadjuvant chemoradiation (external beam radiation therapy with concurrent low-dose chemotherapy) may be used to avoid the need for ultraradical dissections.

Management of the Primary Tumor

In stage III disease, the tumor can sometimes be resected if there is only distal vaginal and/or urethral orifice involvement. A modified radical vulvectomy might allow adequate clearance around the lesion while preserving normal vulva. Historically, the en bloc approach through a trapezoid or butterfly incision was used, but its use has largely disappeared in favor of the separate incision approach involving 3 separate incisions, 1 for the vulvectomy and 1 for each inguinofemoral lymphadenectomy. If resection of the primary tumor is elected, the use of separate incisions for the groin may be possible. The incision should be individualized to the extent of the primary lesion to gain margins of 1 cm or greater.

The incision extends through the fat and superficial fascia to the underlying fascia. The medial incision is extended posteriorly along the labiocrural folds to the perianal area and carried down to the fascia lata. If necessary, a portion of the distal urethra (up to one-half) can be resected without compromising continence. If the tumor involves the urethra or vagina, dissection around the tumor is facilitated by transection of the vulva, thereby improving exposure of the involved area. If necessary, the bulbocavernosus muscle and the vestibular bulb may be resected to ensure a deep margin. This area is vascular and the dissection is best performed by Bovie electrocautery. The vessels supplying the clitoris as well as the internal pudendal vessels posterolaterally should be clamped and tied.

Management of Inguinofemoral Lymph Nodes

The status of the inguinofemoral lymph nodes in advanced-stage disease can first be assessed by clinical examination and CT scan. If there are no clinically or radiologically suspicious nodes, bilateral inguinofemoral lymphadenectomy can be performed through separate groin incisions. Radiation to the groin and pelvis is recommended when there is more than a single lymph node or more micrometastases, or extracapsular spread. In most cases in which there appear to be enlarged suspicious nodes, these nodes can be removed through separate groin incisions. Full pelvic and groin radiation is given after surgery if there are lymph node metastasis.

One study examined the debulking of only the enlarged lymph nodes containing metastatic cancer rather than the performance of a full inguinofemoral lymphadenectomy for patients with advanced vulvar cancer. Seventeen patients who underwent lymph node debulking (in Australia) were compared with 23 similar patients treated by full inguinofemoral lymphadenectomy (in Amsterdam). Both groups received postoperative groin and pelvic radiation. Both disease-specific survival and inguinofemoral lymph node recurrence-free intervals were longer in the group who underwent lymph node debulking.[45] If inguinofemoral lymph nodes appear fixed and unresectable, primary chemoradiation to the groin and pelvis should be considered. It may be appropriate to resect a residual inguinofemoral mass following radiation if there is no other evidence of metastatic disease.

As with early-stage disease, the separate incision technique allows for radical local excision of the primary lesion and inguinofemoral lymph node removal while retaining skin over the groin. This skin bridge decreases risk of postoperative groin wound breakdown and lower extremity lymphedema, and thus improves cosmesis. This operation should be performed in a modified dorsal lithotomy position using Allen stirrups to maximize exposure during each dissection. The surgeon can modify the degree of exposure by adjusting the position when first performing the vulvectomy, and it can then be repositioned for the inguinofemoral lymphadenectomy, which can be performed using separate incisions (see **Fig. 2**).

Chemoradiation for the Primary Vulvar Tumor

Neoadjuvant chemoradiation, with or without surgery, is used as an alternative to radical surgery for patients with locally advanced disease, stage III or IVA, and for inoperable patients. The goal of neoadjuvant chemoradiation is to shrink the primary tumor and either to minimize the extent of surgery to reduce morbidity or to avoid surgery completely.[46,47] Chemotherapy regimens are similar to those used in cervical or anal canal cancer, specifically cisplatin or infusional fluorouracil (5-FU). Most of these studies use either cisplatin or 5-FU as single agents, and the results seem to be the same regardless of which drug is used as the radiosensitizer.[48,49]

A phase II GOG trial showed impressive results after chemoradiation. This trial had 71 women with T3 or T4 primary tumors treated with planned split-course radiation therapy concurrent with cisplatin (50 mg/m^2 as a brief infusion on day 1 of each split-dose course of radiation therapy) and 5-FU (1000 mg/m^2 per day as a 24-hour continuous infusion for the first 4 days of each split-dose course of radiation therapy) followed by surgical excision of any residual primary tumor (incisional biopsy if complete response and additional radiation therapy if no response) and bilateral inguinofemoral lymphadenectomy. Following chemoradiation, 34 of 71 (48%) patients had no visible tumor at the time of surgery and, of these, 70% had no residual microscopic disease. Gross residual disease was present in 38 of 71 (54%) and residual unresectable disease in only 2 of 71 (3%). Seven patients did not undergo a posttreatment surgical procedure. At a median follow-up of 50 months, 40 patients (55%) were alive without evidence of recurrence.

Chemoradiation is a feasible alternative to ultraradical surgery in most patients with locally advanced-stage vulvar cancer. A Cochrane review raised concern about the considerable morbidity associated with chemoradiation and suggested that surgery might be a preferable therapeutic option for some patients.[50] However, preoperative chemoradiotherapy reduces tumor size and improves operability. For most patients with extensive primary lesions that would require full radical vulvectomy or pelvic exenteration, the use of neoadjuvant chemoradiotherapy may be preferable. Specifically in an effort to avoid colostomy and urostomy in patients with anorectal or bladder involvement, or in patients with disease that is fixed to the bone, chemoradiation should be offered. If residual disease remains following chemoradiation, then local resection is indicated.

Intensity-modulated radiation therapy (IMRT) is another modality that can be used for treatment of advanced-stage disease. In a retrospective analysis, 18 patients were treated with twice-daily IMRT and infusional 5-FU/cisplatin during the first and last weeks of therapy. After a median follow-up time of 22 months, 14 patients had surgery performed, with pathologic complete response in 9 (64%) patients and partial response in 5 patients. There were no recurrences in the 9 patients who achieved pathologic complete response. No patient had radiation-related acute or late grade 3 toxicity. The 2-year cause-specific and overall survivals were 75% and 70% respectively.

Pelvic Exenteration

The role of pelvic exenteration in treatment of primary vulvar cancer is limited. For advanced-stage disease, chemoradiation should be the initial treatment. If disease persists after radiation and involves the anus, rectum, rectovaginal septum, or proximal urethra, pelvic exenteration can be considered. Such radical surgery is often inappropriate for elderly patients even in suitable surgical candidates. There is significant morbidity with this approach and a 5-year survival rate of 50%.

Closure of Large Defects

It is usually possible to close the vulvar defect without tension. However, if a more extensive dissection has been required because of a large primary lesion, several options are available. Most can be closed with full-thickness skin flaps, such as a rhomboid flap[51] for covering large defects of the posterior vulva. In more extensive cases of resection, especially in patients in whom surgery is used for resection of persistent or recurrent disease in the vulva or groin after radiation therapy, unilateral or bilateral gracilis myocutaneous grafts have been used. These grafts are most useful when an extensive area from the mons pubis to the perianal area has been resected. The graft brings new blood supply to the area, which is particularly useful for areas that are poorly vascularized from prior surgical resection or radiation.[52] If an extensive defect exists, the tensor fascia lata myocutaneous graft is applicable.[53]

Chemotherapy for Metastatic Disease

The chemotherapy for stage IVB metastatic disease is typically the same as for metastatic cervical cancer.[54–58] Patients are generally treated with platinum-based single-agent or combination regimens that are active for squamous cell cervical cancer. Response rates are 14% to 40% and median progression-free survival ranging from 2.6 months to 10 months.[56,59]

SUMMARY

1. Vulvar cancer is surgically staged.
2. Imaging such as CT of the abdomen and pelvis should be performed for women with tumors 2 cm or larger or to detect lymph node or other metastases.
3. Staging should include evaluation of factors related to prognosis: tumor size, depth of invasion, lymph node involvement, and presence of distant metastases.

4. Inguinofemoral lymph node metastasis is the most important predictor of overall prognosis.
5. Inguinofemoral lymphadenectomy or sentinel lymph node evaluation can be omitted for lesions 2 cm or smaller and depth of invasion less than 1 mm.
6. Sentinel node biopsy seems to be a reliable means to pathologically assess inguinofemoral lymph node metastasis.
7. All tumors larger than 2 cm require pathologic inguinofemoral lymph node evaluation.
8. Radical local excision or modified radical vulvectomy is appropriate for most stage I and II lesions located on the lateral or posterior aspects of the vulva.
9. A tumor-free surgical margin of at least 1 cm decreases the risk of local recurrence.
10. Chemoradiation therapy is the preferred approach for most patients with very advanced vulvar cancer.

REFERENCES

1. Jemal A, Bray F, Center MM, et al. Global cancer statistics. CA Cancer J Clin 2011;61(2):69–90.
2. Way S. Carcinoma of the vulva. Am J Obstet Gynecol 1960;79:692–7.
3. Monaghan JM. Vulvar carcinoma: the case for individualization of treatment. Baillieres Clin Obstet Gynaecol 1987;1(2):263–76.
4. Hoffman JS, Kumar NB, Morley GW. Prognostic significance of groin lymph node metastases in squamous carcinoma of the vulva. Obstet Gynecol 1985;66(3): 402–5.
5. Homesley HD, Bundy BN, Sedlis A, et al. Assessment of current International Federation of Gynecology and Obstetrics staging of vulvar carcinoma relative to prognostic factors for survival (a Gynecologic Oncology Group study). Am J Obstet Gynecol 1991;164(4):997–1003 [discussion: 1003–4].
6. Hildesheim A, Han CL, Brinton LA, et al. Human papillomavirus type 16 and risk of preinvasive and invasive vulvar cancer: results from a seroepidemiological case-control study. Obstet Gynecol 1997;90(5):748–54.
7. Iwasawa A, Nieminen P, Lehtinen M, et al. Human papillomavirus in squamous cell carcinoma of the vulva by polymerase chain reaction. Obstet Gynecol 1997;89(1): 81–4.
8. Sugiyama VE, Chan JK, Shin JY, et al. Vulvar melanoma: a multivariable analysis of 644 patients. Obstet Gynecol 2007;110(2 Pt 1):296–301.
9. de Giorgi V, Salvini C, Massi D, et al. Vulvar basal cell carcinoma: retrospective study and review of literature. Gynecol Oncol 2005;97(1):192–4.
10. Benedet JL, Miller DM, Ehlen TG, et al. Basal cell carcinoma of the vulva: clinical features and treatment results in 28 patients. Obstet Gynecol 1997;90(5):765–8.
11. Felix JC, Cote RJ, Kramer EE, et al. Carcinomas of Bartholin's gland. Histogenesis and the etiological role of human papillomavirus. Am J Pathol 1993;142(3): 925–33.
12. Copeland LJ, Sneige N, Gershenson DM, et al. Bartholin gland carcinoma. Obstet Gynecol 1986;67(6):794–801.
13. Parker LP, Parker JR, Bodurka-Bevers D, et al. Paget's disease of the vulva: pathology, pattern of involvement, and prognosis. Gynecol Oncol 2000;77(1):183–9.
14. Fanning J, Lambert HC, Hale TM, et al. Paget's disease of the vulva: prevalence of associated vulvar adenocarcinoma, invasive Paget's disease, and recurrence after surgical excision. Am J Obstet Gynecol 1999;180(1 Pt 1):24–7.

15. Taussig FJ. Cancer of the vulva: an analysis of 155 cases. Am J Obstet Gynecol 1940;79:692–9.
16. Hacker NF, Berek JS, Lagasse LD, et al. Individualization of treatment for stage I squamous cell vulvar carcinoma. Obstet Gynecol 1984;63(2):155–62.
17. Hacker NF, Leuchter RS, Berek JS, et al. Radical vulvectomy and bilateral inguinal lymphadenectomy through separate groin incisions. Obstet Gynecol 1981;58(5):574–9.
18. Rouzier R, Haddad B, Atallah D, et al. Surgery for vulvar cancer. Clin Obstet Gynecol 2005;48(4):869–78.
19. DeSimone CP, Van Ness JS, Cooper AL, et al. The treatment of lateral T1 and T2 squamous cell carcinomas of the vulva confined to the labium majus or minus. Gynecol Oncol 2007;104(2):390–5.
20. Tantipalakorn C, Robertson G, Marsden DE, et al. Outcome and patterns of recurrence for International Federation of Gynecology and Obstetrics (FIGO) stages I and II squamous cell vulvar cancer. Obstet Gynecol 2009;113(4): 895–901.
21. Farias-Eisner R, Cirisano FD, Grouse D, et al. Conservative and individualized surgery for early squamous carcinoma of the vulva: the treatment of choice for stage I and II (T1-2N0-1M0) disease. Gynecol Oncol 1994;53(1):55–8.
22. Chan JK, Sugiyama V, Pham H, et al. Margin distance and other clinico-pathologic prognostic factors in vulvar carcinoma: a multivariate analysis. Gynecol Oncol 2007;104(3):636–41.
23. Heaps JM, Fu YS, Montz FJ, et al. Surgical-pathologic variables predictive of local recurrence in squamous cell carcinoma of the vulva. Gynecol Oncol 1990;38(3):309–14.
24. Wilkinson EJ, Rico MJ, Pierson KK. Microinvasive carcinoma of the vulva. Int J Gynecol Pathol 1982;1(1):29–39.
25. Magrina JF, Webb MJ, Gaffey TA, et al. Stage I squamous cell cancer of the vulva. Am J Obstet Gynecol 1979;134(4):453–9.
26. Sedlis A, Homesley H, Bundy BN, et al. Positive groin lymph nodes in superficial squamous cell vulvar cancer. A Gynecologic Oncology Group Study. Am J Obstet Gynecol 1987;156(5):1159–64.
27. Hacker NF, Van der Velden J. Conservative management of early vulvar cancer. Cancer 1993;71(Suppl 4):1673–7.
28. Atamdede F, Hoogerland D. Regional lymph node recurrence following local excision for microinvasive vulvar carcinoma. Gynecol Oncol 1989;34(1):125–8.
29. Van Der Velden J, Kooyman CD, Van Lindert AC, et al. A stage Ia vulvar carcinoma with an inguinal lymph node recurrence after local excision. A case report and literature review. Int J Gynecol Cancer 1992;2(3):157–9.
30. Vernooij F, Sie-Go DM, Heintz AP. Lymph node recurrence following stage IA vulvar carcinoma: two cases and a short overview of literature. Int J Gynecol Cancer 2007;17(2):517–20.
31. Stehman FB, Bundy BN, Dvoretsky PM, et al. Early stage I carcinoma of the vulva treated with ipsilateral superficial inguinal lymphadenectomy and modified radical hemivulvectomy: a prospective study of the Gynecologic Oncology Group. Obstet Gynecol 1992;79(4):490–7.
32. Iversen T, Aas M. Lymph drainage from the vulva. Gynecol Oncol 1983;16(2): 179–89.
33. Homesley HD, Bundy BN, Sedlis A, et al. Prognostic factors for groin node metastasis in squamous cell carcinoma of the vulva (a Gynecologic Oncology Group study). Gynecol Oncol 1993;49(3):279–83.

34. Micheletti L, Levi AC, Bogliatto F, et al. Rationale and definition of the lateral extension of the inguinal lymphadenectomy for vulvar cancer derived from an embryological and anatomical study. J Surg Oncol 2002;81(1):19–24.
35. Dardarian TS, Gray HJ, Morgan MA, et al. Saphenous vein sparing during inguinal lymphadenectomy to reduce morbidity in patients with vulvar carcinoma. Gynecol Oncol 2006;101(1):140–2.
36. Zhang X, Sheng X, Niu J, et al. Sparing of saphenous vein during inguinal lymphadenectomy for vulval malignancies. Gynecol Oncol 2007;105(3):722–6.
37. Barton DP, Berman C, Cavanagh D, et al. Lymphoscintigraphy in vulvar cancer: a pilot study. Gynecol Oncol 1992;46(3):341–4.
38. Levenback C, Coleman RL, Burke TW, et al. Intraoperative lymphatic mapping and sentinel node identification with blue dye in patients with vulvar cancer. Gynecol Oncol 2001;83(2):276–81.
39. Van der Zee AG, Oonk MH, De Hullu JA, et al. Sentinel node dissection is safe in the treatment of early-stage vulvar cancer. J Clin Oncol 2008;26(6):884–9.
40. Dhar KK, Woolas RP. Lymphatic mapping and sentinel node biopsy in early vulvar cancer. BJOG 2005;112(6):696–702.
41. de Hullu JA, Hollema H, Piers DA, et al. Sentinel lymph node procedure is highly accurate in squamous cell carcinoma of the vulva. J Clin Oncol 2000;18(15):2811–6.
42. Ansink A, van der Velden J. Surgical interventions for early squamous cell carcinoma of the vulva. Cochrane Database Syst Rev 2000;2:CD002036.
43. Moore RG, DePasquale SE, Steinhoff MM, et al. Sentinel node identification and the ability to detect metastatic tumor to inguinal lymph nodes in squamous cell cancer of the vulva. Gynecol Oncol 2003;89(3):475–9.
44. De Cicco C, Sideri M, Bartolomei M, et al. Sentinel node biopsy in early vulvar cancer. Br J Cancer 2000;82(2):295–9.
45. Hyde SE, Valmadre S, Hacker NF, et al. Squamous cell carcinoma of the vulva with bulky positive groin nodes-nodal debulking versus full groin dissection prior to radiation therapy. Int J Gynecol Cancer 2007;17(1):154–8.
46. Thomas G, Dembo A, DePetrillo A, et al. Concurrent radiation and chemotherapy in vulvar carcinoma. Gynecol Oncol 1989;34(3):263–7.
47. Gerszten K, Selvaraj RN, Kelley J, et al. Preoperative chemoradiation for locally advanced carcinoma of the vulva. Gynecol Oncol 2005;99(3):640–4.
48. Koh WJ, Wallace HJ 3rd, Greer BE, et al. Combined radiotherapy and chemotherapy in the management of local-regionally advanced vulvar cancer. Int J Radiat Oncol Biol Phys 1993;26(5):809–16.
49. Gaffney DK, Du Bois A, Narayan K, et al. Patterns of care for radiotherapy in vulvar cancer: a Gynecologic Cancer Intergroup study. Int J Gynecol Cancer 2009;19(1):163–7.
50. van Doorn HC, Ansink A, Verhaar-Langereis M, et al. Neoadjuvant chemoradiation for advanced primary vulvar cancer. Cochrane Database Syst Rev 2006;3:CD003752.
51. Barnhill DR, Hoskins WJ, Metz P. Use of the rhomboid flap after partial vulvectomy. Obstet Gynecol 1983;62(4):444–7.
52. Ballon SC, Donaldson RC, Roberts JA, et al. Reconstruction of the vulva using a myocutaneous graft. Gynecol Oncol 1979;7(2):123–7.
53. Chafe W, Fowler WC, Walton LA, et al. Radical vulvectomy with use of tensor fascia lata myocutaneous flap. Am J Obstet Gynecol 1983;145(2):207–13.
54. Deppe G, Bruckner HW, Cohen CJ. Adriamycin treatment of advanced vulvar carcinoma. Obstet Gynecol 1977;50(Suppl 1):13s–4s.

55. Gadducci A, Cionini L, Romanini A, et al. Old and new perspectives in the management of high-risk, locally advanced or recurrent, and metastatic vulvar cancer. Crit Rev Oncol Hematol 2006;60(3):227–41.

56. Witteveen PO, van der Velden J, Vergote I, et al. Phase II study on paclitaxel in patients with recurrent, metastatic or locally advanced vulvar cancer not amenable to surgery or radiotherapy: a study of the EORTC-GCG (European Organisation for Research and Treatment of Cancer–Gynaecological Cancer Group). Ann Oncol 2009;20(9):1511–6.

57. Trope C, Johnsson JE, Larsson G, et al. Bleomycin alone or combined with mitomycin C in treatment of advanced or recurrent squamous cell carcinoma of the vulva. Cancer Treat Rep 1980;64(4–5):639–42.

58. Muss HB, Bundy BN, Christopherson WA. Mitoxantrone in the treatment of advanced vulvar and vaginal carcinoma. A Gynecologic Oncology Group study. Am J Clin Oncol 1989;12(2):142–4.

59. Cormio G, Loizzi V, Gissi F, et al. Cisplatin and vinorelbine chemotherapy in recurrent vulvar carcinoma. Oncology 2009;77(5):281–4.

Surgical Management of Cervical Carcinoma

Jessica L. Berger, MD[a],*, Pedro T. Ramirez, MD[b]

KEYWORDS

- Cervical cancer • Radical hysterectomy • Laparoscopy
- Robotics • Trachelectomy • Exenteration

Cervical carcinoma is the second most common cancer worldwide with global estimates exceeding 530,200 new cases and 275,000 deaths in 2010.[1] In developed countries, screening programs have dramatically decreased the incidence of this disease, with estimates of 12,710 new cases and 4290 deaths in the United States in 2011.[2] Improved screening has increased the proportion of early-stage disease amenable to surgical intervention. Although primary chemoradiation achieves equal cure rates to radical hysterectomy with lymphadenectomy for early-stage disease, treatment must be chosen carefully taking into account side effect profiles, medical comorbidities, histopathologic data, reproductive plans, and patient and physician preference.[3] These are important considerations in a population that is generally younger than in other gynecologic malignancies and includes a significant portion of women in their reproductive years. Many of these women with early-stage disease achieve a cure and have a lengthy lifespan, shifting focus of treatment toward quality-of-life issues and maintaining hormone production and reproductive options.

Cervical carcinoma remains a clinically staged disease because of the predominance of patients treated with definitive radiation globally. However, clinical staging is often inaccurate in estimating the true extent of disease, with many patients being upstaged from surgical findings.[4] In developed countries, surgery remains the mainstay of treatment of early disease. The scope of surgical treatment of cervical carcinoma is discussed here and includes conization for the earliest-stage and lowest-risk patients, radical hysterectomy with lymphadenectomy, radical trachelectomy for appropriately selected patients who desire future fertility, and pelvic exenteration for recurrent disease. In addition, current surgical advances such as surgical staging methods and minimally invasive approaches are discussed.

[a] Department of Obstetrics and Gynecology, Banner Good Samaritan Medical Center, 1111 East McDowell Road, Phoenix, AZ 85006, USA
[b] Department of Gynecologic Oncology, University of Texas MD Anderson Cancer Center, Unit 1362, PO Box 301439, Houston, TX 77230, USA
* Corresponding author.
E-mail address: Jessica.Berger@bannerhealth.com

Hematol Oncol Clin N Am 26 (2012) 63–78
doi:10.1016/j.hoc.2011.10.008
0889-8588/12/$ – see front matter © 2012 Elsevier Inc. All rights reserved.

RADICAL HYSTERECTOMY FOR EARLY-STAGE DISEASE

Radical hysterectomy is the standard surgical approach for early-stage cervical cancer, with the exception of the earliest-stage and lowest-risk disease. Stage IA1 squamous cell carcinoma without lymphovascular space invasion (LVSI) carries a small risk of metastatic spread and may be treated with cervical conization or simple hysterectomy alone.[5,6] The risk of lymph node metastasis in this group is less than 1% and does not require lymphadenectomy.[7-9] Patients with IA2, IB1, early IIA, and some IB2 cancers are candidates for radical hysterectomy with pelvic and para-aortic (PA) lymphadenectomy.

The operation originally described by Meigs[10] in 1944 and classified by Piver and colleagues[11] in 1974 involves the en bloc resection of the uterus, parametrium, and upper vagina in varying degrees of radicality. The Piver-Rutledge-Smith classification described 5 types of hysterectomy based on extent of uterine vascular and ligamentous resection as outlined in **Table 1**. The type II and III classification are most commonly performed for cervical carcinoma; however, the degree of vaginal resection has been criticized by some as overly aggressive and rarely necessary. Type IV and type V procedures are rarely performed, and have been largely replaced by radiation therapy and pelvic exenteration.

A new classification was published in 2008 by Querleu and Morrow[12] that describes 4 categories of radical hysterectomy with subcategories, where appropriate, as outlined in **Table 2**. Lymphadenectomy is considered separately, and divided into 4 levels. This simplified classification is based on lateral dissection, and takes into account the curative intent and adverse effects of the procedure, namely bladder dysfunction. Devised in the spirit of international standardization for research and communication purposes, this system can be applied to both fertility-sparing surgery and hysterectomy, and adapted for open, vaginal, laparoscopic, and robotic approaches.

Table 1
Piver-Rutledge-Smith classification of hysterectomy, 1974

Classification	Description	Disease
Type I: extrafascial hysterectomy	Simple hysterectomy	Benign IA1 cervical cancer
Type II: modified radical hysterectomy	Uterine artery ligation at the ureters Proximal cardinal and uterosacral ligaments Upper third vagina	IA2 cervical cancer
Type III: radical hysterectomy	Uterine artery ligation at its origin Entire cardinal and uterosacral ligament Upper half vagina	IA2–IIA cervical cancer
Type IV: extended radical hysterectomy	Dissection of ureter off vesicouterine ligament Resection of superior vesicle artery Upper three-fourths vagina	Central recurrence
Type V: partial exenteration	Resection of portion of bladder or ureter with reimplantation	Central recurrence

Data from Piver M, Rutledge R, Smith J. Five classes of extended hysterectomy for women with cervical cancer. Obstet Gynecol 1974;44:265–72.

Table 2
Querleu and Morrow classification of radical hysterectomy, 2007

	Radical Hysterectomy		Lymphadenectomy
Type A	Extrafascial hysterectomy Paracervix medial to ureter <10 mm vagina	Level 1	External and internal iliac
Type B	Partial uterosacral and vesicouterine ligaments Paracervix at the ureter 10 mm vagina B1: without lateral paracervical lymph nodes B2: with lateral paracervical lymph nodes	Level 2	Common iliac (including presacral)
Type C	Uterosacral ligaments at the rectum Vesicouterine ligaments at the bladder Paracervix at the internal iliac vessels 15–20 mm vagina C1: with hypogastric nerve preservation C2: without hypogastric nerve preservation	Level 3	Inframesenteric PA
Type D	Complete paracervical resection D1: with hypogastric vessels D2: with hypogastric vessels and adjacent fascia and muscular structures	Level 4	Infrarenal PA

Data from Querleu D, Morrow CP. Classification of radical hysterectomy. Lancet Oncol 2008;9: 297–303.

For patients with early-stage disease, definitive chemoradiation achieves equal cure rates to radical hysterectomy and pelvic lymphadenectomy.[3] However, surgical treatment confers several benefits, especially in a younger population with a longer life expectancy if cure is attained. Surgery allows complete assessment of the extent of disease and tailoring of further treatment if necessary. Ovarian function is preserved in premenopausal patients, and if future radiotherapy is anticipated the opportunity is provided to transpose the ovaries out of the radiation field. Although vaginal length is slightly reduced, caliber is maintained and the risk of radiation fibrosis, atrophy, and stenosis avoided.[13] Sexual functioning in general is underreported, and reports vary by radicality of the surgery. However, a retrospective study 5 years out from either radical hysterectomy with lymphadenectomy or radiation therapy reported significantly improved sexual function in the surgical group compared with the radiation group, and was comparable with age-matched controls without a history of cancer.[14]

However, surgical treatment carries its own set of risks, complications, and side effects, many of which are perioperative considerations. Radical surgery naturally carries a risk of intraoperative injuries to pelvic vessels and nerves, the ureters, bladder, and rectum, and blood loss generally ranges from 500 to 1500 mL for open radical procedures.[15,16] The postoperative period is inevitably complicated by voiding dysfunction and prolonged recovery of bowel function. Less common complications include infectious morbidity, venous thromboembolic events, fistula, lymphocysts, and ureteral stricture. Late complications include bladder atony and lymphedema, both of which can prove distressing to patients and significantly affect quality of life. Long-term voiding dysfunction may necessitate timed voiding with accessory muscle use or even intermittent self-catheterization and has been reported in 0.8% to 8.3% of patients.[15,16]

Surgical damage to the pelvic autonomic nerves has been implicated in defecatory, voiding, and sexual dysfunction. In an effort to maintain radical resection and minimize these long-term complications, the nerve-sparing radical hysterectomy was developed.[17,18] The technique as described by Trimbos and colleagues[18] involves dissection of the hypogastric nerve lateral to the uterosacral ligament and underneath the ureter, lateralizing the hypogastric plexus within the parametrium, and preservation of the most distal portion of the nerve in the posterior vesicouterine ligament. Postoperative recovery of bladder function and quality of life 1 year from surgery were found to be significantly improved with nerve-sparing radical hysterectomy in a prospective randomized trial by Wu and colleagues.[19] Oncologic outcomes are likely not affected by the nerve-sparing procedure, but long-term prospective studies are needed.[20]

MINIMALLY INVASIVE APPROACHES TO RADICAL HYSTERECTOMY

In the last 20 years, minimally invasive approaches have been pursued to decrease the morbidity of surgery and improve recovery times, and maintain surgical and oncologic outcomes. With the advent of and subsequent improvement in laparoscopic surgical techniques, minimally invasive approaches became a reality in the treatment of cervical carcinoma. Dargent and Salvat[21] performed the first lymphadenectomy in women with cervical cancer in 1989, and later combined the procedure with radical vaginal hysterectomy. Multiple subsequent reports confirmed decreased blood loss and transfusion rates, shorter hospital stays, less postoperative pain, and similar recurrence rates, but longer operating times with laparoscopic-assisted radical vaginal hysterectomy compared with abdominal radical hysterectomy.[22–24]

With further improvement and acceptance of laparoscopic technologies, total laparoscopic radical hysterectomy has gained momentum. Its safety and feasibility have been well established, with multiple investigators reporting reduced blood loss, shorter hospital stay, maintenance of lymph node counts, and decreased perioperative morbidity.[25–29] One of the largest studies to date by Putambekar and colleagues[29] included 248 patients and reported a median operative time of 92 minutes, median blood loss of 165 mL, median hospital stay of 3 days, and median number of lymph nodes of 18. Other studies have generally reported longer operating times of 203 to 344 minutes and shorter hospital stays of 1 to 2 days.[25–28] Although longer follow-up is needed, intermediate follow-up times have shown similar oncologic outcomes among laparoscopic and abdominal radical hysterectomy. Both Spirtos and colleagues[25] and Putambekar and colleagues[29] report 3-year follow-up data on patients with IA2 to IB cervical cancer treated with laparoscopic radical hysterectomy and lymphadenectomy with recurrence rates of 5.1% and 2.8%, respectively. Pomel and colleagues[30] also reported a 5-year survival rate of 96% in patients with stage IA2 to IB1 cervical cancer treated with laparoscopic radical hysterectomy. Li and colleagues[27] compared laparoscopic and abdominal radical hysterectomy and lymphadenectomy in stage IB to IIA cervical cancer, reporting similar respective recurrence rates (13.75% vs 12%, $P>.05$) and mortality (10% vs 8%, $P>.05$) at 26 months' median follow-up.

Despite the advantages and equivalent outcomes there are still barriers to treating cervical cancer with minimally invasive approaches. Complex radical procedures performed with traditional laparoscopy are associated with long learning curves and increased operating time. They also require an expert assistant and are limited by two-dimensional viewing and lack of dexterity. Furthermore, many practicing gyneco-logic oncologists and fellows, when surveyed, believed that their laparoscopic training was inadequate to perform such procedures.[31]

Recent advances in minimally invasive surgery have incorporated the use of robotic technology. The da Vinci surgical system (Intuitive Surgical, Sunnyvale, CA, USA) is a robotic surgical platform that was approved for gynecologic procedures in 2005. Three-dimensional stereoscopic viewing and wristed instruments provide improved visualization, precision, and dexterity, and allow a single surgeon to perform complex procedures with a less experienced bedside assistant. Robotically assisted laparo-scopic surgery has also been shown to have a shorter learning curve and decreased operating time when compared with conventional laparoscopy.[32]

Several investigators have confirmed the safety and feasibility of robot radical hysterectomy, with operative characteristics similar to traditional laparoscopy.[33–39] A multi-institutional study of 42 patients who underwent robotic-assisted type II or III radical hysterectomy reported favorable operative characteristics and a low complication rate. Overall median operative time was 215 minutes, median estimated blood loss was 50 mL, median lymph node count was 25, and median hospital stay was 1 day. Intraoperative complications included 1 conversion to laparotomy and 1 ureteral injury. The postoperative complication rate was 12% and included infectious morbidity (7.1%), deep venous thrombosis (2.4%), and prolonged catheterization (2.4%).[38] A series by Magrina and colleagues[32] compared 27 patients undergoing robotic radical hysterectomy with matched patients who underwent radical hysterec-tomy by traditional laparoscopic or open approaches. These investigators reported decreased blood loss and shorter hospital stays in the laparoscopic and robotic group compared with the laparotomy group, and decreased operative times in the robotic and laparotomy group compared with the laparoscopic group. The robotic group had no intraoperative complications or conversion to laparotomy.

Recently, oncologic outcomes of robotic-assisted radical hysterectomy have been evaluated. A retrospective analysis was conducted comparing 63 consecutive robotic type III radical hysterectomies for early-stage (IA1–IIB) cervical cancer with a historical cohort of open type III radical hysterectomies. The robotic and open groups did not differ with regards to age, body mass index (calculated as weight in kilograms divided by the square of height in meters), histology, or stage. As with other studies, patients in the robotic group benefited from decreased blood loss, shorter hospital stays, and increased lymph node retrieval. Progression-free survival (94% vs 89%, $P = .27$) and overall survival did not differ between groups at 36 months' follow-up. Although longer follow-up is needed, with clear benefits to minimally invasive surgery and mounting evidence of equivalent surgical and oncologic outcomes, robotics offers a platform to overcome barriers to use of minimally invasive approaches in patients with early-stage cervical cancer. A prospective multicenter trial is under way to estab-lish equivalence of total laparoscopic or robotic radical hysterectomy compared with abdominal radical hysterectomy with respect to disease-free survival. This biphasic trial will enroll 740 patients and evaluate morbidity, cost-effectiveness, recurrence patterns, quality of life, intraoperative sentinel node sampling, and overall survival.

FERTILITY-SPARING RADICAL SURGERY

Cervical cancer affects a significant number of reproductive age women, with 40% of cervical cancer cases diagnosed less than the age of 45 years.[40] Younger women are diagnosed at an earlier stage and with disease amenable to surgical treatment more often than their postmenopausal counterparts.[41] Because many of these patients have yet to complete their childbearing, fertility-sparing options have increasingly been explored and refined. Dargent and colleagues[42] first described the radical vaginal trachelectomy (RVT) in 1994 for fertility-sparing treatment of early cervical cancer. In combination with pelvic lymphadenectomy, it is the most common and accepted fertility-sparing option for cervical cancer, with equivalent surgical and oncologic outcomes compared with radical hysterectomy and acceptable obstetric results.[43]

Patient selection is of particular importance to achieve successful outcomes. Candidates for RVT should undergo preoperative evaluation with magnetic resonance imaging (MRI) to assess endocervical extension in relation to the uterine isthmus. The following selection criteria are generally accepted and have remained essentially unchanged over the last 10 years[43]:

- Desire and capability for future fertility
- Stage IA1 with LVSI, IA2, or IB1
- Squamous, adenocarcinoma, or adenosquamous histology
- Tumor limited to the cervix
- Tumor size ≤2 cm (2.5 cm can be considered in strictly exophytic lesions)
- Limited endocervical extension by MRI or intraoperative frozen section
- Absence of lymph node metastasis or distant metastatic spread.

The procedure entails laparoscopic pelvic lymphadenectomy with frozen section evaluation to rule out lymph node metastasis, followed by removal of the uterine cervix, parametrium, and upper vagina with preservation of the uterine fundus and adnexa. Frozen section of the superior cervical margin is obtained to assure adequate margins of 5 to 8 mm. A permanent cerclage is placed in the uterine isthmus and the vaginal cuff reapproximated to the neoectocervix. Several investigators have reported their experience with RVT for fertility preservation.[44–49] When compared with radical hysterectomy, operative characteristics seem equivalent or better with regards to blood loss and hospital stay. One study reported a longer median operative time in the RVT group because of the long learning curve; however, other studies were equivalent.[50–52] One of the largest series comparing RVT with laparoscopic-assisted radical vaginal hysterectomy reported comparable intraoperative complication rates of 2.5% and 5.8%, respectively.[50] Similar results have been published in other series.[45–49] The most common intraoperative complications were bladder injuries, followed by vascular injuries mainly occurring during the laparoscopic lymphadenectomy. RVT has some postoperative complications unique to this procedure including cervical stenosis, cerclage erosion, dysmenorrhea, menstrual irregularities, and hematometria.[51]

The main concern with fertility-preserving therapy for cervical cancer is whether similar oncologic outcomes can be achieved with conservative surgery with regard to the need for adjuvant therapy, recurrence rates, and mortality. Despite careful selection, 10% to 12% of patients selected to undergo fertility-sparing surgery require adjuvant therapy.[43] The largest series of RVT by Plante and colleagues[53] includes 140 patients, 125 of whom successfully underwent the procedure. The procedure was abandoned in 10 patients for positive lymph nodes on frozen section, and in 5 patients for positive endocervical margins. After routine preoperative MRI was instituted, all abandoned procedures were a result of nodal metastasis rather than close endocervical margins, highlighting the usefulness of preoperative imaging for patient selection. Three patients with high-risk features on final pathology received adjuvant therapy after radical trachelectomy. This group reports favorable oncologic outcomes over a mean follow-up time of 95 months. There were 6 patients (4.8%) who developed a recurrence and 2 patients (1.6%) who died of disease for a 5-year recurrence-free survival of 96%. The only feature significantly associated with recurrence was tumor size greater than 2 cm (P = .002). These results compare favorably with a review of more than 600 cases reporting an overall recurrence rate of 5.3% and mortality of 3.2%.[43] Comparative studies of RVT and radical hysterectomy also show no differences in recurrence rate or 5-year overall survival.[50,52,54] In one of these studies LVSI and depth of invasion correlated with recurrence risk, but not tumor diameter.[54]

In addition to equivalent oncologic outcomes, Plante and colleagues also reported favorable obstetric outcomes with the largest series of pregnancies after RVT. Fifty-eight women in this series conceived a total of 106 pregnancies. Of 125 patients, 15% experienced infertility issues, 40% of which were caused by cervical stenosis. The rate of first-trimester and second-trimester losses, 20% and 3% respectively, were comparable with the general population, and 55% of pregnancies were delivered at term. The rate of significant prematurity (<32 weeks) was only 4%. In a review of more than 250 published pregnancies after RVT, Gien and colleagues[43] report pregnancy rates of 41% to 79%, with 40% of deliveries at term and a 12% rate of significant prematurity (<32 weeks). Infertility rates ranged from 25% to 30%. Possible causes include cervical stenosis, reported to affect 15% of patients who have undergone RVT, decreased cervical mucus, surgical adhesion formation, and subclinical salpingitis. First-trimester loss rates were comparable with the general population at 16% to 20%, and second-trimester loss rates were twice that of the general population at 8% to 10% compared with 4%. This finding may reflect a propensity for ascending infection because of decreased residual cervical length leading to chorioamnionitis or midtrimester premature rupture of membranes. These pregnancies are also at increased risk of preterm delivery, with rates of 20% to 30% compared with the national average of 12.2% in 2009.[55] The superior preterm delivery rates and second-trimester loss rates reported by Plante and colleagues have been attributed to an attempt to leave 1 cm residual cervix as long as margins are adequate. Pregnancies after radical trachelectomy are high risk and should be managed by a maternal fetal medicine specialist.

With equivalent surgical and oncologic outcomes to radical hysterectomy and acceptable reproductive outcomes, RVT has become an accepted treatment option for early-stage cervical cancer in carefully selected young women desiring fertility. Despite hundreds of reported cases, its use has not been implemented widely, perhaps because of a lack of training in radical vaginal surgery. Alternative approaches such as abdominal radical trachelectomy (ART) and robotic radical trachelectomy have been investigated. ART has a more limited experience, with just more than 100 cases reported in the literature.[43] The abdominal approach broadens the scope of fertility-sparing surgery to include patients with restrictive vaginal anatomy or larger tumors (up to 4 cm). The procedure differs slightly in that the round ligaments are divided and the uterine vessels are sacrificed at their origin from the internal iliac vessels. Care is taken to preserve the infundibulopelvic and utero-ovarian ligaments, which provide the sole blood supply to the uterus through the ovarian vessels. The remainder of the procedure is similar to a type III radical hysterectomy. The specimen is transected from the vagina and at the desired length from the uterine isthmus, and sent for frozen section. Again, a cerclage can be placed once an adequate margin is achieved and the vaginal cuff is then reapproximated to the uterus. In 1 comparative study the abdominal approach allowed for a wider parametrial resection (3.97 cm vs 1.45 cm, P<.0001), a shorter operative time (319 minutes vs 363 minutes, P = .01), and a similar complication rate, but resulted in greater blood loss (300 mL vs 100 mL,

$P = .001$).[56] The largest series of 33 patients who underwent ART by Ungar and colleagues[57] reported no recurrences over a median follow-up of 47 months, and 9% of patients needed adjuvant therapy. Another series by Abu-Rustum and colleagues[58] reported a higher adjuvant therapy rate of 32%, but may reflect an inherently higher-risk population because larger tumors were selected for this approach.

Robotic surgery has also been used to perform this procedure with the benefit of improved precision and visualization. Robotic radical trachelectomy for fertility preservation in early cervical cancer has been reported by several investigators as feasible and safe for surgeons trained in laparoscopy and radical pelvic surgery.[59–63] A series of 4 patients reported favorable surgical outcomes, with a median operative time of 339 minutes, estimated blood loss of 62 mL, and hospital stay of 1.5 days; no patient required adjuvant therapy.[62] The fine dissection capability also allows for nerve-sparing and uterine artery preservation as a refinement in the technique and potential for improved outcomes.[63]

Fertility preservation has been a major advancement in the treatment of cervical cancer for young women over the last decade. With comparable morbidity, recurrence, and survival, radical trachelectomy has gained widespread acceptance, and should be offered to appropriately selected women wishing to maintain reproductive options. Future directions will focus on the role of ultraconservative surgery, such as simple trachelectomy or conization for low-risk disease and the role of neoadjuvant chemotherapy to broaden patient eligibility. Further investigation is needed to improve patient selection and preoperative evaluation, define prognostic factors for adjuvant therapy, and improve management of subsequent pregnancies.

SURGICAL STAGING

Cervical cancer is a clinically staged disease because most cases occur in developing countries without access to advanced imaging and surgical techniques and are primarily treated with radiation. This strategy allows uniformity for communication and research purposes globally. The International Federation of Gynecology and Obstetrics (FIGO) allows the following evaluation in the clinical staging of cervical cancer.

- Careful physical examination
- Colposcopy with endocervical curettage
- Conization
- Hysteroscopy
- Cystoscopy
- Proctoscopy
- Intravenous pyelogram
- Plain film radiologic examination of the lungs and skeleton.

Although clinical staging is suitable for locally advanced disease, it is often inaccurate in determining the extent of regional spread. A Gynecologic Oncology Group (GOG) study reported that a significant portion of patients with locally advanced cervical cancer who underwent surgical staging were upstaged from the FIGO clinical stage and most of these were based on pelvic or PA lymph node metastasis.[4] Nodal metastasis is not a component of clinical staging, but significantly affects prognosis and treatment planning. Pelvic lymph nodes are encompassed by external beam radiation fields; however, PA nodes are not. Extended field radiation is of benefit in patients with positive PA lymph nodes, but carries a significant risk of morbidity, particularly in patients with previous abdominal surgery.[64] For this reason, it cannot be used routinely in patients without histologic or radiographic evidence of PA nodal disease. Although these modalities cannot be used in FIGO clinical staging, they can be used for treatment planning.

Conventional imaging techniques can identify enlarged or metabolically active lymph nodes, but are limited in their accuracy, detecting less than 30% of PA nodal disease.[65] This finding led to an interest in surgical staging with PA lymphadenectomy to identify patients who would benefit from extended field radiation. In the 1970s, a study by Berman and colleagues[66] evaluated surgical staging with exploratory laparotomy and pelvic and PA lymphadenectomy in patients with locally advanced cervical cancer. A transperitoneal approach was used in 31 patients and an extraperitoneal approach in 39 patients. These investigators found unacceptable morbidity with the transperitoneal approach because 30% of patients suffered from small bowel complications requiring surgical correction, including small bowel obstruction, enterovaginal fistula, and radiation enteritis. There were 2 deaths related to these complications. The extraperitoneal approach had a 2.5% rate of small bowel complications, none of which was severe or fatal. The open extraperitoneal approach does not delay the initiation of radiotherapy, and with advances in minimally invasive surgery, a laparoscopic or robotic approach is now feasible and safe in the hands of an experienced surgeon.

A prospective study by Ramirez and colleagues[67] enrolled patients with stage IB2 to IVA cervical cancer without evidence of PA lymphadenopathy on computed tomography (CT) or MRI who were candidates for treatment with primary chemoradiation. Sixty patients underwent preoperative positron emission tomography (PET)-CT imaging and laparoscopic extraperitoneal PA lymphadenectomy. Median operative time was 140 minutes, blood loss was 22 mL, hospital stay 1 day, and lymph node retrieval 11. One patient had intraoperative bleeding requiring conversion to laparotomy, and 7 patients (12%) had lymphocysts requiring drain placement. PA nodes were positive in 14 (23%) of patients. Of 26 patients with negative pelvic and PA nodes on PET-CT, 3 (12%) had positive PA nodes on histopathology, and of 27 patients with positive pelvic nodes but negative PA nodes on PET-CT, 6 (22%) had positive nodes on histopathology. Of the 7 patients with positive PA nodes on PET-CT, 5 (71%) had positive PA nodes on final pathology. Treatment modification was made in 11 patients (18.3%) based on surgical findings, and the median time to initiation of radiation therapy was only 10 days.

Another study by Uzan and colleagues[68] reviewed 98 patients with stage IB2 to IVA cervical cancer who had negative PA nodes on PET-CT and underwent laparoscopic extraperitoneal staging PA lymphadenectomy. The median operative time was 185 minutes, hospitalization was 3 days, and lymph node retrieval 13. Postoperative complications included 7 patients (10.7%) with lymphocysts requiring drainage and 1 patient with acute renal failure who fully recovered. Eight patients (8.4%) had PA nodal metastasis without suspicious PA lymph nodes on PET-CT imaging. The risk of PA lymph node metastasis was significantly higher in patients with positive pelvic lymph nodes on PET-CT imaging (24% vs 2.9%, $P = .004$). Median time to initiation of radiation therapy was 18 days and was not statistically different among patients with complications. Both of these studies showed the safety and feasibility of surgical staging with laparoscopic extraperitoneal PA lymphadenectomy and improved sensitivity for detection of PA lymph node metastasis compared with PET-CT imaging, particularly in patients with suspicious pelvic nodes on imaging.

Patient outcomes of surgical staging were evaluated in a retrospective review of 3 phase III GOG studies of patients with cervical cancer who were treated with chemoradiation after exclusion of PA lymph node metastasis by radiographic methods (CT or MRI) compared with surgical methods. The group with radiographic exclusion of PA nodal disease (130 patients) had a worse prognosis compared with the surgical group

(555 patients) on multivariate analysis, with a hazard ratio for disease progression of 1.35, 95% confidence interval (CI) 1.01 to 1.81, and for death 1.46, 95% CI 1.08 to 1.99.[69] A single randomized trial has been performed to evaluate surgical staging compared with clinical staging. This study was stopped early because of a significantly worse progression-free survival (P = .003) and overall survival (P = .024) in the surgical staging group. However, the surgical group in this study had a higher rate of unfavorable histology, a greater delay to start of radiotherapy, and a greater number of patients who did not receive concurrent chemotherapy with radiation compared with the clinically staged group.[70] The therapeutic benefit of surgical staging remains unproved and further investigation with high-quality prospective trials is necessary.

The role of surgical staging remains the subject of debate. Laparoscopic extraperitoneal PA lymphadenectomy is safe in the hands of an experienced surgeon and has a low complication rate. Most morbidity is related to pelvic lymphocysts, which are easily managed with image-guided drainage. Detection of PA nodal disease is improved with surgical evaluation compared with radiographic evaluation alone, and is of particular importance in patients with evidence of pelvic lymph node metastasis on imaging because they have a higher rate of PA nodal disease. PA lymph node status has important prognostic implications, although the therapeutic advantage remains unproved. A randomized clinical trial initiated at MD Anderson Cancer Center is under way to evaluate the progression-free and overall survival of patients with IB2 to IVA cervical cancer who undergo surgical staging compared with the standard of care, radiotherapy with concurrent cisplatin chemotherapy. This study aims to enroll 480 patients and it is to be hoped that it will define the future role of surgical staging in locally advanced cervical cancer.

PELVIC EXENTERATION

Pelvic exenteration is the most radical surgical procedure used in the treatment of cervical carcinoma. First described in 1946 as a palliative procedure, the perioperative mortality was 22.7%.[71] Since that time and with improvements in surgical technique, intensive medical care, blood banking, and antibiotic development, pelvic exenteration has become a successful procedure with curative intent for carefully selected patients. The original procedure described en bloc resection of the gynecologic organs, vagina, bladder, distal ureters, urethra, rectosigmoid colon, and anus. The procedure can be tailored by limiting resection to the anterior or posterior compartment only, depending on the location of disease, and may or may not involve a perineal phase. Sophisticated reconstruction is now used with intestinal diversion or reanastomosis, continent or incontinent urinary diversion, and neovaginal reconstruction. Despite these advances, the procedure carries considerable morbidity, and patients should be thoroughly counseled regarding the prolonged recovery, common complications, and impact on quality of life and sexual functioning.

With the success of chemoradiation for primary treatment of locally advanced cervical cancer, the main indication for exenteration is central pelvic recurrence. Preoperative evaluation should confirm the patient is fit for a prolonged surgical procedure with considerable blood loss, exclude distant metastasis, and provide reasonable assurance that the disease is resectable. Because the intent is curative, the procedure should be abandoned if lymphatic or distant metastases are discovered or if the disease cannot be fully resected. Despite careful patient evaluation, there is still an approximately 30% risk of intraoperative abandonment because of metastatic spread or unresectable disease.[72]

The perioperative mortality has steadily dropped to less than 5% over time, but postoperative morbidity remains a significant problem. A recent study by Maggioni and colleagues[73] reported 1 institution's experience with pelvic exenteration with regards to morbidity, mortality, and survival. Over 10 years 106 patients underwent anterior (49%), posterior (6%), or total (45%) pelvic exenteration for persistent or recurrent gynecologic cancer, 58.5% of which were cervical primaries. Mean estimated blood loss was 1240 mL, median hospital stay was 21.6 days, 61.6% of patients required intraoperative blood transfusion, and 50% required postoperative blood transfusion. There were no perioperative deaths in this series and the overall complication rate was 66%. Reoperation was necessary in 25 patients (23.3%), gastrointestinal complications occurred in 20 patients (18.8%), urinary complications in 50 patients (49.5%), and general postoperative complications in 46 patients (42.9%). Overall survival for patients with cervical cancer was 52%. When cervical and vaginal cancer were considered together, patients with negative margins had imroved 5-year survival (60% vs 25%, $P = .043$), as did patients with negative lymph nodes (60% vs 30%, $P = .045$). Similarly, positive surgical margins and lymph node metastases have been shown to be important prognostic variables in other studies.[74,75] Five-year survival rates have ranged from 20% to 64% in other series, as outlined in **Table 3**.[73,74,76–84] Prognostic factors predictive of survival and recurrence in other studies include length of time from radiation therapy to exenteration, size of central mass, and pelvic side wall fixation by clinical examination.[78]

For patients who achieve cure, quality-of-life issues present significant challenges, including psychosocial conflict, fear of disease recurrence, sexual dysfunction, and self-consciousness regarding physical appearance. Organ reconstruction provides significant benefit in these patients. In 1 study fewer ostomies were associated with better adjustment and improved body image. Likewise vaginal reconstruction was associated with improved overall quality of life, and significantly better sexual functioning.[85] Preoperative counseling is imperative to prepare patients for these struggles, and multidisciplinary care with sexual therapists and oncology-psychologists may be beneficial.

Exenterative surgery carries the risk of significant postoperative morbidity and can drastically alter quality of life, physical appearance, and sexual functioning. It is important that patients are properly selected and counseled preoperatively and that surgery is performed by a skilled multidisciplinary team familiar with the care of these patients.

Table 3
Intraoperative mortality and 5-year survival for pelvic exenteration

Author, Year	N	Operative Mortality (%)	5-Year Survival (%)
Rutledge et al,[76] 1977	296	13.5	42
Soper et al,[77] 1989	69	7.2	40
Shingleton et al,[78] 1989	143	6.3	50
Lawhead et al,[79] 1989	65	9.2	23
Morely et al,[80] 1989	100	2	61
Standhope et al,[81] 1990	133	6.7	41
Berek et al,[82] 2005	75	4	54
Goldberg et al,[83] 2006	103	1	47
Fleisch et al,[74] 2007	203	1.8	21
Maggioni et al,[73] 2009	106	0	52
Benn et al,[84] 2011	54	0	64

With proper planning and experience, the procedure can be accomplished with success, offering curative potential and promising 5-year survival rates to patients without alternative treatment options.

SUMMARY

Surgical management for cervical carcinoma uses a wide variety of procedures for all stages of disease, ranging from the most conservative excisional biopsy to aggressive extirpative surgery with sophisticated reconstruction. Innovative surgical procedures have given fertility-sparing treatment options to women of reproductive age, and refinement and use of minimally invasive surgical approaches have minimized operative morbidity without sacrificing outcomes. Conservative staging procedures are being evaluated to improve survival in locally advanced disease. There have been many breakthroughs in the treatment of cervical carcinoma over recent years, which have improved not only survival but also the quality of ensuing life for women afflicted by this disease.

REFERENCES

1. Ferlay J, Shin HR, Bray F, et al. GLOBOCAN 2008 v1.2, Cancer Incidence and Mortality Worldwide: IARC Cancer Base No. 10. Lyon (France): International Agency for Research on Cancer; 2010. Available at: http://globocan.iarc.fr. Accessed September 25, 2011.
2. American Cancer Society. Cancer Facts and Figures 2011. Atlanta, 2011 Available at: http://www.cancer.org/. Accessed September 25, 2011.
3. Landoni F, Maneo A, Colombo A, et al. Randomized study of radical surgery versus radiotherapy for stage IB-IIa cervical cancer. Lancet 1997;350:535–40.
4. Lagasse LD, Creasman WT, Shingleton HM, et al. Results and complications of operative staging in cervical cancer: experience of the Gynecology Oncology Group. Gynecol Oncol 1986;24:194–9.
5. Roman LD, Felix JC, Muderspach LI, et al. Risk of residual invasive disease in women with microinvasive squamous cancer in a conization specimen. Obstet Gynecol 1997;90:759–64.
6. Phongnarisorn C, Srisomboon J, Khunamornpong S, et al. The risk of residual neoplasia in women with microinvasive squamous cervical carcinoma and positive cone margins. Int J Gynecol Cancer 2006;16:655–9.
7. Sevin BU, Nadji M, Averette HE, et al. Microinvasive carcinoma of the cervix. Cancer 1992;70:2121.
8. Ostor AG. Studies on 200 cases of early squamous cell carcinoma of the cervix. Int J Gynecol Pathol 1993;12:193–207.
9. Elliot P, Coppleson M, Russel P, et al. Early invasive (FIGO IA) carcinoma of the cervix: a clinicopathologic study of 476 cases. Int J Gynecol Cancer 2000;10:42–52.
10. Meigs J. Carcinoma of the cervix: the Wertheim operation. Surg Gynecol Obstet 1944;78:195–9.
11. Piver M, Rutledge R, Smith J. Five classes of extended hysterectomy for women with cervical cancer. Obstet Gynecol 1974;44:265–72.
12. Querleu D, Morrow CP. Classification of radical hysterectomy. Lancet Oncol 2008; 9:297–303.
13. Brand AH, Bull CA, Cakir B. Vaginal stenosis in patients treated with radiation therapy for carcinoma of the cervix. Int J Gynecol Cancer 2006;16:288–93.
14. Frumovitz M, Sun CC, Schover LR, et al. Quality of life and sexual functioning in cervical cancer survivors. J Clin Oncol 2005;23:7428–36.

15. Pikaat DP, Holloway RW, Ahmad S, et al. Clinico-pathologic morbidity analysis of types 2 and 3 abdominal radical hysterectomy for cervical cancer. Gynecol Oncol 2007;107:205–10.
16. Sivanesaratnam V, Sen DK, Jayalakshmi P, et al. Radical hysterectomy and pelvic lymphadenectomy for early invasive cancer of the cervix. Int J Gynecol Cancer 1993;3:231–8.
17. Fujii S, Tanakura K, Matsumura N, et al. Anatomic identification and functional outcomes of the nerve sparing Okabayashi radical hysterectomy. Gynecol Oncol 2007;107:4–13.
18. Trimbos JB, Maas CP, Derviter MC, et al. A nerve sparing radical hysterectomy: guidelines and feasibility in western patients. Int J Gynecol Cancer 2001;11: 180–6.
19. Wu J, Lui X, Hua K, et al. Effect of nerve-sparing radical hysterectomy on bladder function recovery and quality of life in patients with cervical carcinoma. Int J Gynecol Cancer 2010;20:905–9.
20. Londoni F, Maneo A, Cormio G, et al. Class II versus class III radical hysterectomy in stage IB-IIA cervical cancer: a prospective randomized study. Gynecol Oncol 2001;80:3–12.
21. Dargent D. A new future for Schauta's operation through a presurgical retroperitoneal pelviscopy. Eur J Gynecol Oncol 1987;8:292–6.
22. Morgan DJ, Hunter DC, McCracken G, et al. Is laparoscopically assisted radical vaginal hysterectomy for cervical carcinoma safe? A case control study with follow up. BJOG 2007;114:537–42.
23. Jackson KS, Da N, Naik R, et al. Laparoscopically assisted radical vaginal hysterectomy vs. radical abdominal hysterectomy for cervical cancer: a match controlled study. Gynecol Oncol 2004;95:655–61.
24. Steed H, Rosen B, Murphy J, et al. A comparison of laparoscopic-assisted radical vaginal hysterectomy and radical abdominal hysterectomy in the treatment of cervical cancer. Gynecol Oncol 2004;93:588–93.
25. Spirtos NM, Eisenkop SM, Schlaerth JB, et al. Laparoscopic radical hysterectomy (type III) with aortic and pelvic lymphadenectomy in patients with stage I cervical cancer: surgical morbidity and intermediate follow-up. Am J Obstet Gynecol 2002;187:340–8.
26. Ramirez PT, Slomovitz BM, Soliman PT, et al. Total laparoscopic radical hysterectomy and lymphadenectomy: the M.D. Anderson Cancer Center experience. Gynecol Oncol 2006;102:252–5.
27. Li G, Yan X, Shang H, et al. A comparison of laparoscopic radical hysterectomy and pelvic lymphadenectomy and laparotomy in the treatment of Ib-IIa cervical cancer. Gynecol Oncol 2007;105:176–80.
28. Frumovitz M, dos Reis R, Sun CC, et al. Comparison of total laparoscopic and abdominal radical hysterectomy for patients with early-stage cervical cancer. Obstet Gynecol 2007;10:96–102.
29. Puntambekar SP, Palep RJ, Puntambekar SS, et al. Laparoscopic total radical hysterectomy by the Pune technique: our experience of 248 cases. J Minim Invasive Gynecol 2007;14:682–9.
30. Pomel C, Atallah D, Le Bouedec G, et al. Laparoscopic radical hysterectomy for invasive cervical cancer: 8 year experience of a pilot study. Gynecol Oncol 2003; 91:534–9.
31. Frumovitz M, Ramirez PT, Greer M, et al. Laparoscopic training and practice in gynecologic oncology among Society of Gynecologic Oncologists members and fellows-in-training. Gynecol Oncol 2004;94:746–53.

32. Magrina JF, Kho RM, Weaver AL, et al. Robotic radical hysterectomy: comparison with laparoscopy and laparotomy. Gynecol Oncol 2008;109:86–91.

33. Sert B, Abeler V. Robotic radical hysterectomy in early-stage cervical carcinoma patients, comparing results with total laparoscopic radical hysterectomy cases. The future is now? Int J Med Robot 2007;3:224–8.

34. Kim YT, Kim SW, Hyung WJ, et al. Robotic radical hysterectomy with pelvic lymphadenectomy for cervical carcinoma: a pilot study. Gynecol Oncol 2008;108:312–6.

35. Fanning J, Fenton B, Purohit M. Robotic radical hysterectomy. Am J Obstet Gynecol 2008;198:649.e1–4.

36. Nezhat FR, Datta MS, Liu C, et al. Robotic radical hysterectomy versus total laparoscopic radical hysterectomy with pelvic lymphadenectomy for treatment of early cervical cancer. JSLS 2008;12:227–37.

37. Boggess JF, Gehrig PA, Cantrell L, et al. A case-control study of robot-assisted type III radical hysterectomy with pelvic lymph node dissection compared with open radical hysterectomy. Am J Obstet Gynecol 2008;199:357.e1–7.

38. Lowe MP, Chamberlain DH, Kamelle SA, et al. A multi-institutional experience with robotic-assisted radical hysterectomy for early stage cervical cancer. Gynecol Oncol 2009;113:191–4.

39. Cantrell LA, Mendivil A, Gehrig PA, et al. Survival outcomes for women undergoing type III robotic radical hysterectomy for cervical cancer: a 3-year experience. Gynecol Oncol 2010;117:260–5.

40. Surveillance, Epidemiology and End Results. Available at: http://www.seer.cancer.gov/statfacts/html/cervix.html. Accessed September 5, 2011.

41. Surveillance, Epidemiology and End Results. Available at: http://www.seer.cancer.gov/faststats/selections.php?series=cancer. Accessed September 5, 2011.

42. Dargent D, Brun J, Roy M, et al. Pregnancies following radical trachelectomy for invasive cervical cancer [abstract]. Gynecol Oncol 1994;52:105.

43. Gien LT, Covens A. Fertility sparing options for early stage cervical cancer. Gynecol Oncol 2010;117:350–7.

44. Schlaerth JB, Spirtos NM, Schlaerth AC. Radical trachelectomy and pelvic lymphadenectomy with uterine preservation in the treatment of cervical cancer. Am J Obstet Gynecol 2003;188:29–34.

45. Burnett AF, Roman LS, O'Meara AT, et al. Radical vaginal trachelectomy and pelvic lymphadenectomy for preservation of fertility in early cervical carcinoma. Gynecol Oncol 2003;88:419–23.

46. Plante M, Renaud MC, Francois H, et al. Vaginal radical trachelectomy: an oncologically safe fertility-preserving surgery. An updated series of 72 cases and review of the literature. Gynecol Oncol 2004;94:614–23.

47. Chen Y, Xu H, Zhang Q, et al. A fertility-preserving option in early cervical carcinoma: laparoscopy-assisted vaginal radical trachelectomy and pelvic lymphadenectomy. Eur J Obstet Gynecol Reprod Biol 2008;136:90–3.

48. Sonoda Y, Chi DS, Carter J, et al. Initial experience with Dargent's operation: the radical vaginal trachelectomy. Gynecol Oncol 2008;108:214–9.

49. Shepherd JH, Spencer C, Herod J, et al. Radical vaginal trachelectomy as a fertility-sparing procedure in women with early-stage cervical cancer-cumulative pregnancy rate in a series of 123 women. BJOG 2006;113:719–24.

50. Marchiole P, Benchaib M, Buenerd A, et al. Oncological safety of laparoscopic-assisted vaginal radical trachelectomy (LARVT or Dargent's operation): a comparative study with laparoscopic-assisted vaginal radical hysterectomy (LAVRH). Gynecol Oncol 2007;106:132–41.

51. Alexander-Sefre F, Chee N, Spencer C, et al. Surgical morbidity associated with radical trachelectomy and radical hysterectomy. Gynecol Oncol 2006;101:450–4.
52. Beiner ME, Hauspy J, Rosen B, et al. Radical vaginal trachelectomy vs. radical hysterectomy for small early stage cervical cancer: a matched case-control study. Gynecol Oncol 2008;110:168–71.
53. Plante M, Gregoire J, Renaud MC, et al. The vaginal radical trachelectomy: an update of a series of 125 cases and 106 pregnancies. Gynecol Oncol 2011; 121:290–7.
54. Diaz JP, Sonoda Y, Leitao MM, et al. Oncologic outcome of fertility-sparing radical trachelectomy versus radical hysterectomy for stage IB1 cervical carcinoma. Gynecol Oncol 2008;111:255–60.
55. Centers for Disease Control and Prevention. Available at: http://www.cdc.gov/nchs/data/nvsr/nvsr59/nvsr59_03.pdf. Accessed September 10, 2011.
56. Einstein MH, Park KJ, Sonoda Y, et al. Radical vaginal versus abdominal trachelectomy for stage IB1 cervical cancer: a comparison of surgical and pathologic outcomes. Gynecol Oncol 2009;112:73–7.
57. Ungar L, Palfalva L, Hogg R, et al. Abdominal radical trachelectomy: a fertility-preserving option for women with early cervical cancer. BJOG 2005;112:366–9.
58. Abu-Rustum NR, Su W, Levine DA, et al. Surgical and pathologic outcomes of fertility-sparing radical abdominal trachelectomy for FIGO stage Ib1 cervical cancer. Gynecol Oncol 2008;111:261–4.
59. Geisler JP, Orr CJ, Manahan KJ. Robotically assisted total laparoscopic radical trachelectomy for fertility sparing in stage IB1 adenosarcoma of the cervix. J Laparoendosc Adv Surg Tech A 2008;18:727–9.
60. Chuang LT, Lerner DL, Lui CS, et al. Fertility-sparing robotic-assisted radical trachelectomy and bilateral pelvic lymphadenectomy in early-stage cervical cancer. J Minim Invasive Gynecol 2008;15:767–70.
61. Burnett AF, Stone PJ, Duckworth LA, et al. Robotic radical trachelectomy for preservation of fertility in early cervical cancer: case series and description of technique. J Minim Invasive Gynecol 2009;16:569–72.
62. Ramirez PT, Schmeler KM, Malpica A, et al. Safety and feasibility of robotic radical trachelectomy in patients with early-stage cervical cancer. Gynecol Oncol 2010;116:512–5.
63. Hong DG, Lee YS, Park NY, et al. Robotic uterine artery preservation and nerve-sparing radical trachelectomy with bilateral pelvic lymphadenectomy in early-stage cervical cancer. Int J Gynecol Cancer 2011;21:391–6.
64. Rotman M, Pajak TF, Choi K, et al. Prophylactic extended-field irradiation of para-aortic lymph nodes in stages IIB and bulky IB and IIA cervical carcinomas. Ten-year treatment results of RTOG 79-20. JAMA 1995;274:387–93.
65. Leblanc E, Narducci F, Frumovitz M, et al. Therapeutic value of pretherapeutic extraperitoneal laparoscopic staging of locally advanced cervical carcinoma. Gynecol Oncol 2007;105:304–11.
66. Berman MI, Lagasse LS, Watring WG, et al. The operative evaluation of patients with cervical carcinoma by an extraperitoneal approach. Obstet Gynecol 1977; 50:658–64.
67. Ramirez PT, Jhingran A, Macapinlac HA, et al. Laparoscopic extraperitoneal para-aortic lymphadenectomy in locally advanced cervical cancer: a prospective correlation of surgical findings with positron emission tomography/computed tomography findings. Cancer 2011;117:1928–34.
68. Uzan C, Souadka A, Gouy S, et al. Analysis of morbidity and clinical implications laparoscopic para-aortic lymphadenectomy in a continuous series of 98 patients

with advanced stage cervical cancer and negative PET-CT imaging in the para-aortic area. Gynecol Oncol 2011;16:1021–7.

69. Gold MA, Tian C, Whitney CW, et al. Surgical versus radiographic determination of para-aortic lymph node metastases before chemoradiation for locally advanced cervical carcinoma: a Gynecologic Oncology Group study. Cancer 2008;112: 1954–63.

70. Lai CH, Huang KG, Hong JH, et al. Randomized trial of surgical staging (extraperitoneal or laparoscopic) versus clinical staging in locally advanced cervical cancer. Gynecol Oncol 2003;89:160–7.

71. Brunschwig A. Complete excision of pelvic viscera for advanced carcinoma [abstract]. Cancer 1948;1:177–83.

72. Miller B, Morris M, Rutledge F, et al. Aborted exenterative procedures in recurrent cervical cancer. Gynecol Oncol 1993;50:94–9.

73. Maggioni A, Roviglione G, Landoni F, et al. Pelvic exenteration: ten-year experience at the European Institute of Oncology in Milan. Gynecol Oncol 2011;114: 64–8.

74. Fleisch MC, Pantke P, Beckmann MW, et al. Predictors for long-term survival after interdisciplinary salvage surgery for advanced or recurrent gynecologic cancer. J Surg Oncol 2007;95:476–84.

75. Park JY, Choi HJ, Jeong SY, et al. The role of pelvic exenteration and reconstruction for treatment of advanced or recurrent gynecologic malignancies: analysis of risk factors predicting recurrence and survival. J Surg Oncol 2007;96:560–8.

76. Rutledge FN, Smith JP, Wharton JT, et al. Pelvic exenteration: analysis of 296 patients. Am J Obstet Gynecol 1977;129:881–92.

77. Soper JT, Berchuck A, Creasman WT, et al. Pelvic exenteration: factors associated with major surgical morbidity. Gynecol Oncol 1989;35:93–8.

78. Shingleton HM, Soong SJ, Gelder MS, et al. Clinical and histopathologic factors predicting recurrence and survival after pelvic exenteration for cancer of the cervix. Obstet Gynecol 1989;73:1027–34.

79. Lawhead RA, Clard DG, Smith DH, et al. Pelvic exenteration for recurrent or persistent gynecologic malignancies: a 10-year review of the Memorial Sloan-Kettering Cancer Center experience (1972-1981). Gynecol Oncol 1989;33: 279–82.

80. Morley GW, Hopkins MP, Lindenauer SM, et al. Pelvic exenteration, University of Michigan: 100 patients at 5 years. Obstet Gynecol 1989;74:934–43.

81. Stanhope CR, Webb MJ, Podratz KC. Pelvic exenteration for recurrent cervical cancer. Clin Obstet Gynecol 1990;33:897–909.

82. Berek JS, Howe C, Lagasse LD, et al. Pelvic exenteration for recurrent gynecologic malignancy: survival and morbidity analysis of the 45-year experience of UCLA. Gynecol Oncol 2005;99:153–9.

83. Goldberg GL, Sukumvanich P, Einstein MH, et al. Total pelvic exenteration: the Albert Einstein College of Medicine/Montefiore Medical Center experience (1987 to 2003). Gynecol Oncol 2006;101:261–8.

84. Benn T, Brooks PA, Zhang Q, et al. Pelvic exenteration in gynecologic oncology: a single institution study over 20 years. Gynecol Oncol 2011;122:14–8.

85. Hawighorst-Knapstein S, Schonefussrs G, Hoffmann SO, et al. Pelvic exenteration: effects of surgery on quality of life and body image. A prospective longitudinal study. Gynecol Oncol 1997;66:495–500.

Current Surgical Management of Endometrial Cancer

M. Heather Einstein, MD, MS[a],*, Laurel W. Rice, MD[b]

KEYWORDS

- Endometrial cancer • Robotic • Lymphadenectomy
- Cytoreduction

A total of 43,470 women were diagnosed with endometrial cancer in the United States in 2010, and 7950 died of the disease.[1] Surgery plays a vital role in the management of endometrial cancer at all stages, particularly clinically early-stage disease.[2] Despite being the most common gynecologic cancer in developed countries, there are still many unanswered questions regarding optimal surgical management of endometrial cancer, not the least of which is who should undergo surgical staging.[3] There is ample evidence supporting the lower complication rate achieved with laparoscopic surgery compared with traditional open staging,[4,5] and building evidence to support laparoscopic-assisted robotic surgery for early endometrial cancer.[6,7] Surgery plays an important role in the treatment of advanced stage disease as well, with retrospective studies showing some benefit to optimal cytoreduction.[8–12] This review discusses the role of surgery in the management of endometrial cancer, with an emphasis on current controversies.

EARLY-STAGE DISEASE
Surgical Staging of Endometrial Cancer

Surgical staging is performed for prognosis and to direct adjuvant treatment. Endometrial cancer has been staged surgically since 1988. The procedure involves procurement of peritoneal washings (which no longer factor into the staging system but should be reported with the stage), hysterectomy, bilateral salpingo-oophorectomy, and evaluation of the lymph nodes.[13] Internationally, controversy continues as to what constitutes endometrial cancer staging, and even the FIGO (International

---

The authors have nothing to disclose.

[a] Division of Gynecologic Oncology, Hartford Hospital, University of Connecticut, 85 Seymour Street, Suite 705, Hartford, CT 06106, USA

[b] Division of Gynecologic Oncology, Department of Obstetrics and Gynecology, Paul B. Carbone Cancer Center, University of Wisconsin, 1 South Park Street, Suite 555, Madison, WI 53715, USA

* Corresponding author.

E-mail address: heinstein@harthosp.org

Hematol Oncol Clin N Am 26 (2012) 79–91

doi:10.1016/j.hoc.2011.10.005

Federation of Gynecology and Obstetrics) staging booklet is vague.[14] In the United States, the Gynecologic Oncology Group (GOG) generally requires complete pelvic and para-aortic lymphadenectomy in protocols involving clinically early-stage endometrial cancer.[4] Staging can be performed open, laparoscopically, or robotically. The incidence of lymph node metastases in patients with clinical stage I endometrial cancer ranges from 7.4% to 13.3%, with the incidence being significantly higher in patients with poorly differentiated and deeply invasive tumors.[15–17]

The Role of Lymphadenectomy

Two large multicenter randomized control trials have been performed evaluating lymphadenectomy in early-stage endometrial cancer, and both concluded that lymphadenectomy did not change survival.[15,17] The results have been interpreted in various ways, although most agree that these trials indicate that pelvic lymphadenectomy is not a therapeutic procedure.

ASTEC (A Study in the Treatment of Endometrial Cancer) was a multicenter trial in 4 countries involving 1408 women with clinically stage 1 endometrial cancer.[15] Participants were randomized to hysterectomy and bilateral salpingo-oophorectomy (BSO) versus hysterectomy, BSO and pelvic lymphadenectomy, with a primary end point of overall survival. Patients with high-risk uterine factors were then further randomized to adjuvant therapy, regardless of lymph node status. After a median follow-up time of 3 years, there was no statistically significant difference in overall survival with lymphadenectomy (hazard ratio [HR] 1.16 in favor of no lymphadenectomy, 95% confidence interval [CI] 0.81–1.54). Although there appeared to be a trend toward improved survival without lymphadenectomy, the lymphadenectomy group had more patients with aggressive histologies, as well as more patients who were found to have advanced disease (not including lymph node metastases) at the time of surgery.

Concurrently, in Italy, Panici and colleagues[17] performed a similar multicenter trial involving 514 patients with clinical stage 1 endometrial cancer and evidence of myometrial invasion (at least 50% depth if grade 1) on frozen section. Hysterectomy with BSO and pelvic lymphadenectomy was compared with hysterectomy and BSO alone. The primary outcome was overall survival. The Italian trial differed from ASTEC in that adjuvant therapy was administered at the discretion of the treating physician, and the median lymph node count was 20 (as opposed to 12). After a median follow-up of 4 years, there was no statistically significant difference in overall survival with the addition of lymphadenectomy (HR for death 1.2, 95% CI 0.7–2.07), with 5-year overall survivals of 86% (lymphadenectomy) and 90% (no lymphadenectomy).

The ASTEC and the Italian trials show that there is not an independent survival advantage with pelvic lymphadenectomy. However, they do not fully answer the question of whether or not it is beneficial to perform lymphadenectomy because results of the lymphadenectomy were not used to direct treatment. In ASTEC, less than half of the patients who had positive lymph nodes were assigned to radiotherapy, and few patients in the trial received adjuvant chemotherapy or hormonal therapy. In the Italian trial, slightly more than 30% of each arm received adjuvant therapy, showing that lymphadenectomy had not been used specifically to make decisions on adjuvant therapy. These trials confirm the findings of PORTEC 1 (Post Operative Radiation Therapy in Endometrial Carcinoma),[16] which showed that when patients are treated with adjuvant therapy regardless of nodal status, there is no survival benefit.[15,18]

The complications reported in ASTEC[15] and the Italian trial[17] are listed in **Table 1**, as are the complications from LAP-2,[4] a GOG study comparing staging via laparotomy with laparoscopic staging for early endometrial cancer. Data from LAP-2 are included

Table 1
Complications associated with endometrial cancer staging in 3 randomized controlled trials

Complication	ASTEC[15] No LAD (n = 704) (%)	ASTEC[15] LAD (n = 704) (%)	Italian[17] No LAD (n = 250) (%)	Italian[17] LAD (n = 264) (%)	LAP-2[4] Laparotomy[a] (n = 886) (%)	LAP-2[4] Laparoscopy[b] (n = 1630) (%)
Intraoperative	Not reported	Not reported	1	1	8	10
Vascular	Not reported	Not reported	<1	<1	3	5
Bowel	Not reported	Not reported	<1	0	2	2
Bladder/Ureter	Not reported	Not reported	0	0	1	2
Other	Not reported	Not reported	<1	1	1	2
Postoperative	2	6	14	30	21	14
Ileus	1	3	Not reported	Not reported	8	4
Bowel obstruction	Not reported	Not reported	2	2	1	1
Deep vein thrombosis	<1	1	1	1	Not reported	Not reported
Pulmonary embolism	Not reported	Not reported	0	1	1	1
Lymphocyst	<1	1	Included in lymphedema	Included in lymphedema	Not reported	Not reported
Lymphedema[c]	<1	3	2	13	Not reported	Not reported
Wound dehiscence	<1	1	Not reported	Not reported	Not reported	Not reported
Reoperation	Not reported	Not reported	Not reported	Not reported	2	3
Fistula	Not reported	Not reported	0	1	<1	1
Late[c]	12	17	Not reported	Not reported	Not reported	Not reported

a 99% of patients had at least pelvic lymph nodes removed.
b 98% of patients had at least pelvic lymph nodes removed.
c Includes patients who had adjuvant therapy.

to report complications associated with laparoscopic staging, because more than 90% of patients in ASTEC and the Italian trial were staged via laparotomy. (The complications in LAP-2 are reported as intent to treat, meaning the 25.8% of patients who were converted to laparotomy are included in the laparoscopy arm.) Because of differences in reporting and patient populations, it is impossible to compare across studies, even in a hypothesis-generating manner. Overall, the incidence of serious complications was low, although higher with lymphadenectomy than without. Of particular interest is the incidence of lymphedema, which ranged from 3% to 13%. Lymphedema is bothersome to patients, and although it can be treated, it is not curable.[19]

Before prospective trials that documented the incidence of associated complications, lymphadenectomy had been considered a relatively benign procedure, particularly if it saved a patient adjuvant radiation. Now that multiple trials suggest that adjuvant radiation decreases local recurrence without improving overall survival,[16,18,20] fewer patients receive adjuvant therapy even when unstaged. As seen in **Table 1**, although complications are not frequent, the risks of serious complications associated with lymphadenectomy are notable. The question remains "Is the risk of lymphadenectomy more significant than the risk of missing a positive lymph node, which would prompt systemic therapy and possibly improve survival?"

It is a difficult question to answer: how do you weigh the impact of persistent side effects for a large group, versus the cost of 1 or more lives saved? It would require us to know the number of staging procedures that would need to be performed to discover 1 treatable lymph node metastasis, the improvement in median survival expected with systemic therapy for lymph node metastases, and the cost of the complications of staging to patients, in terms of quality-adjusted life-years. In the absence of those data, careful consideration must be given to the risks and benefits of lymphadenectomy to make the best treatment decisions for our patients. In the Italian trial, there were no surgery-related deaths[17]; in ASTEC, there was a 7% to 9% treatment-related death incidence in the lymphadenectomy group, although it is not clear what percentage was related to postoperative adjuvant radiation therapy.[15] In LAP-2, the incidence of postoperative death within 30 days was 0.56% (laparoscopy) to 0.88% (laparotomy).[4] There is no clear evidence-based threshold of risk for lymphatic metastases that should prompt lymphadenectomy; however, in light of the risk of major complications and treatment-related deaths, it seems reasonable to assume that the risk of lymph node metastases should be at least 3% to justify the risks associated with lymphadenectomy. This remains a controversial topic, with some investigators arguing for lower thresholds or systematic staging of all endometrial cancer cases.[21,22]

Several systems have been proposed to identify patients at higher risk for lymph node metastases preoperatively or intraoperatively, all of which have similar limitations. Although it is agreed that grade, depth of invasion,[20,23] and lymph vascular space invasion (LVSI) predict[24–26] lymph node metastases and recurrence, it is difficult to come to consensus on criteria that reliably yield an incidence of lymph node metastases low enough to justify forgoing lymphadenectomy. In GOG 33, the surgical pathology study evaluating clinical stage 1 endometrial cancer, patients with either grade 1 tumors or endometrioid tumors with no myometrial invasion had an incidence of lymph node metastases less than 5%. However, there are several limitations: (1) the study required only a lymph node sampling (not a complete lymphadenectomy), (2) grade and depth from final pathology was used (which does not always concur with intraoperative evaluation), and (3) 2 key groups were underrepresented (grade 1 with deep one-third invasion and grade 3 with no myometrial invasion).

In 2000, surgeons at the Mayo Clinic proposed criteria for identifying patients with low-risk disease that are similar to those of GOG 33, with some modifications. The criteria are: type 1 (grade 1 or 2) endometrial cancer confined to the uterus and with 50% or less myometrial invasion and tumor diameter of 2 cm or less, or any grade with no myometrial invasion.[25] The specification of tumor size resulted from work done by Schink and colleagues[23] reporting a correlation between tumor size and incidence of lymph node metastases. In the original study from the Mayo Clinic, 9 of 187 women (5%) with grade 1 or 2 endometrioid tumors with less than 50% invasion on frozen section had lymph node metastases. Of 59 women who met the same criteria and had tumors 2 cm or less in diameter, 0% had lymph node metastases. Twenty-five percent of these same patients with LVSI had lymph node metastases as opposed to 3% of those without LVSI (P<.0001). Significant limitations of this study included non-standardized lymphadenectomy (many had lymph node sampling) and small sample size.

Other studies have found a low incidence of lymph node metastases with similar criteria. Examples include ASTEC, in which the incidence of metastases to the pelvic lymph nodes in patients with low-risk disease (grade 1 or 2 tumors with less than two-thirds myometrial invasion on final pathology) was 2%,[15] and LAP-2, in which the incidence was 1% in 389 patients with grade 1 or 2 tumors less than 2 cm in diameter with less than 50% invasion.[27] In contrast, a retrospective study of 834 women in Korea noted an incidence of 0.47% in women with grade 1 or 2 tumors with no myometrial invasion, but a higher than 3.5% incidence with any other tumors.[26] This observation is most likely related to the fact that women were included in this study even if they had greater than clinical stage 1 disease on preoperative assessment. The major limitation of all of these studies (except that of Mayo Clinic) is that the correlation between risk factors and lymph node metastases is based on final pathology, whereas it is the frozen pathology report that is used to assess real-time risk of lymph node metastasis, thus the need for lymphadenectomy.

The most significant hurdle to adopting a system for identifying low-risk disease at the time of surgery is the reliability of frozen section. The Mayo Clinic has a sophisticated system for frozen diagnosis, including specialized equipment not universally available. A retrospective study of 24,880 frozen sections performed during 1 year at the Mayo Clinic on all tissue types revealed an accuracy of 97.8%.[28] A recent presentation at the 2011 Annual Meeting of the Society of Gynecologic Oncologists from the Mayo Clinic compared frozen section with final pathology in 809 women having surgery for endometrial cancer. In only 1.4% of patients, final pathology differed from frozen section such that it would have altered surgical management (based on the Mayo criteria).[29] Several studies have looked at the accuracy of intra-operative evaluation of depth (gross or frozen) and grade.[30–33] Reliability varies from institution to institution.[28,34] In 1 study the accuracy of depth by gross inspection was 87.3% for grade 1 lesions, with underestimation 5% of the time. However, with increasing grade the ability to accurately predict depth of invasion decreased, with the depth of invasion underestimated more than 50% of the time in grade 3 tumors.[33]

Convery and colleagues[34] recently performed a retrospective study using data from the University of Virginia and Duke University that validated the Mayo criteria. All patients who had intraoperative frozen pathologic consultation and met Mayo criteria were included in this analysis. Among 110 women meeting criteria who had lymphadenectomy (at least 8 lymph nodes removed), the incidence of lymphatic metastases was 1.8%, which carries a 98.2% negative predictive value. Women with tumors greater than 2 cm who otherwise met the Mayo criteria and had a lymphadenectomy performed were also evaluated (a total of 140 women) and found to have a 2.9% incidence of lymph node metastases. Although this is only 1 study, it lends support to the value of intraoperative pathologic consultation to guide surgical decision making.

Omitting lymphadenectomy in grade 1 or 2 tumors with less than 50% invasion, no LVSI, and a diameter of 2 cm or less on final pathology likely yields an acceptable incidence of undiagnosed lymph node metastases. The predictive value of the Mayo criteria[25] has been reproduced in 1 study[34] and may be an appropriate standard depending on the institution. Gynecologic oncologists need to communicate with their pathologists and perform internal quality assurance to determine what thresholds to use intraoperatively to reliably meet these goals on final pathology at their own institution. When attempting to ascertain depth of myometrial invasion intraoperatively, using a lower threshold may help to avoid underestimation.

Extent of Lymphadenectomy

Both of the randomized controlled trials evaluating lymphadenectomy[15,17] mentioned earlier required only pelvic lymphadenectomy. There has been much discussion about whether or not pelvic lymphadenectomy is appropriate. Metastases to the para-aortic lymph nodes portend worse survival than pelvic lymph node metastases alone, which is reflected in the new FIGO staging system.[35] Many believe that to evaluate the true therapeutic value of lymphadenectomy, a complete lymphadenectomy, including the para-aortics, should have been performed in the randomized controlled trials.[21,36–38] To substantiate this theory, these investigators reference a study from the Mayo Clinic that reported that among 281 women who underwent staging for apparent clinical stage 1 disease, 57 had lymph node involvement, 38 of whom had para-aortic lymph node metastases.[36] To those who believe lymphadenectomy has therapeutic value, that finding means that patients who did not have para-aortic lymphadenectomy could have had disease left behind. In the same study, the incidence of isolated para-aortic lymph node metastases was 2.6% in women with type 1 disease and 4.1% in women with type 2 disease (3.2% overall). Whether one believes para-aortic lymphadenectomy is therapeutic or prognostic, patients with metastases to the para-aortics are the most likely to benefit from systemic therapy.[39] Para-aortic lymphadenectomy is considered by many to be an important component of a complete lymphadenectomy, dictating prognosis and directing treatment.

The debate still remains regarding what the appropriate surgical plan should include if high-risk uterine factors are identified on frozen section analysis, but para-aortic lymph nodes cannot be removed safely. If pelvic lymph nodes are accessible, should they be removed in this situation? Some surgeons believe that after peritoneal washings, hysterectomy, and BSO, no further staging is warranted and decisions should be made on uterine factors. Others believe pelvic lymphadenectomy is better than no evaluation of the lymph nodes. In most cases (pending results of ongoing GOG trials regarding adjuvant chemotherapy), the therapy prescribed based on uterine factors in type 1 disease includes radiation therapy, which does not include the para-aortic region. If the para-aortics are not safely accessible, it is best to perform the pelvic lymphadenectomy and use the pathologic results to guide decisions on adjuvant therapy, especially given that the incidence of isolated para-aortic lymph nodes metastases is only 2% to 2.6% in type 1 disease.[24,26,36]

There are proponents of extending the lymphadenectomy for endometrial cancer above the inferior mesenteric artery (IMA) based on the lymphatic drainage pathway from the fundus toward the renal vessels.[3,36] In recent GOG protocols, the IMA is the upper border of the lymphadenectomy for endometrial cancer.[4] With the value of lymphadenectomy already in question, the increased complication rate associated with extending the dissection above the IMA, with the intent of identifying isolated high para-aortic lymph node metastasis, may outweigh the benefit.

Nonendometrioid Histologies

In patients with clear cell or uterine papillary serous adenocarcinoma, the risk of distant metastases is significantly increased.[24] Whenever possible, patients with these histologies should undergo full surgical staging, not only for prognosis and therapeutic decision making but also for the opportunity to be enrolled in clinical trials. Given the higher incidence of occult metastases, staging usually includes an omental biopsy in addition to the usual staging procedures.

Minimally Invasive Surgical Staging: Laparoscopic and Robotic

The concept of laparoscopic staging of endometrial cancer was introduced in the early 1990s[40–42]; however, staging via minimally invasive techniques has only recently become widely accepted as a fully acceptable therapeutic option.[43] This transition to minimally invasive surgical staging correlates with the approval of the Da Vinci robot for use in gynecologic surgery in 2005 by the US Food and Drug Administration[43] and the adoption of robotic surgery by a few key forward-thinking gynecologic oncologists who popularized the approach.[6,7] Multiple retrospective studies and 3 randomized trials have shown the safety and feasibility of the laparoscopic and robotic surgical approaches.[4–6,43–45]

The GOG conducted LAP-2, the largest randomized trial evaluating laparoscopic versus open staging of endometrial cancer. Initially, LAP-2 was intended to evaluate feasibility and complications associated with the 2 techniques; midtrial the primary end point was changed to median time to recurrence and the sample size was adjusted. There were 1682 women in the laparoscopy arm and 920 in the laparotomy arm. The incidence of conversion to open surgery was 25.8%, with that risk closely correlated with body mass index (BMI, calculated as weight in kilograms divided by the square of height in meters). Patients undergoing laparoscopy had significantly longer operating time (204 vs 167 minutes, $P = .001$) and shorter hospital stay. There was a slightly higher (but not significant) risk of intraoperative complications with laparoscopy as opposed to laparotomy (10% vs 8%, $P = .106$, see **Table 1** for details). Perioperative mortality was similar in the 2 groups (0.59% vs 0.88%, $P = .404$) and mostly attributable to pulmonary embolism. Postoperative complications were significantly increased in the laparotomy group (14% vs 21%, $P<.001$). A study using FACT-G (Functional Assessment of Cancer Therapy: General) and other validated scales in a subset of LAP-2 patients reported a small benefit in quality of life (QoL) in the first 6 weeks after surgery for patients randomized to laparoscopy, although by 6 months postoperatively, QoL was equivalent regardless of surgical approach.[44]

Most patients in LAP-2 successfully underwent pelvic and para-aortic lymphadenectomy; however, a higher percentage of patients were staged in the laparotomy group versus the laparoscopy group (96% vs 92%, $P<.001$). Data on risk of recurrence have not been published, but were preliminarily presented as a late-breaking abstract at the 2010 Annual Meeting of the Society of Gynecologic Oncology by Dr Joan Walker. There is no difference in risk of recurrence and survival at 3 years between patients randomized to laparoscopy versus laparotomy. Provided the final results continue to show no difference in oncologic outcome, minimally invasive surgery should be considered the preferable treatment of endometrial cancer in light of the lower rate of complications and faster recovery. As experience with minimally invasive staging increases, the risk of conversion decreases, which may result in an even lower incidence of postoperative complications.[46] The risk of conversion in the 2 smaller randomized control trials of laparoscopy versus laparotomy for endometrial cancer staging ranged from 0% to 3.8%.[5,45]

Robotic-assisted laparoscopic endometrial cancer staging has been evaluated retrospectively, mostly using historical laparoscopic and laparotomy controls.[43] Although limited by selection bias, such studies are helpful in showing the overall safety and feasibility of the robotic approach. Recurrence and survival data are not evaluated, although if the robot is thought of as a surgical tool that assists in laparoscopy rather than a unique surgical procedure, such evaluation is probably not necessary. In most studies, the risk of conversion to laparotomy was lower with robotic-assisted surgery than laparoscopic staging, even although the median BMI of patients staged robotically was often higher than those staged laparoscopically.[6,40,47]

Determining Surgical Approach

Assessing a patient for a minimally invasive surgical approach requires consideration of 3 categories: patient characteristics, uterine factors, and surgeon experience. Patients who are normal to slightly overweight, with few comorbidities and little to no previous surgery can be staged in any fashion, although data support making every effort to offer those patients a minimally invasive approach.

Obesity and Minimally Invasive Surgery

Obesity is a known risk factor for type 1 endometrial cancer, thus consideration must frequently be given to the best surgical approach for overweight and severely obese patients. Obese patients are more likely to have diabetes and poor nutritional status, placing them at higher risk for multiple postoperative complications, including wound infections. It can be assumed that avoiding a large laparotomy incision is in the patient's best interest.[2]

In LAP-2, the incidence of conversion from laparoscopy to laparotomy correlated with BMI, with a sharp increase when the BMI was greater than 35.[4] That is not surprising: at a certain point, the thickness of the anterior abdominal wall severely limits range of motion. Also, because the fulcrum of the straight stick laparoscopic instrument is wider than in a thinner patient, small, subtle movements are more challenging. Much like driving without power steering, the surgeon must make large, exaggerated movements outside the patient's body to move the instruments intraperitoneally, which decreases precision. Robotic surgery has answered these challenges somewhat with articulating instruments, which allow for range of motion intraperitoneally with minimal movement outside the patient. In addition, the weight of the abdominal wall is borne by the robotic arms, not the surgeon, who is subject to fatigue.[47,48]

Although robotic surgery is often seen as preferable for very overweight and obese patients with endometrial cancer, it is not feasible in all cases. BMI is a valuable tool to guide a surgeon; however, it does not account for other factors that can ultimately lead to conversion to laparotomy. Exposure for lymphadenectomy is obtained by reflecting the small bowel into the upper abdomen. Short mesenteric length can severely limit the ability to stage robotically or laparoscopically because it makes exposure of the aortic bifurcation extremely difficult; this is compounded in obese patients with a thick mesentery and heavy epiploica. Even more important than the amount of adipose is the distribution: centripetal obesity is the most challenging because of mesenteric fat impeding exposure and adipose-laden lymphatic beds that can make blood vessels, nerves, and the ureter more difficult to identify and protect. Patients should be examined sitting and lying down because if the patient's weight falls laterally when she is supine, they may be a better candidate than a smaller patient whose weight remains centrally positioned. It is particularly difficult to perform robotic lymphadenectomy in patients who are short-waisted because there is minimal space in which to retract bowel, which limits visualization.

Despite the objective and subjective data, the decision regarding the best surgical approach is determined by the surgeon, taking multiple factors into consideration. Given that in LAP-2 the conversion rate was 26% and the postoperative complication rate was still significantly lower in the patients assigned to laparoscopy, it is reasonable to attempt a minimally invasive surgical approach in patients who may be borderline in terms of feasibility, recognizing that conversion is more likely.[4] With more and more fellowship graduates being trained robotically, the new generation of gynecologic oncologists may eventually be more comfortable robotically than open, meaning that a patient who may not be a candidate for a robotic lymphadenectomy is not a candidate for lymphadenectomy at all.

ADVANCED-STAGE DISEASE
Surgical Debulking for Advanced-Stage Disease

Multiple retrospective reviews have provided data supporting the role of cytoreductive surgery in the management of endometrial cancer.[8–11] In 2010, Barlin and colleagues reviewed the published data on surgical cytoreduction in uterine cancer. In a univariate analysis combining data from 14 retrospective studies of advanced and recurrent uterine cancer, these investigators[12] reported a relationship between complete cytoreduction and improved median survival, with borderline significance. The data came from a heterogeneous group of studies with variable definitions of optimal cytoreduction and there was not sufficient power for multivariable analysis. Thus, it is difficult to determine the true strength of the findings. The morbidity associated with more aggressive surgical techniques was not addressed.

Complete cytoreduction has also been shown to increase median survival in advanced stage uterine papillary serous carcinoma (UPSC). In a retrospective study of 70 patients with stage IIIC or IV UPSC who underwent surgery with curative intent at the Mayo Clinic, the median overall survival in patients with microscopic disease was 51 months versus 14 months in patients optimally reduced to less than 1 cm of disease and 12 months in those who were suboptimally cytoreduced ($P = .0002$). This finding remained significant when examined only in patients with macroscopic tumor at the start of surgery. Findings were similar regardless of whether or not aggressive surgical techniques were required to reach complete cytoreduction, although the study was underpowered for that comparison. Once again, data on surgical complications were not included.[49] Many studies downplay or ignore the complications associated with cytoreduction.[12,49] In some situations, complete cytoreduction requires more aggressive surgical techniques, which are associated with increased morbidity and mortality. In 1 study of stage IV patients, the perioperative mortality was 7% (as a result of 2 pulmonary emboli).[11] Although this is an overestimation of the true perioperative mortality, we know from the ovarian cancer literature that the morbidity and mortality associated with cytoreduction is significant.[50]

The data on the role of surgical cytoreduction in uterine cancer, all of which are retrospective, are severely limited by selection bias, including performance status, histologic subtype, and the use of various postoperative treatment modalities.

Although in general the data available support an attempt at complete cytoreduction in patients with advanced endometrial cancer and a good performance status, the decision to perform cytoreductive surgery and how aggressive to be is an individual one that takes into account the patient's comorbidities, her performance status, her symptoms, and surgical risks. Intraoperatively, it can be difficult to distinguish between advanced uterine and advanced ovarian cancer. Optimal cytoreduction is strongly associated with improved survival in prospective and retrospective studies of women with ovarian cancer.[50–53] As stated earlier, it is less clear for uterine cancer. Thus, whenever there is doubt on frozen section analysis regarding the origin of the pelvic malignancy, be it ovarian, tubal, or primary peritoneal, there is greater reason to risk morbidity to ensure an optimal cytoreductive procedure.

Neoadjuvant Chemotherapy and Interval Debulking

The data in support of neoadjuvant chemotherapy and interval debulking in endometrial cancer lag behind those in ovarian cancer.[50] Surgical cytoreduction is useful only when it is used in conjunction with effective chemotherapy. Data have shown that chemotherapy is effective in advanced endometrial cancer,[39] although not nearly so effective as it is in ovarian cancer.[8] Identifying patients responsive to chemotherapy could assist in triaging which patients might benefit from extensive cytoreduction. This is an area deserving of further investigation.

Unresectable Disease Because of Patient Factors or Extent of Disease

In patients in whom cytoreductive surgery is deemed impossible or inappropriate, it is often beneficial to perform a palliative hysterectomy using the least invasive approach. Unresected uterine tumor outgrows its blood supply and becomes necrotic, emitting a foul odor and causing bothersome drainage. Tumor can erode into vasculature, causing bleeding and eventually hemorrhage. Pelvic tumor can also be painful, much like advanced cervical cancer. Although many of the same symptoms can occur with pelvic or vaginal recurrence, the likelihood is theoretically higher with the uterus in situ.

SUMMARY

It is reasonable to perform complete lymphadenectomy in patients at significant risk of lymph node metastases, and use the results to guide adjuvant treatment decisions.[24,25] Criteria for staging based on intraoperative pathology should be determined in consultation with the pathologist, preferably with an institution-specific quality-assurance review.[34] Patients with more aggressive histologies should undergo a staging procedure including an omental biopsy whenever possible, with the understanding that most require systemic adjuvant therapy. Minimally invasive surgery is associated with shorter recovery and fewer postoperative complications than open endometrial cancer staging,[4,5,45] with preliminary data showing similar oncologic outcomes (Walker and colleagues, late breaking abstract SGO 2010 Annual Meeting). Whenever feasible, patients should be offered minimally invasive surgery for endometrial cancer staging. Retrospective data support an attempt at complete cytoreduction in patients with advanced endometrial cancer and a good performance status.[8–12] The decision to perform aggressive cytoreductive surgery should be individualized, taking into account the patient's comorbidities, her performance status, her symptoms, and the risks associated with more aggressive surgical procedures.

REFERENCES

1. Jemal A, Siegel R, Xu J, et al. Cancer statistics, 2010. CA Cancer J Clin 2010; 60(5):277–300.
2. Barakat RR, Markman M, Randall M. Principles and practice of gynecologic oncology. 5th edition. Philadelphia: Wolters Kluwer Health/Lippincott Williams & Wilkins; 2009.

3. Soliman PT, Frumovitz M, Spannuth W, et al. Lymphadenectomy during endometrial cancer staging: practice patterns among gynecologic oncologists. Gynecol Oncol 2010;119(2):291–4.

4. Walker JL, Piedmonte MR, Spirtos NM, et al. Laparoscopy compared with laparotomy for comprehensive surgical staging of uterine cancer: Gynecologic Oncology Group Study LAP2. J Clin Oncol 2009;27(32):5331–6.

5. Malzoni M, Tinelli R, Cosentino F, et al. Total laparoscopic hysterectomy versus abdominal hysterectomy with lymphadenectomy for early-stage endometrial cancer: a prospective randomized study. Gynecol Oncol 2009;112(1):126–33.

6. Boggess JF, Gehrig PA, Cantrell L, et al. A comparative study of 3 surgical methods for hysterectomy with staging for endometrial cancer: robotic assistance, laparoscopy, laparotomy. Am J Obstet Gynecol 2008;199(4):360.e1–9.

7. Seamon LG, Cohn DE, Richardson DL, et al. Robotic hysterectomy and pelvic-aortic lymphadenectomy for endometrial cancer. Obstet Gynecol 2008;112(6): 1207–13.

8. Landrum LM, Moore KN, Myers TK, et al. Stage IVB endometrial cancer: does applying an ovarian cancer treatment paradigm result in similar outcomes? A case-control analysis. Gynecol Oncol 2009;112(2):337–41.

9. Bristow RE, Zerbe MJ, Rosenshein NB, et al. Stage IVB endometrial carcinoma: the role of cytoreductive surgery and determinants of survival. Gynecol Oncol 2000;78(2):85–91.

10. Chi DS, Welshinger M, Venkatraman ES, et al. The role of surgical cytoreduction in Stage IV endometrial carcinoma. Gynecol Oncol 1997;67(1):56–60.

11. Goff BA, Goodman A, Muntz HG, et al. Surgical stage IV endometrial carcinoma: a study of 47 cases. Gynecol Oncol 1994;52(2):237–40.

12. Barlin JN, Puri I, Bristow RE. Cytoreductive surgery for advanced or recurrent endometrial cancer: a meta-analysis. Gynecol Oncol 2010;118(1):14–8.

13. Pecorelli S. Revised FIGO staging for carcinoma of the vulva, cervix, and endometrium. Int J Gynaecol Obstet 2009;105(2):103–4.

14. Benedet JL, Bender H, Jones H 3rd, et al. FIGO staging classifications and clinical practice guidelines in the management of gynecologic cancers. FIGO Committee on Gynecologic Oncology. Int J Gynaecol Obstet 2000;70(2):209–62.

15. Kitchener H, Swart AM, Qian Q, et al. Efficacy of systematic pelvic lymphadenectomy in endometrial cancer (MRC ASTEC trial): a randomised study. Lancet 2009; 373(9658):125–36.

16. Creutzberg CL, van Putten WL, Koper PC, et al. Surgery and postoperative radiotherapy versus surgery alone for patients with stage-1 endometrial carcinoma: multicentre randomised trial. PORTEC Study Group. Post Operative Radiation Therapy in Endometrial Carcinoma. Lancet 2000;355(9213):1404–11.

17. Benedetti Panici P, Basile S, Maneschi F, et al. Systematic pelvic lymphadenectomy vs. no lymphadenectomy in early-stage endometrial carcinoma: randomized clinical trial. J Natl Cancer Inst 2008;100(23):1707–16.

18. Blake P, Swart AM, Orton J, et al. Adjuvant external beam radiotherapy in the treatment of endometrial cancer (MRC ASTEC and NCIC CTG EN.5 randomised trials): pooled trial results, systematic review, and meta-analysis. Lancet 2009; 373(9658):137–46.

19. Ryan M, Stainton MC, Jaconelli C, et al. The experience of lower limb lymphedema for women after treatment for gynecologic cancer. Oncol Nurs Forum 2003; 30(3):417–23.

20. Keys HM, Roberts JA, Brunetto VL, et al. A phase III trial of surgery with or without adjunctive external pelvic radiation therapy in intermediate risk endometrial

adenocarcinoma: a Gynecologic Oncology Group study. Gynecol Oncol 2004; 92(3):744–51.

21. Chan JK, Kapp DS. Role of complete lymphadenectomy in endometrioid uterine cancer. Lancet Oncol 2007;8(9):831–41.

22. Shah C, Johnson EB, Everett E, et al. Does size matter? Tumor size and morphology as predictors of nodal status and recurrence in endometrial cancer. Gynecol Oncol 2005;99(3):564–70.

23. Schink JC, Lurain JR, Wallemark CB, et al. Tumor size in endometrial cancer: a prognostic factor for lymph node metastasis. Obstet Gynecol 1987;70(2):216–9.

24. Creasman WT, Morrow CP, Bundy BN, et al. Surgical pathologic spread patterns of endometrial cancer. A Gynecologic Oncology Group Study. Cancer 1987; 60(Suppl 8):2035–41.

25. Mariani A, Webb MJ, Keeney GL, et al. Low-risk corpus cancer: is lymphadenectomy or radiotherapy necessary? Am J Obstet Gynecol 2000;182(6):1506–19.

26. Lee KB, Ki DD, Lee JM, et al. The risk of lymph node metastasis based on myometrial invasion and tumor grade in endometrioid uterine cancers: a multicenter, retrospective Korean study. Ann Surg Oncol 2009;16(10):2882–7.

27. Milam M, Java J, Walker J, et al. Incidence of nodal metastasis in endometrioid endometrial cancer risk groups: a Gynecologic Oncology Group multicenter review. Gynecol Oncol 2011;120(Suppl 1):S4.

28. Ferreiro JA, Myers JL, Bostwick DG. Accuracy of frozen section diagnosis in surgical pathology: review of a 1-year experience with 24,880 cases at Mayo Clinic Rochester. Mayo Clin Proc 1995;70(12):1137–41.

29. Mariani A, Medeiros F, Dowdy S, et al. Reliability of frozen-section examination in endometrial carcinoma at a tertiary care center: is it appropriate for intraoperative guidance of treatment decisions? Gynecol Oncol 2011;120(Suppl 1):S92.

30. Case AS, Rocconi RP, Straughn JM Jr, et al. A prospective blinded evaluation of the accuracy of frozen section for the surgical management of endometrial cancer. Obstet Gynecol 2006;108(6):1375–9.

31. Frumovitz M, Slomovitz BM, Singh DK, et al. Frozen section analyses as predictors of lymphatic spread in patients with early-stage uterine cancer. J Am Coll Surg 2004;199(3):388–93.

32. Neubauer NL, Havrilesky LJ, Calingaert B, et al. The role of lymphadenectomy in the management of preoperative grade 1 endometrial carcinoma. Gynecol Oncol 2009;112(3):511–6.

33. Goff BA, Rice LW. Assessment of depth of myometrial invasion in endometrial adenocarcinoma. Gynecol Oncol 1990;38(1):46–8.

34. Convery PA, Cantrell LA, Di Santo N, et al. Retrospective review of an intraoperative algorithm to predict lymph node metastasis in low-grade endometrial adenocarcinoma. Gynecol Oncol 2011;123(1):65–70.

35. Cooke EW, Pappas L, Gaffney DK. Does the revised International Federation of Gynecology and Obstetrics staging system for endometrial cancer lead to increased discrimination in patient outcomes? Cancer 2011;117(18):4231–7.

36. Mariani A, Dowdy SC, Cliby WA, et al. Prospective assessment of lymphatic dissemination in endometrial cancer: a paradigm shift in surgical staging. Gynecol Oncol 2008;109(1):11–8.

37. Uccella S, Podratz KC, Aletti GD, et al. Lymphadenectomy in endometrial cancer. Lancet 2009;373(9670):1170 [author reply: 1170–1].

38. Mariani A, Webb MJ, Galli L, et al. Potential therapeutic role of para-aortic lymphadenectomy in node-positive endometrial cancer. Gynecol Oncol 2000;76(3): 348–56.

39. Randall ME, Filiaci VL, Muss H, et al. Randomized phase III trial of whole-abdominal irradiation versus doxorubicin and cisplatin chemotherapy in advanced endometrial carcinoma: a Gynecologic Oncology Group Study. J Clin Oncol 2006;24(1):36–44.

40. Hoekstra AV, Jairam-Thodla A, Rademaker A, et al. The impact of robotics on practice management of endometrial cancer: transitioning from traditional surgery. Int J Med Robot 2009;5(4):392–7.

41. Childers JM, Hatch KD, Tran AN, et al. Laparoscopic para-aortic lymphadenectomy in gynecologic malignancies. Obstet Gynecol 1993;82(5):741–7.

42. Childers JM, Spirtos NM, Brainard P, et al. Laparoscopic staging of the patient with incompletely staged early adenocarcinoma of the endometrium. Obstet Gynecol 1994;83(4):597–600.

43. Gaia G, Holloway RW, Santoro L, et al. Robotic-assisted hysterectomy for endometrial cancer compared with traditional laparoscopic and laparotomy approaches: a systematic review. Obstet Gynecol 2010;116(6):1422–31.

44. Kornblith AB, Huang HQ, Walker JL, et al. Quality of life of patients with endometrial cancer undergoing laparoscopic international federation of gynecology and obstetrics staging compared with laparotomy: a Gynecologic Oncology Group study. J Clin Oncol 2009;27(32):5337–42.

45. Kondalsamy-Chennakesavan S, Janda M, Gebski V, et al. Randomized controlled trial of laparoscopic approach to carcinoma of the endometrium (LACE): prevalence and risk factors for surgical complications. Gynecol Oncol 2011;120 (Suppl 1):S10.

46. Boruta DM 2nd, Growdon WB, McCann CK, et al. Evolution of surgical management of early-stage endometrial cancer. Am J Obstet Gynecol 2011. [Epub ahead of print].

47. Seamon LG, Cohn DE, Henretta MS, et al. Minimally invasive comprehensive surgical staging for endometrial cancer: robotics or laparoscopy? Gynecol Oncol 2009;113(1):36–41.

48. Shafer A, Boggess JF. Robotic-assisted endometrial cancer staging and radical hysterectomy with the da Vinci surgical system. Gynecol Oncol 2008; 111(Suppl 2):S18–23.

49. Thomas MB, Mariani A, Cliby WA, et al. Role of cytoreduction in stage III and IV uterine papillary serous carcinoma. Gynecol Oncol 2007;107(2):190–3.

50. Vergote I, Trope CG, Amant F, et al. Neoadjuvant chemotherapy or primary surgery in stage IIIC or IV ovarian cancer. N Engl J Med 2010;363(10):943–53.

51. Hoskins WJ, McGuire WP, Brady MF, et al. The effect of diameter of largest residual disease on survival after primary cytoreductive surgery in patients with suboptimal residual epithelial ovarian carcinoma. Am J Obstet Gynecol 1994; 170(4):974–9 [discussion: 979–80].

52. Ozols RF, Bundy BN, Greer BE, et al. Phase III trial of carboplatin and paclitaxel compared with cisplatin and paclitaxel in patients with optimally resected stage III ovarian cancer: a Gynecologic Oncology Group study. J Clin Oncol 2003; 21(17):3194–200.

53. Winter WE 3rd, Maxwell GL, Tian C, et al. Prognostic factors for stage III epithelial ovarian cancer: a Gynecologic Oncology Group Study. J Clin Oncol 2007;25(24): 3621–7.

Current Surgical Management of Ovarian Cancer

John O. Schorge, MD[a],*, Eric E. Eisenhauer, MD[b],
Dennis S. Chi, MD[c]

KEYWORDS

- Ovarian cancer • Primary debulking surgery
- Interval debulking surgery • Secondary debulking surgery

Ovarian cancer is a heterogeneous disease requiring a disciplined surgical approach to consistently achieve the best possible outcomes. Epithelial ovarian carcinomas, including the more indolent (borderline) tumors with low malignant potential, comprise 90% to 95% of all cases. Sex cord–stromal tumors and malignant ovarian germ cell tumors are rare. However, surgery plays a critical role in all stages of these various subtypes of ovarian malignancy. Moreover, current surgical techniques and recent innovations also apply to peritoneal and fallopian tube cancers because of their clinical similarities.

Comprehensive surgical management of ovarian cancer involves both knowledge of the disease process and mastery of a wide spectrum of different procedures. A newly diagnosed complex adnexal mass with or without carcinomatosis may be detectable before surgery, but the intended operation often needs to be revised based on frozen section histology or other intraoperative findings. The surgeon must strike the perfect balance between being appropriately aggressive and trying to avoid unnecessary morbidity. Postoperative complications, disease relapse, and symptomatic end-stage sequelae are other common situations that may need to be addressed. Again, the surgeon is often faced with making a difficult decision to intervene or to manage nonsurgically. Because of the complexities of providing longitudinal care for patients with ovarian cancer, better outcomes are reported when a subspecialist is overseeing treatment.[1]

Fewer than half of such patients in the United States and Europe are cared for by a gynecologic oncologist.[2,3] Instead, most are managed by physicians not necessarily

No funding disclosures.

[a] Massachusetts General Hospital, Harvard Medical School, 55 Fruit Street, Boston, MA 02114, USA

[b] The Ohio State University, M210 Starling-Loving, 320 West 10th Avenue, Columbus, OH 43210, USA

[c] Memorial Sloan-Kettering Cancer Center, 1275 York Avenue, New York, NY 10065, USA

* Corresponding author.

E-mail address: jschorge@partners.org

Hematol Oncol Clin N Am 26 (2012) 93–109
doi:10.1016/j.hoc.2011.10.004
0889-8588/12/$ – see front matter © 2012 Elsevier Inc. All rights reserved.

hemonc.theclinics.com

intimately familiar with the interplay between medical and surgical management. However, improvements in overall survival depend on the precise coordination of both forms of treatment. When a gynecologic oncologist is involved, patients are more likely to undergo both primary staging and surgical debulking.[4] Thereafter, additional surgery may need to be considered as part of the therapeutic strategy or for palliative purposes. This article provides a comprehensive review of the surgical management of ovarian carcinoma.

SURGICAL STAGING

Typically, an adnexal mass is suspected by symptom history or findings on pelvic examination. Alternatively, it may be discovered by serendipity on sonography or computed tomography (CT) scanning. Proper identification of an ovarian malignancy among patients with a pelvic mass may be aided by imaging characteristics of the mass and the rest of the abdomen, in addition to the preoperative CA125 level. More recently, the human epididymis 4 (HE4) serum marker has been approved for use in helping to effectively triage such patients.[5] The current referral guidelines for a newly diagnosed pelvic mass incorporate several of these features and are listed in **Box 1**.[6]

Because ovarian cancer is surgically staged, every patient who is taken to the operating room with a suspicious adnexal mass should be consented for comprehensive staging if malignancy is found. Ideally, a physician trained to appropriately stage ovarian cancers, such as a gynecologic oncologist, should perform the operation. Moreover, the operation should take place in a hospital facility that has the necessary support and consultative services (ie, frozen section pathology). When a malignant ovarian tumor is discovered and the appropriate operation cannot be properly performed, a gynecologic oncologist should be consulted during surgery if possible.[6] If immediate consultation is not available, or if the diagnosis is only noted on final pathology, a postsurgical referral is mandatory. In these instances, the gynecologic oncologist needs to make a clinical judgment about whether there is enough information to recommend expectant management or chemotherapy. Alternatively, restaging might be advisable to better define the disease process.

The intent of surgical staging is threefold: (1) to establish a diagnosis; (2) to assess the extent of disease; (3) to remove as much gross tumor as possible. Patients who

---

Box 1
Society of Gynecologic Oncology and American College of Obstetrics and Gynecology referral guidelines for a newly diagnosed pelvic mass

Postmenopausal women

    Increased CA125 level

    Ascites

    Nodular or fixed pelvic mass

    Evidence of abdominal or distant metastasis

Premenopausal women

    Very increased CA125 level

    Ascites

    Evidence of abdominal or distant metastasis

undergo comprehensive surgical staging to confirm early-stage disease have a better prognosis than patients who are thought to have early-stage disease but do not undergo comprehensive surgical staging, presumably because occult metastatic disease is not detected.[6]

Epithelial Ovarian Cancer

The consistent inability to reliably detect epithelial ovarian carcinoma before metastasis has occurred has been an ongoing disappointment. Routine screening has not been shown to improve early detection or reduce mortality in either the high-risk or general populations.[6–8] As a result, only one-quarter of newly diagnosed women have disease confined to the ovary. Comprehensive staging results in a shifting of patients with subclinical metastases from early-stage to advanced-stage disease with an improved median survival for both groups. In addition, treatment-related side effects or complications may be avoided. Patients with accurately defined surgical stage I disease may not require any additional treatment, or may safely receive less chemotherapy than otherwise would be the case in inadequately staged patients. When occult stage III disease is detected, patients may be treated more aggressively with intraperitoneal chemotherapy, or be eligible for clinical trial participation.

A conceptual understanding of the spread pattern of epithelial ovarian cancer is valuable to help guide the surgical staging procedure. Epithelial ovarian cancer arises within the ovarian surface epithelium, grows focally, and ultimately breaches the ovarian capsule to metastasize by exfoliation or via the abdominal/pelvic lymphatic system. Peritoneal fluid flows in a clockwise fashion; thus, cancer cells shed into the fluid initially implant throughout the pelvis and right paracolic gutters, across the diaphragm, and on the small or large intestine.[9] Lymphatic spread to the pelvic and para-aortic regions is also commonplace.

Surgical staging for ovarian carcinoma has historically been performed through an abdominal incision that allows exposure of the entire abdomen. On entry into the peritoneal cavity, ascites is aspirated for cytology if present. If there is no ascites, cytologic washings of the pelvis and paracolic gutters are obtained. A total abdominal hysterectomy and bilateral salpingo-oophorectomy is performed in most patients. The contents of the peritoneal cavity, including all organs and peritoneal surfaces, are systematically inspected, and any suspicious-appearing areas are biopsied. Unless these areas are confirmed on frozen section to show malignancy, an omentectomy and peritoneal biopsies are performed.[9,10]

Suspicious lymph nodes should be excised and sent for frozen section; if negative for malignancy, bilateral pelvic and para-aortic lymphadenectomy should be performed to exclude microscopic disease. Even when only 1 ovary is grossly involved, the frequency of having only contralateral nodal metastases ranges from 10% to 30%.[11–13] Chan and colleagues[14] retrospectively analyzed 6686 women with clinical stage I ovarian cancer between 1988 and 2001, observing that most women with stage I epithelial ovarian cancers who underwent lymphadenectomy had a significant improvement in survival. Moreover, the extent of lymphadenectomy (0 nodes, less than 10 nodes, and 10 or more nodes) significantly increased the survival rates from 87% to 92% to 94%, respectively. Because nodal metastases are common above the inferior mesenteric artery, the para-aortic lymphadenectomy should be performed up to the level of the left renal vein.[11]

The importance of a comprehensive initial surgical procedure was first shown by a multicenter national trial in which 100 patients with apparent early-stage disease underwent surgical restaging. Before referral, only 25% of patients had an initial surgical incision that was adequate to allow complete examination of the pelvis and abdominal cavity. One-third of patients were found to have more advanced disease at the second surgery. Furthermore, histologic grade was a significant predictor of occult metastasis: 16% of patients with grade 1 tumors were upstaged, compared with 46% with grade 3 disease.[15] After thorough surgical evaluation, the International Federation of Gynecology and Obstetrics (FIGO) staging system is applied to guide adjuvant therapy decisions (**Table 1**).

Comprehensively staged women with stage IA/IB grade 3 disease or stage IC or greater are typically treated with platinum-based adjuvant therapy. Combining the results of 2 large European trials, patients with stage IA and IB grades 2 and 3, stage IC, and stage II who received adjuvant chemotherapy after surgery had an improved survival compared with patients randomly assigned to observation.[16] However, in an analysis of one of the studies, only the incompletely staged patients benefited.[17] Chan and colleagues[18] further showed the value of comprehensive staging in an exploratory analysis of 427 patients prospectively randomized to 3 or 6 cycles of chemotherapy, observing that only those patients having tumors with serous histology derived any benefit from the additional 3 courses of treatment. Thus, comprehensive surgical staging of apparent early-stage epithelial ovarian cancer is critically important to accurately define the extent of disease and appropriately guide postoperative therapy.

Minimally Invasive Staging

Minimally invasive surgery has revolutionized much of gynecologic oncology. However, because most patients with ovarian cancer are diagnosed with advanced disease, the usefulness of this technology has not been as profound as in cervical or endometrial cancer. In addition, the treating gynecologic oncologist may have other concerns (**Box 2**). As a result, the current literature defining the role of laparoscopy in the diagnosis and treatment of ovarian cancer is limited to case reports, case series, and cohort studies.

Table 1
FIGO surgical staging system for ovarian cancer

Stage	Surgical-Pathologic Findings
IA	Growth limited to 1 ovary
IB	Growth limited to both ovaries
IC	Tumor limited to 1 or both ovaries, but with disease on the surface of 1 or both ovaries; or with capsule(s) ruptured; or with malignant ascites or positive peritoneal washings
IIA	Extension and/or metastases to the uterus and/or tubes
IIB	Extension to other pelvic tissues
IIC	Tumor limited to the genital tract or other pelvic tissues, but with disease on the surface of 1 or both ovaries; or with capsule(s) ruptured; or with malignant ascites or positive peritoneal washings
IIIA	Tumor grossly limited to the true pelvis with negative nodes, but with histologically confirmed microscopic seeding of abdominal-peritoneal surfaces
IIIB	Abdominal implants less than 2 cm in diameter with negative nodes
IIIC	Abdominal implants at least 2 cm in diameter and/or positive pelvic, para-aortic, or inguinal nodes
IV	Distant metastases, including malignant pleural effusion or parenchymal liver metastases

Box 2
Clinical concerns of minimally invasive staging of ovarian cancer
Inability to fully explore the abdomen
Risk of intraoperative rupture
Port-site tumor implantation

One disadvantage of minimally invasive surgery is the inability to fully explore the abdomen in search of tumor implants. There are inherent limitations in accessing the entire peritoneal cavity without a large vertical incision, no matter what other approach is used. In one preliminary analysis, Chi and colleagues[19] showed that patients with apparent stage I ovarian or fallopian tube cancer could safely and adequately undergo laparoscopic surgical staging. They reported no differences in omental specimen size or number of lymph nodes removed. Estimated blood loss and hospital stay were also lower for laparoscopy, but operating time was longer. Overall, the limited data suggest equal efficacy of laparoscopy compared with laparotomy in both early and advanced-stage ovarian cancer.[20] Robotic assistance has also been reported to facilitate comprehensive staging.[21]

Laparoscopic or robotic surgery is postulated to increase the risk of intraoperative rupture of an ovarian cystic mass. The clinical relevance of intraperitoneal spillage is controversial, but this is often the event that triggers the indication for adjuvant chemotherapy when it might not otherwise have been required. Most adnexal masses can be safely detached, placed intact within a specimen retrieval bag, drained or morcellated at the abdominal wall, and removed from a trocar site without spillage. Removal of any suspicious mass without enclosure in a specimen bag is inadvisable because of the possibility of seeding the subcutaneous tissues.

Although clinically relevant, the rate of port-site tumor implantation after laparoscopic procedures in women with malignant disease is low. It usually occurs in the setting of synchronous, advanced intra-abdominal or distant metastatic disease. The presence of port-site implantation is a surrogate for advanced disease and should not be used as an argument against laparoscopic surgery in gynecologic malignancies.[22]

Borderline Tumors

Although formally categorized under the umbrella of epithelial ovarian cancers, low malignant potential (LMP) or borderline tumors have a more indolent biologic behavior. Comprehensive surgical staging of these patients has limited value overall, because most tumors are stage I. Even when stage III microscopic noninvasive implants or nodal metastases are detected, the information is of prognostic value only and adjuvant chemotherapy is not recommended. Thus, routine pelvic and para-aortic lymph node dissection is not necessary in most women with proven ovarian borderline tumors.[23] In summary, when a definitive diagnosis is confirmed, no additional staging is required.[24]

However, invasive carcinoma may not be detected until final pathologic review. About 25% to 30% of patients with an intraoperative frozen section diagnosis of a borderline tumor are ultimately diagnosed with an invasive cancer after additional sectioning. Nonserous tumors are more likely to be misinterpreted.[25] Because of the uncertainty of intraoperative diagnosis, in most circumstances these tumors should be staged as indicated for epithelial ovarian carcinoma.

Rare Ovarian Tumors

Sex cord–stromal, malignant ovarian germ cell tumors and infrequent epithelial types such as mucinous or clear cell carcinomas have unique biologic behaviors that differ from the more common epithelial variants. Although most of the standard staging procedures apply to rare tumors, lymphadenectomy has limited value overall.[14] Lymph node metastases in ovarian sex cord–stromal tumors and mucinous ovarian cancers are so rare that lymphadenectomy may be safely omitted when staging such patients.[26] Because of the chemoresistance of clear cell carcinomas, detection of nodal metastases is often of prognostic value, but does not necessarily lead to a clinical benefit. Moreover, because of unique tumor dissemination patterns, lymphadenectomy is most important for dysgerminomas, whereas only staging peritoneal and omental biopsies are of importance for yolk sac tumors and immature teratomas.

Fertility-sparing Surgery

Approximately 10% of epithelial ovarian cancers develop in women younger than 40 years of age, suggesting that fertility-sparing surgery may need to be considered in selected patients. When the cancer seems confined to 1 ovary, especially if it is low grade, it is appropriate to modify the staging procedure by leaving the uterus and the uninvolved ovary in place for younger women who wish to preserve fertility. Surgical staging otherwise proceeds as described. Although many patients are upstaged, those with surgical stage I disease have an excellent long-term survival with unilateral adnexectomy. Preserving the uterus and contralateral ovary does not seem to compromise the chances of cure. In some cases, postoperative chemotherapy may be required, but patients usually retain their ability to conceive and ultimately carry a pregnancy to term.[27]

Fertility-sparing management of borderline tumors with cystectomy or unilateral adnexectomy may also be appropriate for motivated, reproductive-aged women. Preservation of the contralateral adnexa increases the risk of recurrence, but surgical resection is usually curative.[28] Unilateral adnexectomy may also be considered for patients with sex cord–stromal ovarian tumors in the absence of obvious disease spread to the uterus.[29] Most such tumors turn out to be stage I. Because of the characteristic young age of women diagnosed with malignant ovarian germ cell tumors, fertility-sparing surgery is the norm and does not adversely affect survival.[30]

TUMOR DEBULKING

Ovarian cancer is often portrayed as the disease that whispers because it does not present with dramatic bleeding, excruciating pain, or an obvious lump. Instead, the typical symptoms tend to be indolent. Patients and their health care providers often attribute such nonspecific changes to menopause, aging, dietary indiscretions, stress, depression, or functional bowel problems. Frequently, women are medically managed for indigestion or other presumed ailments without having a pelvic examination. As a result, substantial delays before diagnosis are common. Two-thirds of women who are newly diagnosed with invasive epithelial ovarian cancer still present, as they always have, with advanced disease typically characterized by ascites, carcinomatosis, and omental caking (**Fig. 1**).

Procedures such as radical pelvic surgery, bowel resection, and aggressive upper abdominal surgery are commonly required to achieve optimal cytoreduction. Recent evidence suggests that metastatic ovarian cancers, like other solid tumors, contain a small subpopulation of highly specialized stem cells with self-renewal capacity and the potential to reconstitute the cellular heterogeneity of a tumor. Ovarian cancer

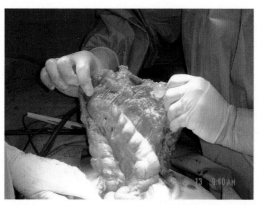

Fig. 1. Omental caking in a patient with stage IIIC epithelial ovarian cancer.

stem cells are thought to be responsible for tumor initiation, maintenance, and growth.[31] Ineffective targeting of this cell population is responsible for the therapeutic failures and tumor recurrences currently observed.[32]

The elimination of potentially chemoresistant cells is one presumed benefit of surgical cytoreduction. The probability of spontaneous mutations to drug-resistant phenotypes increases as tumor size and cell numbers increase according to the Goldie and Coldman[33] hypothesis. Instinctually, cytoreductive surgery should allow removal of existing resistant tumor cells and decrease the spontaneous development of additional resistant cells. Several supportive, but mostly theoretic, additional arguments have been proposed to justify the biologic plausibility of debulking (**Box 3**).[34]

Removal of bulky tumors as part of cancer treatment is an easy concept for patients and their families to understand. The clinical benefits of debulking have been harder to prove. Within the broader field of oncology, the aggressive surgical approach to widely metastatic disease is unique to ovarian cancer. Patients seem to benefit from 1 maximal debulking attempt, but the timing of the procedure and what defines a success have become increasingly controversial.

Primary Debulking

Joe V. Meigs,[35] a gynecologic surgeon at Massachusetts General Hospital, initially described ovarian tumor debulking in 1934. However, the concept was not validated until the mid-1970s.[36] Case series and other retrospective data rapidly accrued thereafter to further establish primary cytoreductive surgery as the de facto standard of care.[37–39]

Box 3
Theoretic arguments for debulking surgery

- Removing large necrotic masses promotes drug delivery to smaller tumors with good blood supply.

- Removing resistant clones decreases the likelihood of early-onset drug resistance.

- Tiny implants have a higher growth fraction that should be more chemosensitive.

- Removing cancer in specific locations, such as tumors causing a bowel obstruction, improves the patient's nutritional and immunologic status.

The success of the operation depends on numerous factors, including patient selection, tumor location, and surgeon expertise. To achieve a survival benefit, an optimal result was initially defined as no residual tumors individually measuring more than 2 cm in size. For purposes of uniformity, the Gynecologic Oncology Group (GOG) redefined optimal debulking as residual implants less than or equal to 1 cm.[10] For the past few decades, this criterion has served as the benchmark of success. Patients undergoing primary optimal cytoreductive surgery (≤1 cm residual disease), followed by intraperitoneal platinum-based chemotherapy have a median overall survival of 66 months, which is the longest duration ever reported in a phase III study.[40] The level of success achieved in this GOG trial (protocol #172) is currently the gold standard for comparisons with any other sequence of treatment.

Despite the accumulated evidence supporting the importance of primary debulking, it remains controversial whether the better outcome is caused by the surgeon's technical proficiency or some ill-defined, intrinsic feature of the cancer that makes the tumor implants easier to remove. In general, extensive upper abdominal disease strongly indicates aggressive tumor biology. Although this is a common location of unresectable disease, optimal debulking may still be achieved in many patients by performing ultraradical procedures, such as splenectomy (**Fig. 2**) or diaphragmatic resection.[41–43] However, it is still unclear what impact ultraradical techniques have on quality of life and morbidity. Furthermore, the cost-effectiveness of this approach has not been investigated.[44] Although these points should be prospectively studied, survival rates have been shown to improve accordingly when the surgical paradigm is revised to a more aggressive philosophy incorporating these and other radical techniques.[45–47] Patients referred to specialized centers where such radical procedures are commonly performed may anticipate higher rates of optimal debulking

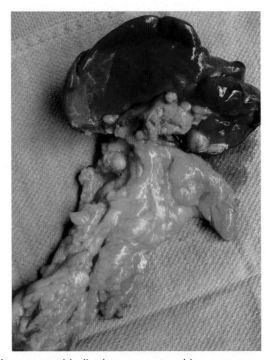

Fig. 2. En bloc splenectomy with distal omentum to achieve no gross residual disease.

and improved survival, without additional surgery necessarily leading to increased major morbidity.

One valid criticism of cytoreductive surgery is the biased, subjective assessment of gross residual disease by the surgeon at the completion of the operation. Because of tissue induration, inadequate exploration, radiologist overestimation, or other factors, inaccuracies of residual tumor size are common.[48] Perhaps because of the inability to reliably quantify the remaining disease, a recent subanalysis of accumulated data from several prospective GOG trials showed that patients with residual disease of 0.1 to 1.0 cm had marginally improved overall survival compared with patients with greater than 1-cm residual disease for stage III ovarian cancer and no improvement in those with stage IV disease. Large survival benefit was only achieved with complete resection to microscopic residual disease.[49,50]

Based on these findings and other similar reports, there is a growing consensus that optimal cytoreduction should be defined using a more stringent criterion. Thus, the current goal of primary debulking is to achieve complete resection with no residual disease. Raising the standard for surgical success accordingly decreases the proportion of patients with stage III to IV ovarian cancer in which this redefined optimal result can be accomplished. For advanced disease, reports range from 15% to 30%.[47,49–53] However, the clinical benefits are substantial. Chi and colleagues[51] analyzed a prospectively kept database for outcomes of 465 women with stage IIIC ovarian cancer who underwent primary cytoreductive surgery. They observed a median overall survival of 106 months for patients with no gross residual disease, 66 months for those with disease less than or equal to 0.5 cm, 48 months with 0.6 to 1.0 cm residual disease, and 33 to 34 months for greater than 1 cm residual disease. As suggested by these data, although complete resection is often not feasible, cytoreduction to as little residual tumor as possible should always be the focus of aggressive surgical efforts, because each incremental decrease in residual disease less than 1 cm may be associated with an incremental improvement in overall survival.

Even when successful, the disadvantage of radical cytoreductive surgery is that it may result in a prolonged postoperative recovery that is fraught with complications. The initiation of chemotherapy may be delayed, or postponed indefinitely.[52,53] Special caution is indicated for women aged 75 years or older, especially in the presence of other significant comorbidities. These patients in particular have an increased 30-day mortality.[54] When an optimal result is not possible, the surgical approach should be limited in scope to avoid unnecessary postoperative morbidity.

Such patients may benefit from attempted cytoreduction by minimally invasive techniques. Recently, laparoscopic and robotic-assisted debulking of advanced ovarian cancer have each been reported with minimal morbidity.[21,55] Although not often feasible because of the disease distribution, such techniques may be warranted in selected circumstances and may be preferable to neoadjuvant chemotherapy (NACT).

Interval Debulking

Preoperative CA125 levels, CT scans, and physical examinations are often not reliable to predict patients who can be optimally debulked. As a result, many patients with advanced ovarian cancers who are taken for surgery cannot be completely resected. Invariably, the final determination cannot be made until abdominal exploration.

Two phase III trials were conducted to determine whether a second interval debulking procedure was worthwhile after an unsuccessful initial attempt followed by a few courses of chemotherapy. A multicenter trial conducted in Europe found a 6-month median survival advantage in patients who were reexplored after 3 cycles of chemotherapy.[56] In contrast, no survival advantage was found when a similar study was conducted in the United States.[57] These conflicting reports are most easily explained by clarifying who performed the first surgery.

In the US trial, virtually all patients had their initial attempt by a gynecologic oncologist, unlike the European study in which few had their first surgery performed by a subspecialist. Thus, interval debulking seems to yield benefit only among patients whose primary surgery was not performed by a gynecologic oncologist, if the first try was not intended as a maximal resection of all gross disease, or if no upfront surgery was performed.

Some patients are too medically ill to initially undergo any type of upfront abdominal operation, whereas others have disease that is too extensive to be resected by an experienced ovarian cancer surgical team. In these circumstances, NACT is routinely used, ideally after the diagnosis has been confirmed by paracentesis, CT-guided biopsy, or laparoscopy.[53] Following 3 to 4 courses of treatment, the feasibility of surgery can be reassessed. In some series, NACT followed by interval debulking has shown comparable survival outcomes with those reported for primary surgery. Fewer radical procedures may be required, the rate of achieving minimal residual disease may be higher, and patients may experience less morbidity.[58,59] However, other reports have suggested that NACT in lieu of primary debulking is associated with an inferior overall survival.[60,61] Direct comparisons have historically been difficult to perform.

In 1986, the GOG and a collaborative group in the Netherlands each opened randomized phase III trials to test the hypothesis that primary debulking was superior to NACT in advanced ovarian cancer. Both studies were closed because of poor accrual. One prevailing opinion at the time was that clinicians did not want to subject their patients to substandard NACT treatment. Until recently, the presumed benefits of primary surgical cytoreduction in advanced ovarian cancer had not been rigorously tested.

The results of a randomized phase III trial conducted in Europe were first presented in October 2008 and subsequently published in September 2010. The data caused a resumption of the debate about how best to initially treat women with advanced ovarian cancer. In the study, 670 patients were randomized to primary debulking surgery versus NACT. After 3 courses of platinum-based treatment, patients receiving NACT who showed a response underwent interval debulking. The investigators reported a median overall survival of 29 to 30 months, regardless of assigned treatment group. In the multivariate analysis, complete resection of all macroscopic disease at debulking surgery was identified as the strongest independent prognostic factor, but the timing of surgery did not seem to matter. Based on the investigators' interpretation of their data, NACT and interval debulking was the preferred treatment.[53]

Despite these findings, most gynecologic oncologists in the United States report that they use NACT for less than 10% of advanced ovarian cancers.[62] Some European gynecologic oncologists have openly questioned what kind of evidence would be needed to convince their US colleagues about the superiority of the NACT approach.[63] At least 2 criticisms of the trial have been suggested as reasons why the results may not be applicable in the United States. First, the duration of patient survival in the study was shorter than expected. The median survival (29–30 months) was less than half that reported for optimally debulked stage III patients receiving postoperative intraperitoneal chemotherapy (66 months).[40] In addition, only 42% of the primary debulking operations resulted in an optimal result with less than or equal to 1 cm of residual disease. Because expert centers in the US often report an optimal result in at least 75% of patients, it is feasible that a more aggressive initial attempt might have led to a better outcome for the group randomized to surgery. A prospective phase III trial conducted within the United States needs to be performed to sway opinion and change the practice of gynecologic oncologists in this country. Meantime, the controversy will persist and individual patterns of care will continue.

Secondary Debulking

Although the rationale for a second debulking operation at the time of relapse is an extrapolation of the rationale for primary surgery, there are several reasons why the certainty of clinical benefit is even more contentious. Recurrent ovarian cancer has a more heterogeneous disease presentation. As a result, treatment is typically more individualized. Secondary debulking is generally considered to be most effective when there is a single isolated relapse, a long disease-free interval after completion of primary therapy (ie, more than 12 months), when the patient is reasonably healthy, and when resection to minimal or no residual disease can be achieved. In contrast, women with symptomatic ascites, carcinomatosis, early relapse (ie, <6 months), and poor conditioning are least likely to benefit.[64–67]

The clinical reality is that most patients are somewhere between these clinical extremes. Chi and colleagues[68] proposed guidelines that are generally accepted (**Table 2**), but, in practice, individual gynecologic oncologists use their own criteria for determining which, if any, patients are good candidates for secondary surgery. The previously reported retrospective series reflect this selection bias. Consequently, the success rates of optimal secondary debulking surgery and the corresponding survival data vary broadly. The potential for significant morbidity, and the notable lack of benefit for patients who are left with residual disease, emphasize the importance of careful counseling and preoperative assessment of patients. Predictably, complete resection seems to be associated with the most prolonged postoperative survival.[69]

Three large, prospective randomized phase III studies are currently underway to evaluate secondary debulking in the treatment of relapsed ovarian cancer. However, it will be years before the results from these trials are finalized. In the meantime, practice patterns will continue to be guided by the results of retrospective studies. Complete resection of disease is most likely to result in prolonged survival. However, because of the wide spectrum of relapsed disease patterns, few women undergo a second debulking operation.

Tertiary Debulking and Beyond

Surgical cytoreduction of a second relapse may offer a survival benefit in a highly select group of patients with recurrent epithelial ovarian, fallopian tube, or peritoneal cancer. Again, the benefits of tertiary debulking seem to be greatest in patients in whom a complete gross resection can be achieved.[70,71] Quaternary, or even

Table 2 Recommendations for secondary cytoreduction			
Disease-Free Interval (mo)	Single Site of Relapse	Multiple Sites but no Carcinomatosis	Carcinomatosis
6–12	Offer SC	Consider SC	No SC
12–30	Offer SC	Offer SC	Consider SC
>30	Offer SC	Offer SC	Offer SC

Abbreviation: SC, secondary cytoreduction.

quinternary, debulking procedures may be reasonable to consider in unique circumstances when there is a single site of recurrent disease.[72]

PALLIATIVE SURGERY

Patients with relapsed ovarian cancer frequently develop bowel obstructions at some point in their treatment course. Bowel obstruction is the most common reason for hospital admission during the last year of life in patients with ovarian carcinoma.[73] Often, patients can initially be managed by nasogastric suction and bowel rest. However, at some point, patients with continued progressive disease will develop worsening symptoms. If not previously addressed, such events should be incorporated into a larger discussion about future goals of care and expectations of continued therapy. Bowel obstruction that does not quickly resolve with nasogastric suction can be managed medically or surgically, but there are limited data to indicate which approach is best. Patients are generally in poor physical condition with a limited life expectancy. Therefore, maintaining their quality of life with effective symptom control is the main purpose of the management of bowel obstruction.[74]

Palliative interventions via endoscopy or surgery have a high likelihood of short-term success in relieving symptoms, although recurrence is common. Gastrostomy tube placement provides the ability to drain accumulated stomach contents intermittently over days or weeks, alleviating nausea or episodes of vomiting. However, plugging or dislodgement is a frequent cause of visits to the emergency room or readmission. Colonic stents may allow patients with large bowel obstruction to avoid major surgery.[75] In some situations, aggressive surgical management is a better option that may provide symptom relief while prolonging survival.[76]

Theoretically, a colostomy, ileostomy, or bowel resection with intestinal bypass should allow return of normal bowel function in a patient with malignant bowel obstruction. However, a satisfactory surgical result is often impossible because of extensive disease, multiple sites of partial or complete obstruction, dense adhesions resulting in visceral injury, or other limiting factors. In addition, successful palliation is rarely achieved when the transit time is prolonged by diffuse peritoneal carcinomatosis or when the anatomy requires a bypass that results in the short bowel syndrome. Furthermore, nearly one-quarter of patients have a grade 3 or 4 complication such as an enterocutaneous fistula, peritonitis, or venous thrombotic events. The perioperative mortality also ranges between 5% and 10%.[77]

Several clinical features have been proposed as contraindications for attempted surgical correction of malignant bowel obstruction (**Box 4**).[78] For many end-stage patients with carcinomatosis refractory to further chemotherapy, the best approach

---

Box 4
Contraindications for attempted surgical correction of malignant bowel obstruction

Ileus secondary to diffuse carcinomatosis

Ascites requiring frequent paracentesis

Diffuse palpable intra-abdominal masses with liver involvement

Recent laparotomy with unsuccessful correction

Previous surgery revealing diffuse metastatic cancer

Involvement of the proximal stomach

may be placement of a palliative gastrostomy tube, pain control, intravenous hydration, and referral to hospice care.

REFERENCES

1. Engelen MJ, Kos HE, Willemse PH, et al. Surgery by consultant gynecologic oncologists improves survival in patients with ovarian carcinoma. Cancer 2006; 106:589–98.
2. Verleye L, Vergote I, van der Zee AG. Patterns of care in surgery for ovarian cancer in Europe. Eur J Surg Oncol 2010;36(Suppl 1):S108–14.
3. Carney ME, Lancaster JM, Ford C, et al. A population-based study of patterns of care for ovarian cancer: who is seen by a gynecologic oncologist and who is not? Gynecol Oncol 2002;84:36–42.
4. Chan JK, Kapp DS, Shin JY, et al. Influence of the gynecologic oncologist on the survival of ovarian cancer patients. Obstet Gynecol 2007;109:1342–50.
5. Moore RG, McMeekin DS, Brown AK, et al. A novel multiple marker bioassay utilizing HE4 and CA125 for the prediction of ovarian cancer in patients with a pelvic mass. Gynecol Oncol 2009;112:40–6.
6. American College of Obstetricians and Gynecologists Committee on Gynecologic Practice. Committee Opinion No. 477: the role of the obstetrician-gynecologist in the early detection of epithelial ovarian cancer. Obstet Gynecol 2011;117:742–6.
7. Schorge JO, Modesitt SC, Coleman RL, et al. SGO White Paper on ovarian cancer: etiology, screening and surveillance. Gynecol Oncol 2010;119:7–17.
8. Buys SS, Partridge E, Black A, et al. Effect of screening on ovarian cancer mortality: the Prostate, Lung, Colorectal and Ovarian (PLCO) cancer screening randomized controlled trial. JAMA 2011;305:2295–303.
9. Fader AN, Rose PG. Role of surgery in ovarian carcinoma. J Clin Oncol 2007;25: 2873–83.
10. Whitney CW, Spirtos N. Gynecologic Oncology Group surgical procedures manual. Philadelphia (PA): Gynecologic Oncology Group; 2009. Available at: www.gog.org. Accessed October 21, 2011.
11. Morice P, Joulie F, Camatte S, et al. Lymph node involvement in epithelial ovarian cancer: analysis of 276 pelvic and paraaortic lymphadenectomies and surgical implications. J Am Coll Surg 2003;197:198–205.
12. Powless CA, Aletti GD, Bakkum-Gamez JN, et al. Risk factors for lymph node metastasis in apparent early-stage epithelial ovarian cancer: implications for surgical staging. Gynecol Oncol 2011;122:536–40.
13. Cass I, Li AJ, Runowicz CD, et al. Pattern of lymph node metastases in clinically unilateral stage I invasive epithelial ovarian carcinomas. Gynecol Oncol 2001;80: 56–61.
14. Chan JK, Munro EG, Cheung MK, et al. Association of lymphadenectomy and survival in stage I ovarian cancer patients. Obstet Gynecol 2007;109:12–9.
15. Young RC, Decker DG, Wharton JT, et al. Staging laparotomy in early ovarian cancer. JAMA 1983;250:3072–6.
16. Trimbos JB, Parmar M, Vergote I, et al. International collaborative ovarian neoplasm trial 1 and adjuvant chemotherapy in ovarian neoplasm trial: two parallel randomized phase III trials of adjuvant chemotherapy in patients with early-stage ovarian carcinoma. J Natl Cancer Inst 2003;95:105–12.
17. Trimbos JB, Vergote I, Bolis G, et al. Impact of adjuvant chemotherapy and surgical staging in early-stage ovarian carcinoma: European Organisation for

Research and Treatment of Cancer-Adjuvant ChemoTherapy in Ovarian Neoplasm trial. J Natl Cancer Inst 2003;95:113–25.

18. Chan JK, Tian C, Fleming GF, et al. The potential benefit of 6 vs. 3 cycles of chemotherapy in subsets of women with early-stage high-risk epithelial ovarian cancer: an exploratory analysis of a Gynecologic Oncology Group study. Gynecol Oncol 2010;116:301–6.

19. Chi DS, Abu-Rustum NR, Sonoda Y, et al. The safety and efficacy of laparoscopic surgical staging of apparent stage I ovarian and fallopian tube cancers. Am J Obstet Gynecol 2005;192:1614–9.

20. Liu CS, Nagarsheth NP, Nezhat FR. Laparoscopy and ovarian cancer: a paradigm change in the management of ovarian cancer? J Minim Invasive Gynecol 2009; 16:250–62.

21. Magrina JF, Zanagnolo V, Noble BN, et al. Robotic approach for ovarian cancer: perioperative and survival results and comparison with laparoscopy and laparotomy. Gynecol Oncol 2011;121:100–5.

22. Zivanovic O, Sonoda Y, Diaz JP, et al. The rate of port-site metastases after 2251 laparoscopic procedures in women with underlying malignant disease. Gynecol Oncol 2008;111:431–7.

23. Rao GG, Skinner E, Gehrig PA, et al. Surgical staging of ovarian low malignant potential tumors. Obstet Gynecol 2004;104:261–6.

24. Wingo SN, Knowles LM, Carrick KS, et al. Retrospective cohort study of surgical staging for ovarian low malignant potential tumors. Am J Obstet Gynecol 2006; 194:e20–2.

25. Houck K, Nikrui N, Duska L, et al. Borderline tumors of the ovary: correlation of frozen and permanent histopathologic diagnosis. Obstet Gynecol 2000;95: 839–43.

26. Brown J, Sood AK, Deavers MT, et al. Patterns of metastasis in sex cord-stromal tumors of the ovary: can routine staging lymphadenectomy be omitted? Gynecol Oncol 2009;113:86–90.

27. Schilder JM, Thompson AM, DePriest PD, et al. Outcome of reproductive age women with stage IA or IC invasive epithelial ovarian cancer treated with fertility-sparing therapy. Gynecol Oncol 2002;87:1–7.

28. Rao GG, Skinner EN, Gehrig PA, et al. Fertility-sparing surgery for ovarian low malignant potential tumors. Gynecol Oncol 2005;98:263–6.

29. Zanagnolo V, Pasinetti B, Sartori E. Clinical review of 63 cases of sex cord stromal tumors. Eur J Gynaecol Oncol 2004;25:431–8.

30. Peccatori F, Bonazzi C, Chiari S, et al. Surgical management of malignant ovarian germ-cell tumors: 10 years' experience of 129 patients. Obstet Gynecol 1995;86: 367–72.

31. Curley MD, Garrett LA, Schorge JO, et al. Evidence for cancer stem cells contributing to the pathogenesis of ovarian cancer. Front Biosci 2011;16: 368–92.

32. Dean M, Fojo T, Bates S. Tumour stem cells and drug resistance. Nat Rev Cancer 2005;5:275–84.

33. Goldie JH, Coldman AJ. A mathematic model for relating the drug sensitivity of tumors to their spontaneous mutation rate. Cancer Treat Rep 1979;63:1727–33.

34. Covens AL. A critique of surgical cytoreduction in advanced ovarian cancer. Gynecol Oncol 2000;78:269–74.

35. Meigs JV. Tumors of the female pelvic organs. New York: Macmillan; 1934.

36. Griffiths CT. Surgical resection of tumor bulk in the primary treatment of ovarian carcinoma. Natl Cancer Inst Monogr 1975;42:101–4.

37. Griffiths CT, Parker LM, Fuller AF Jr. Role of cytoreductive surgical treatment in the management of advanced ovarian cancer. Cancer Treat Rep 1979;63: 235–40.
38. Hacker NF, Berek JS, Lagasse LD, et al. Primary cytoreductive surgery for epithelial ovarian cancer. Obstet Gynecol 1983;61:413–20.
39. Piver MS, Lele SB, Marchetti DL, et al. The impact of aggressive debulking surgery and cisplatin-based chemotherapy on progression-free survival in stage III and IV ovarian carcinoma. J Clin Oncol 1988;6:983–9.
40. Armstrong DK, Bundy B, Wenzel L, et al. Intraperitoneal cisplatin and paclitaxel in ovarian cancer. N Engl J Med 2006;354:34–43.
41. Aletti GD, Dowdy SC, Podratz KC, et al. Surgical treatment of diaphragm disease correlates with improved survival in optimally debulked advanced stage ovarian cancer. Gynecol Oncol 2006;100:283–7.
42. Eisenhauer EL, Abu-Rustum NR, Sonoda Y, et al. The addition of extensive upper abdominal surgery to achieve optimal cytoreduction improves survival in patients with stages IIIC-IV epithelial ovarian cancer. Gynecol Oncol 2006;103: 1083–90.
43. McCann CK, Growdon WB, Munro EG, et al. Prognostic significance of splenectomy as part of initial cytoreductive surgery in ovarian cancer. Ann Surg Oncol 2011;18(10):2912–8.
44. Ang C, Chan KK, Bryant A, et al. Ultra-radical (extensive) surgery versus standard surgery for the primary cytoreduction of advanced epithelial ovarian cancer. Cochrane Database Syst Rev 2011;4:CD007697.
45. Aletti GD, Dowdy SC, Gostout BS, et al. Quality improvement in the surgical approach to advanced ovarian cancer: the Mayo Clinic experience. J Am Coll Surg 2009;208:614–20.
46. Chi DS, Eisenhauer EL, Zivanovic O, et al. Improved progression-free and overall survival in advanced ovarian cancer as a result of a change in surgical paradigm. Gynecol Oncol 2009;114:26–31.
47. Wimberger P, Lehmann N, Kimmig R, et al. Prognostic factors for complete debulking in advanced ovarian cancer and its impact on survival. An exploratory analysis of a prospectively randomized phase III study of the Arbeitsgemeinschaft Gynaekologische Onkologie Ovarian Cancer Study Group (AGO-OVAR). Gynecol Oncol 2007;106:69–74.
48. Chi DS, Ramirez PT, Teitcher JB, et al. Prospective study of the correlation between postoperative computed tomography scan and primary surgeon assessment in patients with advanced ovarian, tubal, and peritoneal carcinoma reported to have undergone primary surgical cytoreduction to residual disease 1 cm or less. J Clin Oncol 2007;25:4946–51.
49. Winter WE III, Maxwell GL, Tian C, et al. Prognostic factors for stage III epithelial ovarian cancer: a Gynecologic Oncology Group Study. J Clin Oncol 2007;25: 3621–7.
50. Winter WE III, Maxwell GL, Tian C, et al. Tumor residual after surgical cytoreduction in prediction of clinical outcome in stage IV epithelial ovarian cancer: a Gynecologic Oncology Group Study. J Clin Oncol 2008;26:83–9.
51. Chi DS, Eisenhauer EL, Lang J, et al. What is the optimal goal of primary cytoreductive surgery for bulky stage IIIC epithelial ovarian carcinoma (EOC)? Gynecol Oncol 2006;103:559–64.
52. Rauh-Hain JA, Growdon WB, Rodriguez N, et al. Primary debulking surgery versus neoadjuvant chemotherapy in stage IV ovarian cancer. Gynecol Oncol 2011;120:S12–3.

53. Vergote I, Trope CG, Amant F, et al. Neoadjuvant chemotherapy or primary surgery in stage IIIC or IV ovarian cancer. N Engl J Med 2010;363:943–53.
54. Thrall MM, Goff BA, Symons RG, et al. Thirty-day mortality after primary cytoreductive surgery for advanced ovarian cancer in the elderly. Obstet Gynecol 2011;118:537–47.
55. Fanning J, Yacoub E, Hojat R. Laparoscopic-assisted cytoreduction for primary advanced ovarian cancer: success, morbidity and survival. Gynecol Oncol 2011;123:47–9.
56. van der Burg ME, van LM, Buyse M, et al. The effect of debulking surgery after induction chemotherapy on the prognosis in advanced epithelial ovarian cancer. Gynecological Cancer Cooperative Group of the European Organization for Research and Treatment of Cancer. N Engl J Med 1995;332:629–34.
57. Rose PG, Nerenstone S, Brady MF, et al. Secondary surgical cytoreduction for advanced ovarian carcinoma. N Engl J Med 2004;351:2489–97.
58. Hou JY, Kelly MG, Yu H, et al. Neoadjuvant chemotherapy lessens surgical morbidity in advanced ovarian cancer and leads to improved survival in stage IV disease. Gynecol Oncol 2007;105:211–7.
59. Kang S, Nam BH. Does neoadjuvant chemotherapy increase optimal cytoreduction rate in advanced ovarian cancer? Meta-analysis of 21 studies. Ann Surg Oncol 2009;16:2315–20.
60. Bristow RE, Chi DS. Platinum-based neoadjuvant chemotherapy and interval surgical cytoreduction for advanced ovarian cancer: a meta-analysis. Gynecol Oncol 2006;103:1070–6.
61. Bristow RE, Eisenhauer EL, Santillan A, et al. Delaying the primary surgical effort for advanced ovarian cancer: a systematic review of neoadjuvant chemotherapy and interval cytoreduction. Gynecol Oncol 2007;104:480–90.
62. Dewdney SB, Rimel BJ, Reinhart AJ, et al. The role of neoadjuvant chemotherapy in the management of patients with advanced stage ovarian cancer: survey results from members of the Society of Gynecologic Oncologists. Gynecol Oncol 2010;119:18–21.
63. Vergote I, Amant F, Leunen K. Neoadjuvant chemotherapy in advanced ovarian cancer: what kind of evidence is needed to convince US gynaecological oncologists? Gynecol Oncol 2010;119:1–2.
64. Bristow RE, Puri I, Chi DS. Cytoreductive surgery for recurrent ovarian cancer: a meta-analysis. Gynecol Oncol 2009;112:265–74.
65. Bristow RE, Peiretti M, Gerardi M, et al. Secondary cytoreductive surgery including rectosigmoid colectomy for recurrent ovarian cancer: operative technique and clinical outcome. Gynecol Oncol 2009;114:173–7.
66. Fotiou S, Aliki T, Petros Z, et al. Secondary cytoreductive surgery in patients presenting with isolated nodal recurrence of epithelial ovarian cancer. Gynecol Oncol 2009;114:178–82.
67. Schorge JO, Wingo SN, Bhore R, et al. Secondary cytoreductive surgery for recurrent platinum-sensitive ovarian cancer. Int J Gynaecol Obstet 2010;108:123–7.
68. Chi DS, McCaughty K, Diaz JP, et al. Guidelines and selection criteria for secondary cytoreductive surgery in patients with recurrent, platinum-sensitive epithelial ovarian carcinoma. Cancer 2006;106:1933–9.
69. Harter P, Du BA, Hahmann M, et al. Surgery in recurrent ovarian cancer: the Arbeitsgemeinschaft Gynaekologische Onkologie (AGO) DESKTOP OVAR trial. Ann Surg Oncol 2006;13:1702–10.

70. Fotopoulou C, Richter R, Braicu IE, et al. Clinical outcome of tertiary surgical cytoreduction in patients with recurrent epithelial ovarian cancer. Ann Surg Oncol 2011;18:49–57.

71. Shih KK, Chi DS, Barakat RR, et al. Tertiary cytoreduction in patients with recurrent epithelial ovarian, fallopian tube, or primary peritoneal cancer: an updated series. Gynecol Oncol 2010;117(2):330–5.

72. Shih KK, Chi DS, Barakat RR, et al. Beyond tertiary cytoreduction in patients with recurrent epithelial ovarian, fallopian tube, or primary peritoneal cancer. Gynecol Oncol 2010;116:364–9.

73. von Gruenigen VE, Frasure HE, Reidy AM, et al. Clinical disease course during the last year in ovarian cancer. Gynecol Oncol 2003;90:619–24.

74. Kucukmetin A, Naik R, Galaal K, et al. Palliative surgery versus medical management for bowel obstruction in ovarian cancer. Cochrane Database Syst Rev 2010;7:CD007792.

75. Caceres A, Zhou Q, Iasonos A, et al. Colorectal stents for palliation of large-bowel obstructions in recurrent gynecologic cancer: an updated series. Gynecol Oncol 2008;108:482–5.

76. Chi DS, Phaeton R, Miner TJ, et al. A prospective outcomes analysis of palliative procedures performed for malignant intestinal obstruction due to recurrent ovarian cancer. Oncologist 2009;14:835–9.

77. Pothuri B, Vaidya A, Aghajanian C, et al. Palliative surgery for bowel obstruction in recurrent ovarian cancer: an updated series. Gynecol Oncol 2003;89:306–13.

78. Ripamonti C, Bruera E. Palliative management of malignant bowel obstruction. Int J Gynecol Cancer 2002;12:135–43.

Current Management of Gestational Trophoblastic Neoplasia

Donald Peter Goldstein, MD[a],*, Ross S. Berkowitz, MD[b]

KEYWORDS

- Gestational trophoblastic neoplasia • Invasive mole
- Choriocarcinoma • Human chorionic gonadotropin

Gestational trophoblastic neoplasms (GTN) are malignant lesions that arise from placental villous and extravillous trophoblast. Four clinicopathologic conditions make up this entity: (1) invasive mole, which follows either complete hydatidiform mole (CHM) or partial hydatidiform mole (PHM), (2) choriocarcinoma (CCA), (3) placental-site trophoblastic tumor (PSTT), and (4) epithelioid trophoblastic tumor (ETT). Each of these conditions can perforate the uterine wall, metastasize, and lead to death if left untreated. Approximately 50% of cases of GTN arise from molar pregnancy, 25% from miscarriage or tubal pregnancy, and 25% from term or preterm pregnancy.[1] Invasive mole and CCA, which make up the majority of these tumors, always produce easily detectable amounts of human chorionic gonadotropin (hCG) and are highly responsive to chemotherapy with an overall cure rate exceeding 90%, making it usually possible to achieve cure while preserving reproductive function. This success is attributable to several factors, the most important of which are the unique sensitivity of these two trophoblastic neoplasms to chemotherapeutic agents and the use of hCG as a tumor marker for diagnosis, monitoring treatment, and follow-up. By contrast, PSTT and ETT, which rarely occur, produce scant amounts of hCG and are relatively resistant to chemotherapy, making surgery the primary treatment modality. Chemotherapy is used for PSTT and ETT only when the disease has metastasized.

[a] Division of Gynecologic Oncology, New England Trophoblastic Disease Center, Dana Farber/Brigham and Women's Cancer Center, Harvard Medical School, 75 Francis Street, Boston, MA 02115, USA
[b] Harvard Medical School, Brigham and Women's Hospital and Dana Farber Cancer Institute, 75 Francis Street, Boston, MA 02115, USA
* Corresponding author.
E-mail address: dgoldstein@partners.org

Hematol Oncol Clin N Am 26 (2012) 111–131
doi:10.1016/j.hoc.2011.10.007   hemonc.theclinics.com
0889-8588/12/$ – see front matter © 2012 Elsevier Inc. All rights reserved.

EPIDEMIOLOGY

The incidence and etiologic risk factors that contribute to the development of GTN have been difficult to characterize because of problems in accumulating reliable epidemiologic data, bias, and interpretation and differing methods of expressing incidences in terms of hospital-based versus population-based data. Despite these problems, there are sufficient data to indicate that there are wide regional variations in the incidence of CHM.[2,3] Estimates from North America, Australia, New Zealand, and Europe have shown the incidence of CHM to range from 0.57 to 1.1 per 1000 pregnancies, whereas studies from Southeast Asia and Japan report an incidence approaching 2.0 per 1000 pregnancies.[2–6] Similarly there are data that show an increased incidence of CHM among American Indians, Eskimos, Hispanics, and African Americans as well as various Asian populations.[7] There is no conclusive evidence that genetic traits, cultural factors, or differences in reporting account for this increase. The etiologic risk factors that have been linked to the development of CHM are advanced maternal age (>40 years) and prior molar pregnancy.[8,9] Familial clusters of biparental CHM have been associated with NLRP7 gene mutations on chromosome 19q.[10] In addition, well-documented nutritional studies have shown an inverse relationship between β-carotene and animal dietary fat intake and the incidence of CHM.[11,12] In this regard, it is of interest that the documented decrease in the incidence of CHM in South Korea has been associated with a gradual Westernization of the Korean diet.[13]

Determining the incidence rate of CCA is even more problematic because of the rarity of this condition and the difficulty in clinically distinguishing postmolar CCA from metastatic mole. In Europe and North America CCA affects approximately 1 in 40,000 pregnancies, whereas in Southeast Asia and Japan CCA rates are higher at 9.2 and 3.3 per 40,000 pregnancies, respectively. The incidence of both CHM and CCA has gradually declined over the past 30 years.[14,15]

Risk factors for CCA include prior CHM, ethnicity, and advanced maternal age. CCA is 1000 times more likely to occur after CHM than after another type of pregnancy. The risk is also increased in women of Asian, American Indian, and African descent.[15]

PATHOLOGY

Invasive mole develops when molar villi invade the myometrium. Metastases of invading molar villi occur via direct extension through venous channels. Approximately 15% of CHM will result in local invasion, and 5% will develop metastases usually to the lungs or vagina.[16] The development of local invasion after PHM occurs in only 3% to 5% of patients, and metastatic disease is rare.[16] The diagnosis of postmolar GTN is based on a plateau or elevation of hCG levels after molar evacuation rather than on pathology. Therefore, treatment with chemotherapy is frequently initiated without a histopathologic diagnosis other than the antecedent pregnancy.[17]

CCA is a highly malignant disease characterized by hyperplastic and anaplastic syncytioblasts and cytotrophoblasts, absence of chorionic villi, hemorrhage, and tissue necrosis. CCA spreads by directly invading the myometrium and vascular channels, resulting in involvement at distant sites, most commonly the lungs, adnexa, vagina, brain, liver, kidney, intestines, and spleen. In contrast to invasive mole, the vast majority of cases of CCA arise following a nonmolar pregnancy.

PSTT is an extremely rare tumor that arises from the placental implantation site and consists of mononuclear intermediate trophoblasts without chorionic villi that infiltrates between myometrial fibers in sheets or chords. PSTT is associated with less vascular invasion, necrosis, and hemorrhage than CCA. Unlike CCA, PSTT has a propensity for lymphatic metastases. Immunohistochemical staining reveals the diffuse presence of cytokeratin and human placental lactogen (hPL), whereas hCG is only present focally. Because of its slow growth, paucity of symptoms, and low hCG production, early detection is the exception rather than the rule. Most PSTTs follow nonmolar gestations.[18] Because of their relative insensitivity to chemotherapy, the mortality rate of PSTT exceeds that of CCA.

ETT is a rare variant of PSTT that develops from neoplastic transformation of chorionic-type extravillous trophoblast. Like PSTTs, ETTs can present many years after a term delivery. When diagnosed these tumors appear grossly as nodular infiltrates in the myometrium.[19,20]

CLINICAL PRESENTATION

GTN has a varied presentation depending on the antecedent pregnancy, extent of disease, and histopathology. Postmolar GTN (usually invasive mole, occasionally CCA) most commonly presents following evacuation of CHM whose preevacuation uterine size is larger than dates and/or whose hCG level is greater than 100,000 mIU/mL.[21] Bilateral ovarian enlargement is frequently present when the hCG level is markedly elevated. Signs suggestive of persistent disease are an enlarged uterus, irregular bleeding, and persistent bilateral enlarged ovaries. Rarely a metastatic nodule will be present in the vagina, which can bleed vigorously, particularly if biopsied. The Cancer Committee of the International Federation of Gynecologists and Obstetricians (FIGO) has established the following guidelines for the diagnosis of postmolar GTN[22]:

1. Four values or more of hCG plateaued over at least 3 weeks
2. An increase in hCG of 10% or greater for 3 or more values over at least 2 weeks
3. The histologic diagnosis of CCA
4. Persistence of hCG 6 months after molar evacuation.

CCA, the most common histopathologic type of GTN that develops following term pregnancies or miscarriages, may present with nonspecific signs and symptoms, making the diagnosis difficult; this frequently accounts for a delay in diagnosis that often adversely affects prognosis. Therefore, GTN should be considered and an hCG test performed in any woman in the reproductive age group who presents with abnormal uterine bleeding or unexplained metastatic disease. GTN following a term or preterm gestation usually presents with uterine bleeding due to invasion of tumor, or bleeding from a metastatic site. Bleeding from uterine perforation or metastatic lesions may result in abdominal pain, hemoptysis, or melena. Patients with central nervous system metastases often exhibit evidence of increased intracranial pressure from intracerebral hemorrhage, leading to headaches, dizziness, seizures, or hemiplegia. Patients who develop extensive pulmonary metastases may present with dyspnea, cough, or chest pain. PSTTs and ETTs almost always cause irregular bleeding or amenorrhea, frequently long after the antecedent pregnancy. There are rare reported cases of nephrotic syndrome and virilizing syndrome associated with these conditions.[18–20]

WORKUP

Once the diagnosis of GTN is suspected or established, a metastatic workup should be undertaken to determine the extent of disease. Selection of appropriate therapy for patients with GTN is based on both the anatomic staging system adopted by FIGO and the Prognostic Scoring System adopted by the World Health Organization (WHO).[23]

The workup needed to adequately stage and score GTN should include:

1. History and physical examination, baseline (pretreatment) serum quantitative hCG level, complete blood and platelet count, and tests of hepatic and renal function
2. Review of all available pathologic specimens.
3. Pelvic ultrasonography to detect the extent and nature of uterine involvement to help identify patients with deep uterine wall involvement who are at risk of uterine perforation, or who would benefit from a tumor-debulking hysterectomy.
4. Chest radiograph to determine the presence of lung metastases. If the chest radiograph is negative a computed tomography (CT) scan of the chest may be obtained because approximately 40% of patients with negative chest radiographs have metastatic lesions on CT scan. Controversy exists as to the significance of these micrometastases with regard to the patient's response to chemotherapy.[24] In the absence of chest metastases, imaging of other organs may not be necessary because distant metastases are then rarely encountered.
5. Magnetic resonance imaging (MRI) of the brain and abdominopelvic CT scan or MRI are indicated to identify lesions in the brain, liver, and other abdominal organs if the chest radiograph or chest CT indicates the presence of lung metastases.
6. Repeat curettage after molar evacuation is not indicated unless there is excessive uterine bleeding associated with retained molar tissue. Controversy exists as to whether repeat dilation and curettage reduces the incidence of persistent postmolar GTN.[25,26]
7. Cerebrospinal fluid/plasma hCG ratio is sometimes used to confirm cerebral involvement.[27,28]
8. Additional imaging such as ^{18}F-fluorodeoxyglucose positron emission tomography (FDG-PET) may be useful to accurately identify sites of metabolically active disease or viable metastases and to help determine the potential for tumor resectability.[29]

STAGING AND RISK ASSESSMENT

In 2002, the FIGO adopted a combined anatomic staging (**Box 1**) and modified WHO risk-factor scoring system (**Table 1**) for GTN. The FIGO stage is designated by a Roman numeral followed by the modified WHO score designated by the Arabic number separated by a colon.[22] PSTTs and ETTs are classified separately. Treatment is based on the total score, which signifies the risk of the patient developing drug resistance. Patients whose WHO scores are less than 7 are considered to be at low risk,

---

Box 1
FIGO staging of gestational trophoblastic neoplasia

Stage I

   Disease confined to the uterus

Stage II

   Disease extends to the outside of the uterus, but is limited to the genital structures

Stage III

   Disease extends to the lungs, with or without genital tract involvement

Stage IV

   All other metastatic sites

Table 1
World Health Organization risk scoring system based on prognostic factors

Prognostic Factors	Score			
	0	1	2	4
Age (y)	<40	>39	—	—
Antecedent pregnancy	Mole	Abortion	Term	—
Interval (mo)[a]	<4	>3, <7	>6, <13	>12
Pretreatment serum hCG (mIU/mL)	<10^3	10^3 to <10^4	10^4 to <10^5	>10^5
Largest tumor, including uterine (cm)	—	3 to <5	>4	—
Site of metastases	Lung	Spleen, kidney	Gastrointestinal tract	Brain, liver
Number of metastases	—	1–4	5–8	>8
Prior failed chemotherapy	—	—	Single drug	Two drugs

[a] Interval (in months) between end of antecedent pregnancy (where known) or onset of symptoms.

and patients with scores greater than 6 are considered to be at high risk of developing drug resistance. Patients with nonmetastatic disease (Stage I) and low-risk metastatic GTN (Stages II and III, score <7) can be treated initially with single-agent chemotherapy with cure rates approaching 80% to 90%. On the other hand, patients classified as having high-risk metastatic disease (Stage IV and Stages II–III with scores >6) require multiagent chemotherapy, possibly with adjuvant radiation and/or surgery, as indicated, to achieve similar cure rates.[1] There is growing evidence that patients with low-risk GTN who have a large tumor burden reflected in hCG levels of greater than 100,000 mIU/mL and/or prognostic scores of 5 to 6 are associated with an increased risk of initial drug resistance and, therefore, should be treated initially with multiagent chemotherapy.[30] The use of the FIGO staging/scoring system has become the accepted basis for determining the optimal initial therapy that affords the patient the best outcome with the least morbidity.

TREATMENT OF LOW-RISK GTN

Patients with nonmetastatic (Stage 1) and low-risk metastatic GTN (Stages II–III, score <7) should be treated initially with single-agent methotrexate (Mtx) or actinomycin D (actD).[31] Several different outpatient protocols have been used and have yielded fairly comparable results (**Box 2**). The variability in primary remission rates reflect differences in drug dosages, schedules, and routes of administration, as well as patient selection criteria. In general, the weekly intramuscular (IM)[32–34] and intermittent intravenous (IV) infusion of Mtx[35–37] and the biweekly single-dose actD[38–42] protocols are less effective than the 5-day Mtx or actD protocols and the 8-day Mtx/folinic acid (FA) regimen.[43–47] Despite these differences in primary remission rates, all patients with low-risk GTN are eventually cured, with preservation of fertility when desired.

At the New England Trophoblastic Disease Center (NETDC), the initial regimen consists of the sequential use of 8-day Mtx/FA and 5-day actD regimens. A recent study from NETDC found the 8-day Mtx/FA protocol to be not only a highly effective regimen but the most cost-effective as well. Most patients are treated initially with Mtx because it has fewer side effects than actD.[47–49] actD should be used as first-line therapy in patients with evidence of preexisting or chemotherapy-related hepatic

---

Box 2
Single-agent regimens for low-risk gestational trophoblastic neoplasms

Mtx Regimens

1. Mtx: 0.4–0.5 mg/kg IV or IM daily for 5 days

2. Mtx: 30–50 mg/m² IM weekly

3. Mtx/FA:

    a. Mtx 1 mg/kg IM or IV on days 1, 3, 5, 7

    b. FA 10 mg PO days 2, 4, 6, 8

4. High-dose Mtx/FA

    a. Mtx 100 mg/m² IV bolus

    b. Mtx 200 mg/m² 12 h infusion

    c. FA 15 mg every 12 h in 4 doses IM or PO beginning 24 h after starting Mtx

Actinomycin D Regimens

1. actD 10–12 µg/kg IV push daily for 5 days

2. actD 1.25 mg/m² IV push every 2 weeks

Abbreviations: actD, actinomycin D (Cosmegan); FA, folinic acid (calcium leucovorin); IM, intramuscular; IV, intravenous; Mtx, methotrexate; PO, by mouth.

---

dysfunction, or who have had a known adverse reaction to Mtx, and as sequential therapy if the patient exhibits Mtx resistance. Unlike Mtx, which can be given IM or IV, actD must be administered through an adequate vein to reduce the risk of local tissue injury due to extravasation. The most bothersome side effects of actD are severe nausea and vomiting (which is rarely encountered with Mtx), hair loss, and a pruritic acneiform rash. Treatment is usually continued at 2- to 3-week intervals until the hCG level becomes undetectable. One or two courses of consolidation therapy are administered after gonadotropin remission (3 consecutive weekly undetectable hCG titers) is achieved in patients with Stage I GTN who require sequential or multiagent therapy, and in all patients with low-risk Stage II and III metastatic GTN. The authors usually do not administer consolidation therapy to patients with FIGO Stage I GTN (nonmetastatic disease) who respond completely to the initial single-agent regimen. In select patients with Stage I GTN and low FIGO scores (<3), it is their practice to closely monitor the hCG level after the first course of therapy and administer additional courses only if the hCG level fails to decline by 1 log within 18 days, if the hCG level plateaus or rises.

If the hCG level declines by less than 1 log, the patient is considered to be relatively resistant to that drug, and either an alternative agent is considered or the dose of the original drug is escalated, toxicity permitting. In general, patients with low-risk GTN should be treated with the least toxic effective therapy. When resistance to single-agent therapy is encountered for both Mtx and actD, combination chemotherapy with either MAC (Mtx, actD, and cyclophosphamide) or EMA/CO (etoposide, Mtx, actD, cyclophosphamide, and vincristine) is initiated. Factors found to be associated with resistance to initial Mtx chemotherapy were high pretreatment hCG levels, nonmolar antecedent pregnancy, and clinicopathologic diagnosis of CCA.[50] The use of etoposide as in EMA/CO in GTN patients has been associated with an increased risk of secondary tumors including leukemia, breast and colon carcinoma, and melanoma.[51] For that reason it is the authors' policy to use MAC as the combination chemotherapy in patients with low-risk GTN who become resistant to single-agent therapy.

Regardless of the treatment protocol used, chemotherapy should be continued until the hCG level becomes undetectable. At that point consolidation therapy may be indicated, as discussed earlier. Chemotherapy is changed to an alternative singe-agent regimen if the hCG level plateaus above normal during treatment, or if toxicity precludes adequate dose or frequency of treatment. Multiagent therapy should be initiated promptly if resistance to sequential single-agent chemotherapy develops as reflected by inadequate hCG response or disease progression.

Table 2 summarizes the authors' experience with the treatment of low-risk GTN patients at the NETDC. A total of 745 women with low-risk GTN were treated between 1965 and 2010. Complete remission was achieved with single-agent chemotherapy in 501 of 588 patients (85.2%) with Stage I GTN, 17 of 21 patients (81%) with low-risk Stage II disease, and 108 of 136 patients (79.4%) with low-risk Stage III GTN. All 118 patients (15.8%) with low-risk GTN who developed resistance to initial single-agent therapy achieved remission with combination chemotherapy with or without surgery.

Hysterectomy was used as initial therapy in 33 patients with Stage I GTN who no longer wished to preserve fertility. Because of the risk of occult metastatic disease, it is the authors' practice to administer adjunctive chemotherapy with either high-dose

Table 2
Results for patients with low-risk gestational trophoblastic neoplasia treated at the NETDC, 1995–2010

Stage	No. of Patients	No. of Remissions
I	588	588 (100%)
Initial Therapy		502 (85.4%)
Sequential Mtx/actD		459
Combination chemotherapy[a]		1
Hysterectomy[b] (with adjunctive chemotherapy)		33
Local resection[b] (with adjunctive chemotherapy)		9
Resistant Therapy		86 (14.6%)
Combination chemotherapy[a]		71
Hysterectomy/local resection[b]		14
Pelvic infusion		1
II	21	21 (100%)
Initial Therapy		17 (81%)
Sequential Mtx/actD		17
Resistant Therapy		4 (19%)
Combination chemotherapy[a]		4
III	136	136 (100%)
Initial Therapy		108 (79.4%)
Sequential Mtx/actD		108
Resistant Therapy		28 (20.6%)
Combination chemotherapy[a]		28

[a] Includes MAC (methotrexate, actinomycin D, cyclophosphamide), EMA (etoposide, methotrexate, actinomycin D), EMA/CO (EMA, cyclophosphamide, vincristine), EMA/EP (EMA, cisplatin).
[b] With adjunctive chemotherapy.

IV Mtx/FA or bolus actD at the time of surgery. Hysterectomy should also be considered when the uterus is extensively involved with tumor to prevent or treat hemorrhage, perforation, and/or infection. Under these circumstances, hysterectomy may shorten the duration of treatment with multiagent chemotherapy in patients with resistance to single-agent therapy.

In summary, cure rates for both nonmetastatic and low-risk metastatic GTN should approach 100% with the use of single-agent Mtx and actD administered sequentially and the use of multiagent protocols when resistance to single agents develops. Approximately 10% to 30% of low-risk patients will develop resistance to the initial agent used and thus require a second drug, and 15% to 20% will require multiagent chemotherapy with or without hysterectomy to achieve remission. The patients most likely to prove resistant to single-agent therapy are those with higher risk scores.

TREATMENT OF HIGH-RISK GTN

Patients with high-risk metastatic GTN (FIGO Stage IV and Stages II–III, score >6) should be treated initially with multiagent chemotherapy with or without adjuvant radiation therapy and/or surgery. During the 1970s and 1980s the preferred first-line multiagent regimen consisted of Mtx, actD, and cyclophosphamide or chlorambucil (MAC), which achieved cure rates in this group of patients of 50% to 71%.[52–54] In the 1980s etoposide was found to be a highly effective agent for GTN when used as a single agent in patients with low-risk disease[55] and in combination with Mtx, actD, cyclophosphamide, and vincristine (EMA/CO). EMA/CO is now the preferred primary combination chemotherapy regimen in high-risk metastatic GTN with an 80% to 90% remission rate.[56–58] **Tables 3** and **4** summarize the most commonly used multiagent protocols for patients with high-risk GTN and low-risk GTN who are resistant to single agents.

Table 5 summarizes the experience at the NETDC of 115 patients with high-risk GTN. Six of 8 patients (75%) with high-risk Stage II disease, and 55 of 64 patients (85.9%) with high-risk Stage III GTN achieved remission with their initial therapy. All but one of the 11 remaining patients with high-risk Stage II and III GTN who were resistant to their initial regimen ultimately achieved remission. Of the 23 patients with Stage IV disease treated after 1975 when initial multiagent chemotherapy became standard procedure, 18 (78.3%) were cured. The only patients who died in this series were 14 Stage IV patients treated before 1975 initially with single-agent regimens, and 5 Stage IV patients treated after 1975 with initial multiagent regimens. Most reports concur that mortality occurs almost exclusively in those patients with high-risk scores characterized by a histopathologic diagnosis of CCA who present with brain and/or liver metastases.[59]

In patients with high-risk GTN, optimal cure rates are achieved by the intermittent intensive administration of chemotherapy at 2- to 3-week intervals, toxicity permitting. Medications to support blood cell production should be used as necessary. However, the regimens are generally well tolerated. No treatment-related deaths or life-threatening toxicity should occur if marrow, renal, and hepatic function are monitored carefully. Neutropenia necessitating a 1-week delay of treatment, anemia requiring blood transfusions, and grades 3 to 4 neutropenia without thrombocytopenia are reported to occur in only 14%, 5.8%, and 1.9% of treatment cycles, respectively.[60–64] Patients who develop resistance to EMA/CO can be treated with EMA/EP, a regimen that substitutes cyclophosphamide and vincristine on day 8 with cisplatin or carboplatin and etoposide.[65–67] In patients with EMA/CO resistance, EMA/EP induced

Table 3
Protocols for EMA/CO and EMA/EP regimens

Day	Drug	Dose
Protocol for EMA/CO		
1	Etoposide	100 mg/m^2 by infusion in 200 mL saline over 30 min
	actD	0.5 mg IVP
	Mtx	100 mg/m^2 IVP
		200 mg/m^2 by infusion over 12 h
2	Etoposide	100 mg/m^2 by infusion in 200 mL saline over 30 min
	actD	0.5 mg IVP
	Folinic acid	15 mg every 12 h × 4 doses IM or
		PO beginning 24 h after starting Mtx
8	Cyclophosphamide	600 mg/m^2 by infusion in saline over 30 min
	Vincristine	1 mg/m^2 IVP
Protocol of EMA/EP		
1	Etoposide	100 mg/m^2 by infusion in 200 mL saline over 30 min
	actD	0.5 mg IVP
	Mtx	100 mg/m^2 IVP
		200 mg/m^2 by infusion over 12 h
2	Etoposide	100 mg/m^2 by infusion in 200 mL saline over 30 min
	actD	0.5 mg IVP
	Folinic acid	15 mg every 12 h × 4 doses IM or PO
8	Cisplatin	60 mg/m^2 IV with prehydration
	Etoposide	100 mg/m^2 by infusion in 200 mL saline over 30 min

Abbreviations: actD, actinomycin (Cosmegan); EMA/CO, etoposide, actinomycin D, methotrexate, cyclophosphamide, vincristine; EMA/EP, etoposide, methotrexate, actinomycin D, cisplatin; FA, folinic acid; IM, intramuscular; IVP, intravenous push; Mtx, methotrexate; PO, by mouth.

remission, sometimes with surgical intervention, in 9 of 12 (75%) patients.[67] In contrast to the management of patients with low-risk GTN, it is mandatory to continue chemotherapy for high-risk disease for at least 2 to 3 courses after the first normal hCG in order to reduce the likelihood of relapse.

MANAGEMENT OF CENTRAL NERVOUS SYSTEM METASTASES

When central nervous system metastases are present, either whole brain irradiation (3000 cGy in 200 cGy fractions) or surgical excision with stereotactic irradiation in selected patients is usually given simultaneously with the initiation of systemic chemotherapy.[68–71] During radiotherapy, it is advisable to increase the Mtx infusion dose to 1 g/m^2 with 30 mg of FA every 12 hours for 3 days starting 32 hours after the start of the infusion, to facilitate passage of the drug through the blood-brain barrier.[72] An alternative to brain irradiation is surgical excision, particularly in those patients whose lesion is solitary and located peripherally.[72]

MANAGEMENT OF PULMONARY METASTASES

Surgery is also an important adjunct to chemotherapy in the management of solitary pulmonary nodules, particularly if they prove resistant to chemotherapy.[73–78] Tomoda and colleagues[73] reported on 19 patients with chemoresistant GTN who were treated with adjuvant thoracotomy. Based on their experience they proposed the following criteria to predict successful outcome: (1) patient is a good surgical candidate; (2)

Table 4
Protocol for MAC regimen

Day	Drug	Dose
1	Mtx	1 mg/kg IM
	actD	0.5 mg IVP
	Cyclophosphamide	3 mg/kg IVB over 45–60 min
2	FA	0.1 mg/kg PO[a]
	actD	0.5 mg IVP
	Cyclophosphamide	3 mg/kg IVB over 45–60 min
3	Mtx	1 mg/kg IM
	actD	0.5 mg IVP
	Cyclophosphamide	3 mg/kg IVB over 45–60 min
4	FA	0.1 mg/kg PO[a]
	actD	0.5 mg IVP
	Cyclophosphamide	3 mg/kg IVB over 45–60 min
5	Mtx	1 mg/kg IM
	actD	0.5 mg IVP
	Cyclophosphamide	3 mg/kg IVB over 45–60 min
6	FA	0.1 mg/kg PO[a]
7	Mtx	1 mg/kg IM
8	FA	0.1 mg/kg PO[a]

Abbreviations: actD, actinomycin D; FA, folinic acid (calcium leucovorin); IM, intramuscular; IVB, intravenous bolus; IVP, intravenous push; Mtx, methotrexate; PO, by mouth.
[a] Administer as either 5-mg or 10-mg tablets.

primary malignancy is controlled; (3) no evidence of other metastatic sites; (4) pulmonary metastasis is limited to one lung; (5) hCG level is less than 1000 mIU/mL. Complete remission was achieved in 14 of 15 (93%) patients who met all 5 criteria, but in none of 4 patients who met only 4 or fewer. Similar findings were reported from the NETDC by Fleming and colleagues,[74] who noted that 10 of 11 (90.9%) carefully selected patients with drug- resistant pulmonary metastases achieved remission following resection of the solitary pulmonary tumor. An undetectable hCG level within 2 weeks of resection of a solitary nodule is highly predictive of a favorable outcome. Pulmonary resection can also establish the diagnosis of GTN in cases where a histopathologic diagnosis is desired. An example of this would be a patient with an elevated hCG level and no history of a recent antecedent pregnancy. Although pulmonary resection can be useful, it must be noted that thoracotomy is seldom necessary and should be undertaken in carefully selected cases, because most lung lesions are successfully treated with chemotherapy.

MANAGEMENT OF HEPATIC METASTASES

Although hepatic involvement poses perhaps the most serious problem, successful treatment with chemotherapy alone has been reported by both Wong and colleagues[79] and Bakri and colleagues,[80] who reported 90% and 62.4% complete remission, respectively, with primary intensive chemotherapy. Surgical intervention is limited to patients with acute bleeding, or for peripheral lesions that are drug resistant. Embolization has also been reported to be effective in controlling hemorrhage, although its use in the management of resistant disease has not been reported.[81,82]

Table 5
Results for patients with high-risk gestational trophoblastic neoplasia treated at the NETDC, 1995–2010

Stage	No. of Patients	No. of Remissions
II	8	8 (100%)
Initial Therapy		6 (75%)
Sequential Mtx/actD		2
Combination chemotherapy[a]		4
Resistant Therapy		2 (25%)
Combination chemotherapy[a]		2
III	64	63 (98.4%)
Initial Therapy		55 (85.9%)
Sequential Mtx/actD		14
Combination chemotherapy[a]		41
Resistant Therapy		8 (12.5%)
Combination chemotherapy[a]		8
IV		
Before 1975	20	6 (30%)
Initial Therapy		5 (25%)
Sequential Mtx/actD		5
Resistant Therapy		1 (5%)
Combination chemotherapy[a]		1
After 1975	23	18 (78.3%)
Initial Therapy		4 (17.4%)
Sequential Mtx/actD		2
Combination chemotherapy[a]		2
Resistant Therapy		14 (60.9%)
High-dose Mtx/actD		4
Combination chemotherapy[a]		10

[a] Includes MAC, EMA, EMA/CO, EMA/EP.

MANAGEMENT OF RECURRENT AND CHEMORESISTANT GTN

Chemoresistant disease poses a significant treatment challenge, which is most likely to occur in patients with Stage IV or high-risk Stage III GTN. Despite the use of multimodal primary therapy, up to 40% of patients will have an incomplete response to first-line chemotherapy or relapse after remission.[83–85] Most of these patients will have multiple metastatic sites to organs other than the lungs, pelvis, and vagina, and many will have had inadequate prior chemotherapy. Patients who relapse or develop resistance to multiagent chemotherapy should be restaged to determine the site of metastases and the feasibility of surgical resection or radiation. The use of FDG-PET imaging may be useful in detecting otherwise occult metastases. Mutch and colleagues[86] reported recurrence rates of 13% in patients with high-risk disease. At the NETDC recurrence rates range from 2.9% in Stage I, 8.3% in Stage II, 4.2% in Stage III, to 9.1% in Stage IV.[23] Several salvage regimens in addition to EMA/EP have been shown to be capable of inducing remission in selected patients. Osborne and colleagues[87] described a novel, 3-drug doublet regimen consisting of paclitaxel, etoposide, and cisplatin (TP/TE) that induced complete remission in 2 patients. Wang and colleagues[88] further studied this regimen in 16 patients with chemoresistant disease, including 6 patients previously treated with a platinum-based regimen. Of the 16 patients, 3 (19%) achieved a complete and 5 (31%) a partial response. Wan and colleagues[89] reported 100% efficacy of a floxuridine-containing regimen when given to 21 patients with drug resistance. Matsui and colleagues[90] found that 5-fluorouracil in combination with actD induced complete remission in 9 of 11 cases (82%). Gordon and colleagues,[91] DuBeshter and colleagues,[92] and Azab and colleagues[93] reported on the efficacy of cisplatin, vinblastine, and bleomycin (PVB), which achieved remission in 2 of 11 patients (18%), 4 of 7 patients (57%) and 5 of 8 patients (62%), respectively. Regimens containing ifosfamide and paclitaxel have also been shown to have some success anecdotally in patient reports.[94,95] Autologous bone marrow transplantation or stem cell support concurrent with high-dose chemotherapy have also been used, with mixed success.[96,97] Because the number of truly resistant patients is small, it is difficult to study any of these regimens with any degree of statistical accuracy.

In summary, cure rates for high-risk GTN of 80% to 90% are now achievable with intensive multimodal therapy, with EMA/CO in conjunction with adjuvant radiotherapy and/or surgery when indicated. Recently, Alifrangis and colleagues from Charing Cross noted that survival for GTN patients who relapsed following EMA/CO improved significantly from 87% to 98%, when they were treated with 2 cycles of low-dose EP-induction chemotherapy (etoposide 100 mg/m^2 and cisplatin 20 mg/m^2) on days 1 and 2, repeated weekly × 2 before commencing EMA/CO.[98] This regimen is highly successful because its relatively low toxicity allows for adherence to the treatment schedule, high complete response rates, and overall high survival. Approximately 20% of high-risk patients will fail therapy or relapse from remission. Salvage therapy with platinum-containing drug combinations such as EMA/EP, often in conjunction with surgical resection of resistant sites, will result in cure of most high-risk patients with resistant disease. Even those patients with brain, liver, and gastrointestinal involvement now have a 75%, 73%, and 50% survival rate, respectively.[99]

MANAGEMENT OF COMPLICATIONS

Women with GTN may present with complications related to their disease, which may necessitate urgent management, including surgical or radiologic intervention. Bleeding from the uterus or metastatic sites is by far the most common complication. Hysterectomy may be necessary to control profuse bleeding or, occasionally, sepsis.[100–102] Cagayan and Suyen Magallanes[100] reported that of 134 women with GTN, 13 (9%) underwent hysterectomy for profuse bleeding, whereas 31 (24%) underwent hysterectomy for uterine rupture. Patients in whom preservation of fertility is a goal and who are hemodynamically stable may be candidates for angiographic uterine artery embolization.[81]

Vaginal metastases should not be biopsied because they are highly vascular and can bleed profusely. When bleeding cannot be controlled by a simple measure such as packing, embolization of pelvic vessels or wide local excision can be performed.[103] Bleeding from hepatic metastases are more problematic, sometimes requiring either local resection or selective hepatic arterial occlusion.[82]

MANAGEMENT OF PSTT AND ETT

Patients diagnosed with PSTT and ETT are managed similarly. Hysterectomy rather than chemotherapy is the first-line treatment in nonmetastatic disease because these neoplasms are relatively chemoresistant. At the time of surgery pelvic lymph nodes should be sampled because, in contrast to CCA, these tumors may spread via lymphatics. The survival rate for patients with nonmetastatic disease treated with hysterectomy alone is approximately 100%. Patients with metastatic disease may still achieve remission with intensive multiagent chemotherapy, particularly when they are diagnosed within 4 years of the antecedent pregnancy.[104–106] The risk factors for metastatic disease in patients with PSTT include interval from previous pregnancy of longer than 2 years, deep myometrial invasion, tumor necrosis, and mitotic count of more than 6 of 10 high-power fields. At present a platinum-containing regimen, such as EMA/EP, is the treatment of choice, with survival rates approaching 50% to 60%.[106–108]

FOLLOW-UP AFTER TREATMENT OF GTN

After achieving 3 consecutive weekly undetectable hCG levels and completion of chemotherapy, serum quantitative hCG levels should be obtained at monthly intervals for 12 months for patients with Stage I to III GTN, and 24 months for patients with Stage IV GTN, before allowing pregnancy. In general, the overall risk of relapse is about 3% to 9% in the first year after completing therapy, but is uncommon after 12 months of normal hCG levels. Physician examinations should be performed at intervals of 3 months during the period of hCG testing. Other tests such as radiographs or scans are indicated for special circumstances only. Contraception is mandatory during treatment and for the 12 (or 24) months of follow-up after completing chemotherapy, preferably by the use of oral contraceptives. Intrauterine devices should not be inserted until the hCG level becomes undetectable. Because of the 1% to 2% risk of another gestational trophoblastic event in a subsequent pregnancy, a pelvic ultrasound scan is recommended in later conceptions at 10 weeks to assure normal fetal development. The products of conception from future miscarriages should be reviewed by pathologists, and the placentas of future pregnancies should be examined grossly for abnormal areas which, if noted, should be reviewed pathologically. Finally, a serum hCG level should be obtained 6 weeks after completion of all future pregnancies, at which point it should be undetectable. Postterm or postabortal CCA should be considered if a patient with a history of molar pregnancy or GTN presents with unusual bleeding or signs of metastatic disease after a term pregnancy or miscarriage.

The introduction of etoposide-containing drug combinations for treatment of GTN in the 1980s has been reported to increase the risk of secondary malignances including acute myelogenous leukemia (1%), colon cancer, melanoma, and breast cancer.[51] This increased susceptibility appears to be dose-related, affecting primarily those patients whose total dose of etoposide exceeds 2 g. Heightened awareness of these conditions should be part of the health care surveillance in susceptible patients.

PERSISTENT LOW LEVELS OF HCG (QUIESCENT GTN)

There is a subset of patients with a history of GTN or molar pregnancy in whom the hCG level plateaus at very low levels for several weeks or months. Metastatic workup in these patients is usually negative. Real hCG is present but is predominantly the non-hyperglycosylated form.[109–112] These patients are characterized as having "quiescent GTN." The source of the hCG is presumably dormant though viable trophoblastic tissue that is resistant to chemotherapy. In most of these patients, the hCG level ultimately becomes undetectable spontaneously. Close follow-up is required, however, because 6% to 19% of women with quiescent GTN will eventually develop active progressing chemosensitive disease as reflected by rising hCG levels, which is now characterized by a high percentage of the hyperglycosylated form of hCG.[113,114]

In addition to persistent low levels of real hCG, patients occasionally present with an elevated hCG level without a clear antecedent pregnancy. False-positive hCG levels are caused by several conditions, including the presence of circulating heterophilic antibodies or elevated cross-reacting luteinizing (LH) hormone levels in perimeno-pausal/menopausal women. Most of the currently available hCG platforms correct for heterophilic antibodies and false-positive hCG levels due to LH cross-reaction in the perimenopause or menopause can be suppressed with oral contraceptives.[110] Furthermore, low levels of real hCG are produced in the menopause by the pituitary gland.[110] Of importance is that if the patient has false-positive hCG due to heterophile antibodies (phantom hCG), the hCG will not be detectable in the urine.

SUBSEQUENT PREGNANCY EXPERIENCE

The most common concern patients express when diagnosed with molar pregnancy or GTN has to do with the effect of this disease on future reproductive function. Patients with a history of molar pregnancy have an increased risk of developing a second molar pregnancy of from approximately 1 in 1000 to 1 in 100 in subsequent pregnancies.[115] This increased risk can even occur with a different partner, suggesting that the ovum holds the key to this disease. Despite an increased risk for developing a second molar pregnancy, patients with a history of a mole or GTN can generally anticipate normal future reproductive outcomes. Summarizing the experience from the NETDC (**Table 6**) and 9 other centers, data have been reported concerning the outcomes of 2657 later pregnancies in women treated with chemotherapy for GTN.[115–123] These subsequent pregnancies resulted in 76.7% live births at or near term, 5.3% premature births, 1.3% stillbirths, 14.2% miscarriages, and congenital malformations in 1.8%. These rates are comparable with those in the general popula-tion except for the increased risk of stillbirths. The secondary infertility rate among women receiving chemotherapy was only 7%. Woolas and colleagues[122] reported no difference in conception rates or pregnancy outcomes between women treated with single-agent chemotherapy and those on multiagent chemotherapy.

Patients occasionally become pregnant before the recommended 12-month follow-up period has elapsed. When a patient's hCG level reelevates after completing chemotherapy, an ultrasound examination enables the clinician to distinguish between a concurrent new pregnancy and disease recurrence. Matsui and colleagues[123] has shown that pregnancies that occur within 6 months following remis-sion are at increased risk of abnormalities including spontaneous miscarriages, still-births, and repeat moles.

Table 6 Subsequent pregnancy outcomes following chemotherapy at the NETDC, 1965–2010		
Outcome	N	%
Total pregnancies	759	100
Total deliveries	593	
Term live	441	58.1
Preterm live	44	5.8
Stillbirth	10	1.3
Congenital anomalies	11	1.4
Cesarean section	87	17.6
Spontaneous miscarriage	122	16.1
Induced abortion	28	3.7
Ectopic	7	0.9
Repeat molar pregnancy	9	1.2

PSYCHOSOCIAL CONSEQUENCES OF GTN

Women who develop GTN may experience significant mood disturbance and marital and sexual problems, in addition to their concerns over future fertility.[124,125] Because GTN is a result of pregnancy, patients and their partners must confront the loss of a pregnancy at the same time they face the threat of malignancy. Significant levels of anxiety, fatigue, anger, confusion, sexual problems, and concern for future pregnancy may last for protracted periods of time. Patients with metastatic disease and active disease who are particularly at risk for severe psychosocial reactions should be provided with psychosocial assessments and interventions. At the time of clinic visits, patients and their partners should be reassured that many patients experience psychosocial distress requiring support and counseling services. The psychological and social stresses related to persistent GTN may last for many years beyond remission. A study conducted at the NETDC and in England revealed that even 5 to 20 years after attaining remission, 51% of patients indicated that they would be "somewhat likely" to "very likely" to participate in a counseling program to discuss issues raised by having GTN.[124]

REFERENCES

1. Berkowitz RS, Goldstein DP. Current management of gestational trophoblastic disease. Gynecol Oncol 2009;112:654–62.
2. Bracken MB. Incidence and aetiology of hydatidiform mole: an epidemiologic review. Br J Obstet Gynaecol 1987;94:1123–35.
3. Palmer JR. Advances in the epidemiology of gestational trophoblastic disease. J Reprod Med 1994;39:155–62.
4. Atrash HK, Hogue CJ, Grimes DA. Epidemiology of hydatidiform mole during early gestation. Am J Obstet Gynecol 1986;154:906–9.
5. Bagshawe KD, Dent J, Webb J. Hydatidiform mole in England and Wales 1973-83. Lancet 1986;2:673–7.
6. Takeuchi S. Incidence of gestational trophoblastic disease by regional registration in Japan. Hum Reprod 1987;2:729–34.
7. Smith HO. Gestational trophoblastic disease. Epidemiology and trends. Clin Obstet Gynecol 2003;46:541–56.
8. Parazzini F, Mangili G, LaVecchia C, et al. Risk factors for gestational trophoblastic disease: a separate analysis of complete and partial hydatidiform moles. Obstet Gynecol 1991;78:1039–45.
9. Sebire NJ, Foskett M, Fisher RA, et al. Risk of partial and complete molar pregnancy in relation to maternal age. Br J Obstet Gynaecol 2002;109:99–102.
10. Wang CM, Dixon PH, Decordova S, et al. Identification of 13 novel NLRP7 mutations in 20 families with recurrent hydatidiform mole; missense mutations cluster in the leucine-rich area. J Med Genet 2009;46:569–75.
11. Berkowitz RS, Cramer DW, Bernstein MR, et al. Risk factors for complete molar pregnancy from a case-control study. Am J Obstet Gynecol 1985;152:1016–20.
12. Parazzini F, LaVecchia C, Mangili G, et al. Dietary factors and risk of trophoblastic disease. Am J Obstet Gynecol 1988;158:93–9.
13. Martin BH, Kim JM. Changes in gestational trophoblastic tumors over four decades: a Korean experience. J Reprod Med 1998;43:60–8.
14. Brinton LA, Bracken MB, Connelly RR. Choriocarcinoma incidence in the United States. Am J Epidemiol 1986;123:1094–100.

15. Smith HO, Qualls CR, Prarie BA, et al. Trends in gestational choriocarcinoma: a 27-year perspective. Obstet Gynecol 2003;102:978–87.
16. Berkowitz RS, Goldstein DP. Molar pregnancy. N Engl J Med 2009;360:1639–45.
17. Lurain JR, Brewer JI. Invasive mole. Semin Oncol 1982;9:174–80.
18. Baergen RN, Rutgers JL, Young RH, et al. Placental site trophoblastic tumor: a study of 55 cases and review of the literature emphasizing factors of prognostic significance. Gynecol Oncol 2006;100:511–20.
19. Shih IM, Kurman RJ. Epithelioid trophoblastic tumor: a neoplasm distinct from choriocarcinoma and placental site trophoblastic tumour simulating carcinoma. Am J Surg Pathol 1998;22:1393–403.
20. Allison KH, Love JE, Garcia RL. Epithelioid trophoblastic tumor: review of a rare neoplasm of the chorionic-type intermediate trophoblast. Arch Pathol Lab Med 2006;130:1875–7.
21. Soto-Wright V, Bernstein MR, Goldstein DP, et al. The changing clinical presentation of complete molar pregnancy. Obstet Gynecol 1995;86:775–9.
22. Kohorn EI. Negotiating a staging and risk factor scoring system for gestational trophoblastic neoplasia. A progress report. J Reprod Med 2002;47:445–50.
23. Goldstein DP, Zanten-Przybysz IV, Bernstein MR, et al. Revised FIGO staging system for gestational trophoblastic tumors; recommendations regarding therapy. J Reprod Med 1998;43:37–43.
24. Garner EI, Garrett A, Goldstein DP, et al. Significance of chest computed tomography findings in the evaluation and treatment of persistent gestational trophoblastic neoplasia. J Reprod Med 2004;49:411–4.
25. Van Trommel NE, Massuger LF, Verheijen RH, et al. The curative effect of a second curettage in persistent trophoblastic disease: a retrospective cohort study. Gynecol Oncol 2005;99:6–13.
26. Garner EI, Feltmate CM, Goldstein DP, et al. The curative effect of a second curettage in persistent trophoblastic disease: a retrospective cohort study. Gynecol Oncol 2005;99:3–5.
27. Bagshawe KD, Harland S. Immunodiagnosis and monitoring of gonadotropin-producing metastases in the central nervous system. Cancer 1976;38:112–8.
28. Bakri YN, Al-Hawashim N, Berkowitz RS. Cerebrospinal fluid/serum beta subunit human chorionic gonadotropin ratio in patients with brain metastases of gestational trophoblastic tumor. J Reprod Med 2000;45:94–6.
29. Dhillon T, Palmieri C, Sebire NJ, et al. Value of whole body 18 FDG-PET to identify the active site of gestational trophoblastic neoplasia. J Reprod Med 2006;51:879–87.
30. Lurain JR. Pharmacotherapy of gestational trophoblastic disease. Expert Opin Pharmacother 2003;4:1–13.
31. Alazzam M, Tidy JA, Hancock BW, et al. First line chemotherapy in low risk gestational trophoblastic neoplasia. Cochrane Database Syst Rev 2009;1:CD007102.
32. Homesely HD, Blessing JA, Rettenmaier M, et al. Weekly intramuscular methotrexate for nonmetastatic gestational trophoblastic disease. Obstet Gynecol 1988;72:413–8.
33. Homesley HD, Blessing JA, Schlaerth J, et al. Rapid escalation of weekly intramuscular methotrexate for nonmetastatic gestational trophoblastic disease. A Gynecologic Oncology Group study. Gynecol Oncol 1990;39:305–8.
34. Hoffman MS, Fiorica JV, Gleeson NC, et al. A single institution experience with weekly intramuscular methotrexate for nonmetastatic gestational trophoblastic disease. Gynecol Oncol 1996;60:292–4.

35. Berkowitz RS, Goldstein DP, Bernstein MR. Methotrexate infusion with folinic acid in primary therapy of nonmetastatic trophoblastic tumors. Gynecol Oncol 1990;36:56–9.
36. Elit L, Coven A, Osborne R, et al. High-dose methotrexate for gestational trophoblastic disease. Gynecol Oncol 1994;54:282–7.
37. Wong LC, Ngan HY, Cheng DK, et al. Methotrexate infusion in low-risk gestational trophoblastic disease. Am J Obstet Gynecol 2000;183:1579–82.
38. Schlaerth JB, Morrow CP, Nalick RH, et al. Single-dose actinomycin D in the treatment of postmolar trophoblastic disease. Gynecol Oncol 1984;19:53–6.
39. Petrilli ES, Twiggs LB, Blessing JA, et al. Single-dose actinomycin D treatment for nonmetastatic gestational trophoblastic disease; a prospective phase II trial of the Gynecologic Oncology Group. Cancer 1987;60:2173–6.
40. Gilani MM, Yarandi F, Eftekhar Z, et al. Comparison of pulse methotrexate and pulse actinomycin D in the treatment of low-risk gestational trophoblastic neoplasia. Aust N Z J Obstet Gynecol 2005;45:161–4.
41. Yerandi F, Eftekhar Z, Shojaei H, et al. Pulse methotrexate versus pulse actinomycin D in the treatment of low-risk gestational trophoblastic neoplasia. Int J Gynaecol Obstet 2008;103:33–7.
42. Osborne R, Filiaci V, Schink J, et al. A randomized phase III trial comparing weekly parental methotrexate and pulsed dactinomycin as primary management of low-risk gestational trophoblastic neoplasia: A Gynecologic Oncology Group study. J Clin Oncol 2011;29:825–31.
43. Smith EB, Weed JC Jr, Tyrey L, et al. Treatment of nonmetastatic gestational trophoblastic disease: results of methotrexate alone versus methotrexate-folinic acid. Am J Obstet Gynecol 1982;144:88–92.
44. Gleeson NC, Finan MA, Fiorica JV, et al. Non-metastatic gestational trophoblastic disease: Weekly methotrexate compared with 8-day methotrexate-folinic acid. Eur J Gynaecol Oncol 1993;14:461–5.
45. Lertkhachonsuk A, Israngura N, Wilailak S, et al. Actinomycin D versus methotrexate-folinic acid as the treatment of stage I, low-risk gestational trophoblastic neoplasia. A randomized controlled trial. Int J Gynecol Cancer 2009;19:985–8.
46. Kohorn EI. Decision making for chemotherapy administration in patients with low-risk gestational trophoblastic neoplasia. Int J Gynecol Oncol 1996;6:279–85.
47. Berkowitz RS, Goldstein DP, Jones MA, et al. Methotrexate with citrovorum factor rescue: reduced chemotherapy toxicity in the management of gestational trophoblastic neoplasms. Cancer 1980;45:423–6.
48. Petrilli ES, Morrow CP. Actinomycin D toxicity in the treatment of trophoblastic disease. A comparison of the 5-day course to single dose administration. Gynecol Oncol 1980;9:18–22.
49. Growdon WB, Wolfberg AJ, Goldstein DP, et al. Evaluating methotrexate therapy in patients with low-risk post-molar gestational trophoblastic neoplasia. Gynecol Oncol 2009;112:353–7.
50. Hammond CB, Borchert LG, Tyrey L, et al. Treatment of metastatic trophoblastic disease: good and poor prognosis. Am J Obstet Gynecol 1973;115:451–7.
51. Rustin GJ, Newlands ES, Lutz JM, et al. Combination but not single-agent methotrexate chemotherapy for gestational trophoblastic tumors increases the incidence of second tumors. J Clin Oncol 1996;14:2769–73.
52. Dubeshter B, Berkowitz RS, Goldstein DP, et al. Metastatic gestational trophoblastic disease: Experience at the New England Trophoblastic Disease Center, 1965-1985. Obstet Gynecol 1987;69:390–5.

53. Begent RH, Bagshawe KD. The management of high- risk choriocarcinoma. Semin Oncol 1982;9:198–203.
54. Curry SL, Blessing JA, DiSaia PJ, et al. A prospective randomized comparison of methotrexate, dactinomycin and chlorambucil versus methotrexate, dactinomycin, cyclophosphamide, doxorubicin, melphalan, hydroxyurea, and vincristine in poor prognosis metastatic gestational trophoblastic disease: a Gynecologic Oncology Group study. Obstet Gynecol 1989;73:357–62.
55. Wong LC, Choo YC, Ma HK. Primary oral etoposide therapy in gestational trophoblastic disease, an update. Cancer 1986;58:14–7.
56. Newlands ES, Bagshawe KD, Begent RH, et al. Results with EMA/CO (etoposide, methotrexate, actinomycin D, cyclophosphamide, vincristine) regimen in high-risk gestational trophoblastic tumors, 1979-1989. Br J Obstet Gynaecol 1991;98:550–7.
57. Bolis G, Bonazzi C, Landoni F, et al. EMA/CO regimen in high-risk gestational trophoblastic tumor (GTT). Gynecol Oncol 1988;31:439–44.
58. Bower M, Newlands ES, Holden L, et al. EMA/CO for high-risk gestational trophoblastic tumors: results from a cohort of 272 patients. J Clin Oncol 1997; 15:2636–43.
59. Kim SJ, Bae SN, Kim JH, et al. Risk factors for the prediction of treatment failure in gestational trophoblastic tumors treated with EMA/CO regimen. Gynecol Oncol 1998;71:247–53.
60. Matsui H, Suzuka K, Litsika Y, et al. Combination chemotherapy with methotrexate, etoposide and actinomycin D for high-risk gestational trophoblastic tumors. Gynecol Oncol 2000;78:28–31.
61. Escobar PF, Lurain JR, Singh DK, et al. Treatment of high-risk gestational trophoblastic neoplasia with etoposide, methotrexate actinomycin D, cyclophosphamide, and vincristine chemotherapy. Gynecol Oncol 2003;91:552–7.
62. Lurain JR, Singh DK, Schink JC. Primary treatment of metastatic high-risk gestational trophoblastic neoplasia with EMA-CO chemotherapy. J Reprod Med 2006; 51:767–72.
63. Turan T, Karacay O, Tulunay G, et al. Results with EMA/CO (etoposide, methotrexate, actinomycin D, cyclophosphamide, vincristine) chemotherapy in gestational trophoblastic neoplasia. Int J Gynecol Oncol 2006;16:1432–8.
64. Lu WG, Ye F, Shen YM, et al. EMA-CO chemotherapy for high-risk gestational trophoblastic neoplasia: a clinical analysis of 54 patients. Int J Gynecol Oncol 2008;18:357–62.
65. Lurain JR, Nejad B. Secondary chemotherapy for high-risk gestational trophoblastic neoplasia. Gynecol Oncol 2005;97:618–23.
66. Mao Y, Wan X, Lv W, et al. Relapsed or refractory gestational trophoblastic neoplasia treated with etoposide and cisplatin/etoposide, methotrexate, and actinomycin D (EP-EMA) regimen. Int J Gynecol Oncol 2007;98:44–7.
67. Newlands ES, Mulholland PJ, Holden L, et al. Etoposide and cisplatin/etoposide, methotrexate and actinomycin D (EMA) for patients with high-risk gestational trophoblastic tumors refractory to EMA/cyclophosphamide and vincristine and patients presenting with metastatic placental site tumors. J Clin Oncol 2000;18:854–9.
68. Evans AC Jr, Soper JT, Clarke-Pearson DL, et al. Gestational trophoblastic disease metastatic to the central nervous system. Gynecol Oncol 1995;59: 226–30.
69. Small W Jr, Lurain JR, Shetty RM, et al. Gestational trophoblastic disease metastatic to the brain. Radiology 1996;200:277–80.

70. Rustin GJ, Newlands ES, Begent RH, et al. Weekly alternating etoposide, methotrexate, and actinomycin/vincristine and cyclophosphamide chemotherapy for the treatment of CNS metastases of choriocarcinoma. J Clin Oncol 1989;7:900–3.

71. Bakri YN, Berkowitz RS, Goldstein DP, et al. Brain metastases of gestational trophoblastic tumor. J Reprod Med 1994;39:179–84.

72. Newlands ES, Holden L, Seckl MJ, et al. Management of brain metastases in patients with high risk gestational trophoblastic tumors. J Reprod Med 2002; 47:465–71.

73. Tomoda Y, Arii Y, Kaseki S, et al. Surgical indications for resection in pulmonary metastases of choriocarcinoma. Cancer 1980;46:2723–30.

74. Fleming EL, Garrett LA, Growdon WB, et al. The changing role of thoracotomy in gestational trophoblastic neoplasia at the New England Trophoblastic Disease Center. J Reprod Med 2008;53:493–8.

75. Edwards JL, Makey AR, Bagshawe KD. The role of thoracotomy in the management of pulmonary metastases of gestational choriocarcinoma. Clin Oncol 1975; 1:329–39.

76. Shirley RL, Goldstein DP, Collins JJ Jr. The role of thoracotomy in management of patients with chest metastases from gestational trophoblastic disease. J Thorac Cardiovasc Surg 1972;63:545–50.

77. Wang Y, Song HZ, Xia Z. Drug resistant pulmonary choriocarcinoma metastasis treated by lobectomy. Chin Med J 1980;93:758–66.

78. Sink JD, Hammond CB, Young WG. Pulmonary resection in the management of metastases from choriocarcinoma. J Thorac Cardiovasc Surg 1981;81:830–4.

79. Wong LC, Choo JC, Ma HK. Hepatic metastases in gestational trophoblastic disease. Obstet Gynecol 1986;67:107–11.

80. Bakri YN, Subhi J, Amer M, et al. Liver metastases of gestational trophoblastic tumor. Gynecol Oncol 1993;48:110–3.

81. Tse KY, Chan KK, Tam KF, et al. 20-year experience of managing profuse bleeding in gestational trophoblastic disease. J Reprod Med 2007;52:397.

82. Grumbine FC, Rosenshein NB, Brereton HD, et al. Management of liver metastases from gestational trophoblastic neoplasia. Am J Obstet Gynecol 1980;137: 959–61.

83. Yang J, Xiang Y, Wan X, et al. Recurrent gestational trophoblastic tumor: management and risk factors for recurrence. Gynecol Oncol 2006;103:587–90.

84. Ngan HY, Tam KF, Lam KW, et al. Relapsed gestational trophoblastic neoplasia: a 20-year experience. J Reprod Med 2006;51:829–34.

85. Powles Y, Savage PM, Stebbing J, et al. A comparison of patients with relapsed and chemo-refractory gestational trophoblastic neoplasia. Br J Cancer 2007;96:732–7.

86. Mutch DG, Soper JT, Babcock CJ, et al. Recurrent gestational trophoblastic disease. Experience of the Southeastern Regional Trophoblastic Disease Center. Cancer 1990;66:978–82.

87. Osborne R, Covens A, Merchandani DE, et al. Successful salvage of relapsed high-risk gestational trophoblastic neoplasia patients using a novel paclitaxel-containing doublet. J Reprod Med 2004;49:655–61.

88. Wang J, Short D, Sebire J, et al. Salvage chemotherapy of relapsed or high- risk gestational trophoblastic neoplasia (GTN) with paclitaxel/cisplatin alternating with paclitaxel/etoposide(TP/TE). Ann Oncol 2008;19:1578–83.

89. Wan X, Yang Y, Wu Y, et al. Floxuridine-containing regimens in the treatment of gestational trophoblastic tumor. J Reprod Med 2004;49:453–6.

90. Matsui H, Iitsuka Y, Suzuka K, et al. Salvage chemotherapy for high-risk gestational trophoblastic tumor. J Reprod Med 2004;49:438–42.

91. Gordon AN, Kavanagh JJ, Gershenson DM, et al. Cisplatin, vinblastine, and bleomycin combination chemotherapy in resistant gestational trophoblastic disease. Cancer 1986;58:1407–10.
92. DuBeshter B, Berkowitz RS, Goldstein DP, et al. Vinblastine, cisplatin and bleomycin as salvage therapy for refractory high-risk metastatic gestational trophoblastic disease. J Reprod Med 1989;34:189–92.
93. Azab M, Droz JP, Theodore C, et al. Cisplatin, vinblastine and bleomycin combination in the treatment of resistant high-risk gestational trophoblastic tumors. Cancer 1989;64:1829–32.
94. Sutton GP, Soper JT, Blessing JA, et al. Ifosfamide alone and in combination in the treatment of refractory malignant gestational trophoblastic disease. Am J Obstet Gynecol 1992;167:489–95.
95. Jones WB, Schneider J, Shapiro F, et al. Treatment of resistant gestational trophoblastic choriocarcinoma with taxol: a report of two cases. Gynecol Oncol 1996;61:126–30.
96. Giacalone PL, Benos P, Donnadio D, et al. High-dose chemotherapy with autologous bone marrow transplantation for refractory metastatic gestational trophoblastic disease. Gynecol Oncol 1995;58:383–5.
97. Van Besien K, Verschraegen C, Mehra R, et al. Complete remission of refractory gestational trophoblastic disease with brain metastases treated with multicycle ifosfamide, carboplatin, and etoposide (ICE) and stem cell rescue. Gynecol Oncol 1997;65:366–9.
98. Tewari KS, Monk BJ. American Society of Clinical Oncology 2011 Annual Meeting Update: Summary of selected gynecologic cancer abstracts. Gynecol Oncol 2011;122:211–2.
99. Hoekstra AV, Lurain JR, Rademaker AW, et al. Gestational trophoblastic neoplasia: treatment outcomes. Obstet Gynecol 2008;112:251–8.
100. Cagayan MS, Suyen Magallanes M. The role of adjuvant surgery in the management of gestational trophoblastic neoplasia. J Reprod Med 2008;53:513–8.
101. Clark R, Nevadunsky N, Ghosh E, et al. The evolving role of hysterectomy in gestational trophoblastic neoplasia at the New England Trophoblastic Disease Center. J Reprod Med 2010;55:194–8.
102. Lurain JR, Singh DK, Schink JC. Role of surgery in the management of high-risk gestational trophoblastic neoplasia. J Reprod Med 2006;51:773–6.
103. Yingna S, Yang X, Xiuyu Y, et al. Clinical characteristics and treatment of gestational trophoblastic tumor and vaginal metastasis. Gynecol Oncol 2002;84:416–9.
104. Feltmate CM, Genest DR, Goldstein DP, et al. Advances in the understanding of placental site trophoblastic tumor. J Reprod Med 2002;47:337–41.
105. Palmer JE, Macdonald M, Wells M, et al. Epithelioid trophoblastic tumor: a review of the literature. J Reprod Med 2008;53:465–75.
106. Papadopoulos AJ, Foskett M, Seckl MJ, et al. Twenty- five years' clinical experience with placental site trophoblastic tumors. J Reprod Med 2002;47:460–4.
107. Hassaida A, Gillespie A, Tidy J. Placental site trophoblastic tumor: clinical features and management. Gynecol Oncol 2005;99:603–7.
108. Schmid P, Nagai Y, Agarwal R, et al. Prognostic markers and long-term outcome of placental-site trophoblastic tumors: a retrospective observational study. Lancet 2009;374:48–55.
109. Khanlian SA, Cole LA. Management of gestational trophoblastic disease and other cases with low serum levels of human chorionic gonadotropin. J Reprod Med 2006;51:812–8.

110. Cole LA, Yasushi S, Muller CY. Normal production of human chorionic gonado-tropin in menopause. N Engl J Med 2007;356:1184–6.
111. Cole LA, Butler S. Detection of hCG in trophoblastic disease. The USA hCG Reference Service experience. J Reprod Med 2002;47:433–44.
112. Cole LA, Kohorn EI. The need for an hCG assay that appropriately detects trophoblastic disease and other hCG- producing tumors. J Reprod Med 2006; 51:793–811.
113. Kohorn EI. What we know about low-level hCG: definition, classification and management. J Reprod Med 2004;49:433–7.
114. Hwang D, Hancock BW. Management of persistent, unexplained, low-level human chorionic gonadotropin elevation: a report of 5 cases. J Reprod Med 2004;49:559–62.
115. Garrett LA, Garner EI, Feltmate CM, et al. Subsequent pregnancy outcomes in patients with molar pregnancy and persistent gestational trophoblastic neoplasia. J Reprod Med 2008;53:481–6.
116. Ayhan A, Ergeneli MH, Yuce K, et al. Pregnancy after chemotherapy for gesta-tional trophoblastic disease. J Reprod Med 1990;35:522–4.
117. Kim JH, Park DC, Bae SN, et al. Subsequent reproductive experience after treat-ment for gestational trophoblastic disease. Gynecol Oncol 1998;71:108–12.
118. Kjer JJ, Iversen T. Malignant trophoblastic tumors in Norway: fertility rate after chemotherapy. Br J Obstet Gynaecol 1990;97:623–5.
119. Kobayashi O, Matsui H, Takamizawa H. Analysis of pregnancy outcome after chemotherapy for trophoblastic disease. Nippon Sanka Fujinka Gakkai Zasshi 1986;38:181–6.
120. Ngan HYS, Wong LC, Ma HK. Reproductive performance of patients with gesta-tional trophoblastic disease in Hong Kong. Acta Obstet Gynecol Scand 1988; 67:11–4.
121. Song HZ, Wu PC, Wang Y, et al. Pregnancy outcome after successful chemo-therapy for choriocarcinoma and invasive mole: long-term follow-up. Am J Ob-stet Gynecol 1988;158(3 Pt 1):538–45.
122. Woolas RP, Bower M, Newlands ES, et al. Influence of chemotherapy for gesta-tional trophoblastic disease on subsequent pregnancy outcome. Br J Obstet Gynaecol 1998;105:1032–5, 9:1326–7.
123. Matsui H, Iitsuka Y, Suzuka K, et al. Early pregnancy outcome after chemo-therapy for gestational trophoblastic tumor. J Reprod Med 2004;49:531–4.
124. Wenzel L, Berkowitz RS, Newlands E, et al. Quality of life after gestational trophoblastic disease. J Reprod Med 2002;47:387–94.
125. Cagayan MS, Llarena RT. Quality of life of gestational neoplasia survivors: a study of patients at the Philippine General Hospital Trophoblastic Disease Section. J Reprod Med 2010;55:321–6.

New Biologic Agents for the Treatment of Gynecologic Cancers

Neil Horowitz, MD[a], Ursula A. Matulonis, MD[b],*

KEYWORDS

- Ovarian cancer • Endometrial cancer • Cervical cancer
- Antiangiogenesis inhibitors
- Poly-ADP-ribose polymerase inhibitors
- Phosphoinositide 3-kinase inhibitors

With the development of molecularly targeted therapies, the availability of faster and less expensive technologies for genetic analysis of cancers, and the increasing molecular understanding of gynecologic malignancies, novel targeted biologic approaches are being tested in patients with gynecologic cancers, representing an exciting chapter in the treatment of gynecologic cancers. This article discusses several new areas of therapeutics in gynecologic malignancies: antiangiogenesis agents, poly-ADP-ribose polymerase (PARP) inhibitors, hedgehog (Hh) inhibitors, folate receptor (FR) antagonists, phosphoinositide 3-kinase (PI3K) pathway inhibitors, and inhibitors of the epidermal growth factor receptor (EGFR) family.

ANTIANGIOGENESIS THERAPIES

Antiangiogenic therapies have been tested in ovarian, endometrial, and cervical cancer, and these agents have demonstrated antitumor activity as monotherapy and combined with cytotoxic chemotherapy.

Ovarian Malignancies

Angiogenesis has an important role in ovarian cancer pathogenesis.[1] Epithelial ovarian cancer overexpresses proangiogenic factors, such as vascular endothelial growth factor (VEGF), fibroblast growth factor, platelet-derived growth factor (PDGF), and

Author disclosures: Ursula Matulonis has participated in advisory boards for Clovis Pharmaceuticals, Boehringer Ingelheim, Sanofi-Aventis, and Merck and serves on the Clinical Advisory Board for Pathway Therapeutics. Neil Horowtiz has received research support from Genentech.
[a] Division of Gynecologic Oncology, Department of Obstetrics and Gynecology, Brigham and Women's Hospital, 75 Francis Street, Boston, MA 02115, USA
[b] Medical Gynecologic Oncology, Department of Medical Oncology, Dana-Farber Cancer Institute, 450 Brookline Avenue, Boston, MA 02215, USA
* Corresponding author.
E-mail address: Ursula_matulonis@dfci.harvard.edu

Hematol Oncol Clin N Am 26 (2012) 133–156
doi:10.1016/j.hoc.2011.11.002
0889-8588/12/$ – see front matter © 2012 Published by Elsevier Inc.

hemonc.theclinics.com

angiopoietin, supporting the role of angiogenesis in this cancer.[1] In preclinical models, the expression of VEGF provides a survival advantage to transformed cells of the ovary.[2] Several studies have found an association between higher preoperative serum VEGF and decreased overall survival (OS).[3,4]

Several antiangiogenic agents have been studied in ovarian cancer; these agents are divided into tyrosine kinase inhibitors (TKIs) targeting VEGF receptor (VEGFR), and other kinases and antibody-based approaches, such as bevacizumab and VEGF-Trap.

Single-agent phase II studies of antiangiogenic agents for ovarian cancer

Table 1 lists single-agent antiangiogenic agents that have been tested in recurrent ovarian cancer and results of these studies. Bevacizumab, a recombinant humanized monoclonal IgG1 anti-VEGF antibody, has been studied in two separate single-agent phase II trials for recurrent ovarian cancer. In a Gynecologic Oncology Group (GOG) study, 62 patients with recurrent platinum-resistant or -sensitive (up to 12 months platinum-free interval) ovarian cancer received bevacizumab, 15 mg/kg intravenously (IV) once every 3 weeks.[5] A total of 21% of patients achieved a clinical response, and 40.3% patients had a progression-free survival (PFS) of greater than or equal to 6 months. Median PFS was 4.7 months, and OS was 16.9 months. Clinical activity was observed in platinum-resistant and -sensitive tumors. Toxicities included 9.7% grade 3 hypertension, 22.6% grade 2 proteinuria, and 1.6% grade 3 venous thromboembolism, and there were no reports of gastrointestinal (GI) perforation. A second study that enrolled patients with platinum-resistant ovarian cancer who had received two or three prior lines of therapy tested bevacizumab, 15 mg/kg IV once every 3 weeks.[6] The response rate was 15.9%, median PFS was 4.4 months, OS was 10.7 months, and the 6-month PFS was 27.8%. However, this study was stopped early because of an 11.4% GI perforation rate. Risks for GI perforation included receipt of more than two lines of therapy in the recurrent setting; bowel wall thickening on radiographic imaging or bowel obstruction were also identified as potential risk factors, but the association was not statistically significant. Grade 3 and 4 toxicities included 9.1% hypertension and 15.9% proteinuria. Three patients died on this study with toxicities related to bevacizumab including one episode each of myocardial infarction and cerebrovascular ischemia, intestinal perforation, and convulsion and hypertensive encephalopathy. Additional toxicities observed in single-agent bevacizumab studies were consistent with known bevacizumab toxicities.[7] Aflibercept (VEGF-Trap), a fusion protein that acts as a VEGF sink by combining the Fc portion of human IgG1 with the principal extracellular ligand-binding domains of VEGFR, demonstrated a response rate of 11% in a phase II trial.[8]

Multiple single-agent TKIs have been tested in recurrent ovarian cancer and single-agent results are listed in **Table 1**. Agents that have been tested include cediranib (targets VEGFR and c-Kit); sunitinib (targets VEGFR, c-Kit, PDGFR, RET, and FLT-3); sorafenib (targets VEGFR, c-Kit, RAF, and PDGFR-β); ENMD2076 (targets VEGFR and aurora A); pazopanib (targets VEGFR, PDGFR, and c-Kit); and cabozantinib (targets VEGFR and c-MET).[9–14] These studies have demonstrated response rates between 3% and 29% in recurrent platinum-resistant ovarian cancer. In a recent study of cabozantinib (XL184), which targets VEGFR and c-MET, there was a 29% confirmed partial response (PR) rate in platinum-resistant or -refractory ovarian cancer and 40% response rate in platinum-sensitive cancers.

Randomized phase II studies have also been performed. Ledermann and colleagues[15] conducted a randomized double-blind phase II study of maintenance BIBF 1120 (which has activity against VEGFR, PDGFR, and fibroblast growth factor receptor) versus placebo for up to 9 months in 83 patients with recurrent ovarian cancer who had experienced response to their last chemotherapy in the second-line or greater setting. Thirty-six–week PFS rates were 16.3% and 5% in the BIBF 1120 and placebo groups, respectively (hazard ratio [HR] = 0.65; 95% confidence interval [CI], 0.42–1.02; P = .06), suggesting that maintenance antiangiogenic therapy can delay disease progression in this setting. These positive results have led to the testing of this drug combined with carboplatin and paclitaxel in the newly diagnosed setting, and this study is described next.

Combination chemotherapy plus antiangiogenic agents for ovarian cancer

Phase II studies Single-agent phase II studies of combination chemotherapy with anti-angiogenic drugs have been performed.[16,17] These include combinations of bevacizumab with oral cyclophosphamide, bevacizumab with carboplatin and paclitaxel, bevacizumab with docetaxel and oxaliplatin, bevacizumab with nab-paclitaxel, cediranib with carboplatin and paclitaxel, and aflibercept plus docetaxel.[18–23] Certain combinations (ie, carboplatin, paclitaxel and bevacizumab) have been or are being tested in randomized phase II or III studies. A recent report testing cediranib added to carboplatin-based chemotherapy in recurrent ovarian cancer resulted in acceptable toxicities.[22] In the safety portion of ICON6, 60 patients were enrolled and subsequently randomized (2:3:3) to receive six cycles of carboplatin-based chemotherapy with placebo followed by placebo maintenance, carboplatin-based chemotherapy plus cediranib with placebo maintenance, or carboplatin-based chemotherapy plus cediranib with cediranib maintenance. Grade 3 and 4 toxicities were observed in 50% and 5% of patients, respectively, and no GI perforations were observed. The investigators concluded that the addition of cediranib to platinum-based chemotherapy was tolerable enough to expand the ICON6 trial to stage II.

AMG386 is a selective angiopoietin 1/2-neutralizing peptibody that inhibits angiogenesis by targeting a parallel angiogenic pathway from VEGFR. AMG386 was tested in a randomized phase II study of weekly paclitaxel plus AMG386 versus weekly paclitaxel alone in patients with recurrent platinum-resistant ovarian cancer.[24] The results of this study demonstrated a nonsignificant prolongation of PFS from 4.6 months for paclitaxel and placebo to 7.2 months observed for paclitaxel and AMG386 at a dose of 10 mg/kg (P = .23). These results have led to a phase III study, described next. The activity of sorafenib as a maintenance therapy is also being studied in a phase II study comparing a regimen of carboplatin, paclitaxel, and sorafenib for six cycles followed by 12 months of sorafenib maintenance to carboplatin and paclitaxel alone[25]; results of this study are currently pending.

Phase III studies Bevacizumab combined with carboplatin and paclitaxel chemotherapy has been tested in two separate randomized phase III trials in newly diagnosed advanced ovarian cancer (**Table 2**).[26,27] GOG218 is a double-blind placebo-controlled trial that enrolled 1873 advanced FIGO stage III or IV patients (optimal or suboptimally debulked) who were randomized in a 1:1:1 ratio to one of three arms: Arm 1 (control) consisted of carboplatin AUC 6, paclitaxel, 175 mg/m^2, and placebo every 3 weeks × six cycles, followed by maintenance placebo every 3 weeks for an additional 16 cycles; Arm 2 consisted of carboplatin AUC 6, paclitaxel, 175 mg/m^2, and bevacizumab, 15 mg/kg every 3 weeks × 6 cycles, followed by maintenance placebo; and Arm 3 consisted of carboplatin AUC 6, paclitaxel, 175 mg/m^2, and bevacizumab, 15 mg/kg every 3 weeks, followed by maintenance bevacizumab, 15 mg/kg every 3 weeks.[26] The original endpoint of this study was OS, but this was changed to PFS midway through the study. When Arm 2 was compared with Arm 1, no significant benefit in PFS was seen (median PFS 10.3 months control vs 11.2 months treatment; HR = 0.908; P = .080). However,

Table 1
Selected single-agent phase 2 studies of antiangiogenic agents in recurrent ovarian cancer

Agent Tested	Regimen/Schedule	Patient Population	Outcomes	Notable Toxicities
Bevacizumab[5,6]	15 mg/kg q 3 wk IV	Platinum-free interval <12 mo	CR 3% PR 18% SD 52% Median PFS 4.7 mo 6-mo PFS 40.3%	9.7% grade 3 HTN 22.6% grade 2 proteinuria 1.6% grade 3 venous thromboembolism No episodes of GIP
	15 mg/kg q 3 wk IV	Platinum resistant	PR 16% SD 61% Median PFS 4.4 mo 6-mo PFS 27.8%	11.4% risk of GIP Grades 3 and 4 toxicities: 9.1% HTN 15.9% proteinuria 2.3% bleeding and wound healing complications
Aflibercept[8]	Either 2 or 4 mg/kg q 2 wk	Platinum-resistant, two or three prior lines for recurrence allowed	RR 11%	9% grades 3 and 4 HTN 4% proteinuria 2% renal failure and encephalopathy 2 patients had GIP
Cediranib[9]	45 mg PO daily; dose reduced to 30 mg daily for toxicity	Platinum resistant	PR 17% SD 13% Median PFS 5.2 mo 6-mo PFS 17%	No GIP or fistulas 46% grade 3 HTN 24% grade 3 fatigue 13% grade 3 diarrhea 43% grade 2 hypothyroidism Grade 4: one episode each of CNS bleed, dehydration, elevated cholesterol
Sorafenib[10]	400 mg PO BID	Platinum-free interval <12 mo	PR 3.4% SD 34% Median PFS 2.1 mo 6-mo PFS 24%	19.7% grade 3 dermatologic 14% grade 3 metabolic 1.4% grade 3 HTN 25% grade 2 GI

Drug	Dose	Population	Response	Toxicity
Sunitinib[11]	Stage 1 (17 patients): 50 mg daily 4 wk on/2 wk off; Stage 2 (14 patients): 37.5 mg daily	Platinum sensitive or resistant	RR 3.3% SD 53% Median PFS 4.1 mo	No incidence of GIP 10% grade 3 for each granulocytes, platelets, hemoglobin Fatigue, diarrhea, hand-foot
Pazopanib[12]	800 mg daily	Platinum sensitive or resistant; must have had CA125 CR to initial platinum-based chemotherapy	CA125 response 31% RR by RECIST 18% 6-mo PFS 17%	8% grade 3 ALT elevation 11% grade 3 fatigue 11% grade GGT elevation 8% grade 3 diarrhea
ENMD2076[13]	Starting dose of 375 mg/day was reduced to 275 mg/day	Platinum resistant	PR 7% SD 30% 6-mo PFS 19%	Grade 3 hypertension (46%) Grade 3+ fatigue (24%) Grade 3+ diarrhea (13%) One grade 4 CNS hemorrhage
Cabozantinib (XL184)[14]	100 mg PO q day	Platinum sensitive or resistant	Platinum sensitive: (10 patients) PR 40%, SD 60% Platinum resistant/refractory: (17 patients) PR 29%, SD 41%	Toxicities ≥ grade 3: 12% PPE syndrome 7% diarrhea 5% fatigue 5% vomiting 3% HTN

Abbreviations: ALT, alanine aminotransferase; CNS, central nervous system; CR, complete response; GGT, γ-glutamyltransferase; GI, gastrointestinal; GIP, gastrointestinal perforation; HTN, hypertension; PFS, progression-free survival; PPE, palmar-plantar erythrodysesthesia; PR, partial response; RR, response rate; SD, stable disease.

Table 2
Results of phase III studies testing bevacizumab in ovarian cancer

Setting	Study	Accrual	Dose of Bev	Treatment Regimens	Primary Endpoint	Results
First-line	GOG218[26]	N = 1873	15 mg/kg q 3 wk	C/P/placebo plus maintenance placebo C/P/bev plus maintenance placebo C/P/bev plus maintenance bev	PFS	PFS arm 3: 14.1 mo PFS arm 1: 10.3 mo (HR = 0.717; P<.0001). OS not different
	ICON7[27,28]	N = 1528	7.5 mg/kg q 3 wk	C/P C/P/bev plus maintenance bev	PFS	PFS arm 1: 17.3 mo PFS arm 2: 19 mo (HR = 0.81; P = .0041) OS not different
Recurrent	OCEANS[33]	N = 484	15 mg/kg q 3 wk	C/G/placebo plus maintenance placebo C/G/bev plus maintenance bev	PFS	PFS arm 1: 8.4 mo PFS arm 2: 12.4 mo (HR = 0.484; P<.0001) OS not different

Abbreviations: bev, bevacizumab; C, carboplatin; P, paclitaxel.

when Arm 3 was compared with Arm 1 (prespecified comparisons), Arm 3 showed a statistically significant improvement in PFS compared with Arm 1 (median PFS 10.3 months control vs 14.1 months treatment; HR = 0.717; P<.0001). OS data are not yet mature, but to date no OS benefit has been noted in any of the arms; OS is 39.3 months in Arm 1, 38.7 months in Arm 2, and 39.7 months in Arm 3. Grade 2 or higher hypertension and GI fistula and perforation were higher in the bevacizumab arms compared with Arm 1, which did not contain bevacizumab.

ICON7 is a randomized open-label phase III trial that randomized 1528 women 1:1 to either carboplatin AUC 6 and paclitaxel, 175 mg/m^2, every 3 weeks for six cycles or carboplatin AUC 6 and paclitaxel, 175 mg/m^2, every 3 weeks for six cycles, with the addition of bevacizumab, 7.5 mg/kg, every 3 weeks starting in cycle 2 and continuing for an additional 12 cycles of maintenance therapy.[27] Eligible patients included FIGO stages I or IIA (grade 3), IIB or C, III, and IV. PFS was improved in the bevacizumab arm with a median PFS of 17.3 months in the nonbevacizumab control arm and 19 months in the treatment arm (HR = 0.81; P = .0041). As in GOG218, OS was not significantly different between the two arms in ICON7. In an updated analysis of ICON7, a significant OS benefit was observed with bevacizumab treatment in patients who were suboptimally cytoreduced (>1 cm of cancer remaining at initial cytoreductive surgery) or had stage IV cancer (median OS 28.8 vs 36.6 months; HR = 0.64; P = .002).[28]

Results are pending in other phase III studies of antiangiogenic drugs in newly diagnosed patients. A placebo-controlled randomized phase III trial investigating the antiangiogenic small molecule BIBF 1120 with carboplatin and paclitaxel is ongoing with PFS as the primary endpoint.[29] Pazopanib is being tested in a randomized placebo-controlled phase III study as maintenance after initial surgical debulking and chemotherapy.[30] Two additional ongoing phase III trials are incorporating bevacizumab with different chemotherapy strategies (ie, IP and dose-dense chemotherapy), but neither of these studies is testing the benefit of adding bevacizumab to front-line chemotherapy.[31,32] GOG252 is open to patients with stages II, III, or IV cancer that is either optimally (≤1 cm residual cancer) or suboptimally (>1 cm residual cancer) cytoreduced, randomizes patients to one of three arms, and all of these arms contain bevacizumab followed by maintenance bevacizumab therapy: (1) IV carboplatin AUC 6 Day 1 and IV paclitaxel, 80 mg/m^2, Days 1, 8, and 15; (2) IP carboplatin AUC 6 Day 1 and IV paclitaxel, 80 mg/m^2, Days 1, 8, and 15; or (3) IV paclitaxel, 135 mg/m^2 over 24 hours Day 1, IP cisplatin, 75 mg/m^2, Day 2, and IP paclitaxel, 60 mg/m^2, Day 8.[31] GOG262 is open to suboptimally debulked stages III or IV patients and randomizes patients to either IV carboplatin AUC 6 and IV paclitaxel, 175 mg/m^2, Day 1 or IV carboplatin AUC 6 Day 1 and IV paclitaxel, 80 mg/m^2, Days 1, 8, and 15.[32] In this study, the use of bevacizumab is optional, and if used, is continued until either disease progression or unacceptable toxicity occurs.

Several randomized phase III trials have been performed and others are ongoing that test the role of antiangiogenic agents in recurrent ovarian cancer. The OCEANS study tested bevacizumab in combination with platinum-based chemotherapy in patients with recurrent platinum-sensitive ovarian cancer (see **Table 2**).[33] In this trial, 484 women with platinum-sensitive ovarian cancer with no prior chemotherapy for recurrent cancer were randomized to receive carboplatin AUC 4 Day 1 and gemcitabine, 1000 mg/m^2, Days 1 and 8 with either bevacizumab, 15 mg/kg, or placebo given IV every 3 weeks. The primary endpoint was PFS, and median PFS was 8.4 months in the control arm and 12.4 months with the addition of bevacizumab (HR = 0.484; P<.0001). Response rates were 57.4% in the control group and 78.5% in the treatment arm (P<.0001). OS data are not yet mature, but OS was not statistically significant between the groups. Increased toxicities observed in patients receiving bevacizumab included hypertension, proteinuria, bleeding, and thromboembolic events. No GI perforations were observed during the study, but two patients developed GI perforations after completion of bevacizumab.

Other phase III studies are ongoing in recurrent ovarian cancer. GOG213 is testing the roles of secondary cytoreductive surgery and bevacizumab in combination with carboplatin and paclitaxel in recurrent platinum-sensitive ovarian cancer.[34] ICON6 is testing the role of cediranib in recurrent platinum-sensitive ovarian cancer, described previously.[35] AMG386 is being tested along with chemotherapy in a phase III study in the partially platinum-sensitive or in platinum-resistant patients.[36] Patients are being randomized to either AMG386 with weekly paclitaxel or weekly paclitaxel alone.

Endometrial Cancer

Angiogenesis also has a role in endometrial cancer, and elevated levels of VEGF and other markers of angiogenesis have correlated with a poorer outcome in patients with endometrial cancer.[37] To date, however, treatment of recurrent endometrial cancer with antiangiogenic agents has revealed mixed results. Agents that have been tested include bevacizumab, sunitinib, sorafenib, and thalidomide. Bevacizumab was studied as part of a GOG study in patients with recurrent or persistent endometrial cancer after receiving one or two prior cytotoxic regimens with measurable cancer.[38] Fifty-two patients met eligibility and were evaluable. A total of 13.5% of patients had an objective response (one complete response and six PRs); 40.4% of patients survived progression-free for at least 6 months. Median PFS was 4.2 months, and OS was 10.5 months. No GI perforations or fistulas were reported. Two episodes of grades 3 and 4 hemorrhage were reported and two episodes of grades 3 or 4 thrombosis and embolism.

Other antiangiogenic agents have been tested with less positive results. Sunitinib was tested in patients with recurrent or metastatic endometrial cancer who have received up to one prior chemotherapy regimen for metastatic disease, and sunitinib was given at 50 mg daily for 4 consecutive weeks followed by 2 weeks off.[39] Of the 20 patients evaluable for response, PR was achieved by three patients (overall response rate [ORR] = 15%) and four of these patients remained progression-free for greater than or equal to 6 months (20%). Sorafenib was tested in a cohort of 39 patients with endometrial cancer with the starting sorafenib dose of 400 mg orally twice daily.[40] Two (5%) patients had a PR and 17 (42.5%) achieved stable disease (SD). The 6-month PFS rate for patients with carcinoma was 29%, and the median OS was 11.4 months. The authors concluded that sorafenib had minimal activity in endometrial cancer. Thalidomide was tested in a GOG study in patients with recurrent endometrial cancer using a thalidomide dose of 200 mg orally each day and dose escalated up to 1000 mg/day if tolerated.[41] Response rate was 12.5%, and 8.3% of patients had SD. The investigators believe that thalidomide is an inactive drug in endometrial cancer.

Cervical Cancer

Angiogenesis has several roles in cervical cancer pathogenesis including the finding of elevated intratumoral levels of VEGF, human papilloma virus enhancement of VEGF production by upregulation of the E6 oncoprotein, and VEGF expression and increased vascularization predicts poorer outcomes in cervical cancer.[42–46]

Single-agent bevacizumab has been studied in patients with recurrent or persistent squamous cell carcinoma of the cervix who received one or two prior cytotoxic regimens.[47] Of 46 patients enrolled, 11 (23.9%) survived progression free for at least 6 months, and five patients (10.9%) had a response, all PRs. Toxicities were as expected and included grades 3 or 4 hypertension (N = 7), thromboembolism (N = 5), GI (N = 4), anemia (N = 2), cardiovascular (N = 2), vaginal bleeding (N = 1), neutropenia (N = 1), and fistula (N = 1), with one grade 5 infection observed. Median PFS was 3.40 months. An ongoing phase III study in recurrent cervical cancer through the GOG is testing the efficacy of adding bevacizumab to chemotherapy, and patients are being randomized to one of four arms: (1) pacliltaxel and cisplatin, (2) paclitaxel/cisplatin and bevacizumab, (3) paclitaxel and topotecan, and (4) paclitaxel/topotecan and bevacizumab.[48] OS is the primary endpoint of this study.

Other oral TKIs have been tested in cervical cancer. Single-agent sunitinib was tested in 19 patients with locally advanced or metastatic cervical carcinoma.[49] No objective responses were observed but 84% of patients had SD (median duration, 4.4 months). Four patients developed fistulae while receiving sunitinib, and an additional patient developed a fistula 3.5 months after she had discontinued therapy. The authors concluded that the 26.3% rate of fistula formation was higher than expected and concerning and sunitinib as a single agent had insufficient activity to warrant further exploration of this drug in cervical cancer.

In a randomized phase II study testing the TKI pazopanib in advanced cervical cancer, pazopanib was given either alone or in combination with lapatinib, a combined inhibitor of EGFR and HER2.[50] Patients with measurable persistent or recurrent cervical carcinoma who had received at least one prior regimen in the metastatic setting were randomized in a ratio of 1:1:1 to pazopanib, 800 mg once daily, lapatinib, 1500 mg once daily, or a combination of lapatinib plus pazopanib in one of two regimens: lapatinib at 1000 mg plus pazopanib at 400 mg once daily; or lapatinib at 1500 mg plus pazopanib at 800 mg once daily. The primary end point was PFS. Interim analysis revealed an imbalance of toxicities in the combination arm and this arm was dropped. Median PFS for lapatinib was shorter compared with pazopanib (median PFS, 17.1 weeks vs 18.1 weeks; HR = 0.66; 90% CI, 0.48–0.91; P<.013). Grade 3 adverse events were 13% grade 3 diarrhea and 5% anemia in the lapatinib arm, 11% grade 3 diarrhea and 5% alkaline phosphatase elevation in the pazobanib arm, and 20% grade 3 diarrhea and 5% anemia in the combination arm. Grades 1 and 2 toxicities were not reported.

PARP INHIBITORS

One of the most promising advances in targeted therapy in ovarian cancer has been the discovery and use of PARP inhibitors. **Table 3** lists selected PARP inhibitors currently undergoing testing. These agents inhibit the enzyme PARP and work synergistically with the deficiencies of DNA repair seen in cancers occurring in patients with germline BRCA1 or BRCA2-mutations.[51] In addition, these agents also show activity in high-grade serous ovarian cancer in patients who do not harbor a germline BRCA1 or BRCA2 mutation likely because of the loss of BRCA function from deletion, somatic mutations, or methylation.[52]

Olaparib (AZD2281) is an oral PARP inhibitor that has undergone the most extensive investigation thus far of PARP inhibitors in ovarian cancer, in patients with germline BRCA mutations and in those with no mutations. Initial phase I testing of olaparib using doses from 10 mg orally daily 2 out of 3 weeks up to 600 mg twice a day dosed daily continuously demonstrated a maximally tolerated dose of 400 mg twice a day.[53] Clinical benefit was demonstrated in 12 of 19 patients who were BRCA carriers with ovarian, breast, or prostate cancer. **Table 4** lists selected studies of single-agent olaparib for the treatment of recurrent ovarian cancer, and phase II studies have demonstrated overall response rates up to 41% in patients with germline BRCA-1 or -2 associated cancers and 24% in sporadic high-grade serous cancers (HGSC) using the maximally tolerated dose of olaparib of 400 mg twice a day (capsule formulation).[54,55] Toxicities of olaparib include fatigue, nausea, vomiting, decreased appetite, and myelosuppression.

Table 3
List of selected PARP inhibitors currently in clinical trials

Name of Agent	Company	Route of Administration	Examples of Ongoing Studies
Olaparib (AZD2281) AZD2461	AstraZeneca	Both PO	Olaparib: single-agent studies and combination with chemotherapy AZ2461: single-agent phase I
MK4827	Merck	PO	Single-agent and in combination with chemotherapy
Veliparib (ABT888)	Abbott	PO	Combination with chemotherapy
Rucaparib (PF-01367338)	Clovis	PO, IV	Single-agent and combination studies with chemotherapy
CEP-9722	Cephalon	PO	Single-agent and in combination with chemotherapy
BMN673	BioMarin	PO	Single-agent
E7016	Eisai	PO	Combination with temozolomide

Olaparib has been compared with liposomal doxorubicin in patients who have recurrent ovarian cancer, a known germline BRCA mutation, and have never received pegylated liposomal doxorubicin (PLD).[56] Patients were randomized 1:1:1 to PLD; olaparib, 200 mg twice a day; or olaparib, 400 mg twice a day. No significant differences in PFS were observed between PLD and the combined olaparib arms.

Olaparib has also been explored as maintenance therapy after patients with platinum-sensitive recurrent ovarian HGSC attained a clinical remission after platinum-based chemotherapy.[57] After completion of platinum-based chemotherapy, patients were randomized to either placebo or olaparib, 400 mg twice a day, in this double-blinded study with PFS as the primary endpoint. There was a statistically significant difference between the PFS of the two groups in favor of olarapib compared with placebo (8.4 months vs 4.8 months; HR = 0.35; 95% CI, 0.25–0.49; $P<.00001$).

Olaparib has also been combined with chemotherapy and other studies are ongoing. In addition to PARP inhibitors, other agents are under development that inhibit various aspects of DNA repair pathways.[58]

HH PATHWAY INHIBITORS

The Hh pathway is one that plays a major role in cell differentiation, growth, and proliferation. Not surprisingly, it is involved in embryonic development and in adults presents a novel and potentially beneficial target for cancer therapy. There are several proteins in the signaling process of the Hh pathway including sonic Hh, Indian Hh, and desert Hh. The main extracellular receptor of the Hh pathway is PATCHED1 (PTCH1), a 12-pass transmembrane receptor on the surface of cells. Binding of Hh relieves the inhibitory effect of PTCH1 on SMOOTHENED (SMO), a seven-pass transmembrane domain protein and member of the G-protein–coupled receptor superfamily. Signal transduction by SMO leads to the activation and nuclear localization of GLI1 transcription factors and the induction of Hh target genes, many of which are involved in proliferation, survival, and angiogenesis. Mutated PTCH1 or SMO or overexpression of ligand can lead to uncontrolled cell proliferation.[59] Several Hh inhibitors are in development, but only a few have been tested in ovarian cancer.

Table 4
Results of selected olaparib trials in recurrent ovarian cancer

Study	No. of Patients	Study Design	Patient Population	Primary Outcome	Results
Audeh et al[54]	57	1st cohort: olaparib, 400 mg BID 2nd cohort: olaparib, 100 mg BID	All germline BRCA-1 or -2 mutation carriers	RR	33% RR for 400-mg BID dose 13% RR for 100-mg BID dose
Gelmon et al[55]	65	Phase II of olaparib, 400 mg BID	HGSC, ± germline BRCA mutation	RR	41% RR in germline mutation carriers 24% RR in patients without mutations
Kaye et al[56]	97	Randomized phase II to olaparib, 200 BID, 400 BID, or PLD 50 mg/m^2 (1:1:1 ratio)	All germline BRCA mutation carriers, recurrence within 12 mo of prior platinum, no prior anthra or PARP i	PFS	PFS not significant for olaparib arms vs PLD
Ledermann et al[57]	250	Phase II randomized, double-blinded to either olaparib or placebo. Both penultimate and most recent platinum regimen showed platinum sensitivity	± germline BRCA mutation. All patients had HGSC	PFS	8.4 mo (olaparib) vs 4.8 mo (placebo) ($P<.00001$)

Abbreviations: anthra, anthracycline; HGSC, high-grade serous cancers; PARP i, PARP inhibitor; PLD, pegylated liposomal doxorubicin; RR, response rate.

Ovarian Cancer

Ovarian cancer is the only gynecologic malignancy in which Hh inhibitors have been investigated. Part of the enthusiasm is because a large percentage of ovarian cancers showed Hh overexpression and there is an upregulation of a variety of Hh pathway components.[59] GDC-0449 is an orally bioavailable, well tolerated, and potent antagonist of the Hh pathway. This agent was recently evaluated as maintenance therapy for women with platinum-sensitive ovarian cancer who had achieved second or third remission.[60] One hundred and four women were randomized to GD-0449, 150 mg orally a day, versus placebo. Approximately 80% of women were in second remission. Median time to progression was 7.5 months for GDC-0449 versus 5.8 months for placebo (HR = 0.791; 95% CI, 0.463–1.353). Hh ligand expression in archival tissue was lower than expected with only 26% noted by immunohistochemistry or 13% by quantitative reverse-transcriptase polymerase chain reaction.[60] This low rate of Hh ligand expression may account for the relative lack of improvement with GDC-0449.

FR INHIBITORS

Folic acid is an essential vitamin and its metabolite folate is critical in the synthesis of nucleic acids and the methylation process. There is an increased expression of α-FR in a variety of malignancies including ovarian (90% of nonmucinous histologies), endometrial, and breast cancer. The reason for this is not entirely understood but may increase folate availability to rapidly dividing cells.[61]

There are several strategies to target the FR but leading approaches have been the development of anti–α-FR antibodies; conjugating chemotherapeutic agents to folate; or development of antifolate antineoplastic agents, such as pemetrexed (Alimta). Examples of agents in this class include farletuzumab (MORAb-003) and EC145. Farletuzumab is a monoclonal antibody to α-FR that activates cell- and complement-mediated cytotoxicity.[62] EC145 is a drug that is made from a conjugate of folate with a potent vica alkaloid, desacetylvinblastine hydrazide. In the bloodstream, EC145 is stable and only activated once taken into the cells by endocytosis by the membrane-bound FR. EC145 does not enter cells through the reduced folate carrier and as such is only active in cancer cells, thus theoretically minimizing toxicity. Pemetrexed, however, enters cells through the reduced folate carrier and is converted to a polyglutamated form that has an increased intracellular half-life in malignant cells and acts to inhibit folate-dependent enzymes with resultant interruption of DNA synthesis.

Ovarian Cancer

In a recent phase II trial evaluating 54 women with recurrent, platinum-sensitive ovarian cancer, farletuzumab was able to lengthen the second remission compared with the first.[63] Additionally, there is an ongoing phase III trial investigating carboplatin and paclitaxel with or without farletuzumab in women with first recurrence, platinum-sensitive ovarian cancer and a phase II trial of paclitaxel with and without farletuzumab in women with platinum-resistant or -refractory disease. Promising results were recently published for EC145. In a randomized phase II trial evaluating pegylated doxorubicin with or without EC145 in women with platinum-resistant ovarian cancer, the addition of EC145 improved PFS from 12 to 22 weeks (HR = 0.626; P = .03).[64] This was the first report of a randomized trial in platinum-resistant ovarian cancer where the experimental arm produced an increase in PFS. Mature survival data are pending to confirm the positive results. As part of the trial, optional scans with EC20, an imaging agent that identifies folate-positive tumors, were performed. Approximately 80% of patients were noted to have all or part of their tumors being folate positive. For those patients with folate-positive tumors, the improvement in PFS was even more dramatic (HR = 0.38; P = .018).[64] Pemetrexed has been evaluated as a single agent in platinum-resistant[65] and in combination with carboplatin[66] in platinum-sensitive recurrent ovarian cancer. As a single agent a response rate of 21% and PFS and OS of 2.9 months and 11.4 months were observed. When combined with platinum in platinum-sensitive patients, response rates were more than 50% (all PRs) and SD rates were 30%, whereas the median PFS was 7.57 months (95% CI, 6.44–10 months).

Endometrial Cancer

Pemetrexed has also been evaluated by the GOG in patients with advanced or recurrent endometrial carcinoma. Unfortunately, the activity seen in ovarian cancer was not duplicated in endometrial cancer. Twenty-five patients were treated using a dose of 900 mg/m^2 every 21 days. Seven patients (28%) received five or more cycles. It was well tolerated but grades 3 and 4 toxicities were seen including anemia (20%); leukopenia (40%); neutropenia (48%); and constitutional (16%). Unfortunately, only one patient (4%) had a PR and 11 patients (44%) had SD. Median PFS was 2.7 months and OS was 9.4 months. Based on these results, pemetrexed was deemed inactive and not pursued further in this disease.[67]

Cervical Cancer

Again, led by the GOG, twenty-seven women with recurrent or persistent cervical cancer were treated with pemetrexed, 900 mg/m^2 every 3 weeks. The treatments were well tolerated with similar toxicities as seen in the management of patients with endometrial cancer. Four patients (15%) had a PR and 16 (59%) had SD with a median response duration of 4.4 months. Response rates were different when comparing those who had and had not received prior radiation treatment, 7% versus 25%, respectively. Median PFS was 3.1 months and OS was 7.4 months. Because of the moderate activity seen in this trial combination therapies with pemetrexed are being pursued.[68] Very similar results were reported by the MITO group, who evaluated pemetrexed in patients with cervical cancer at a similar dose and schedule.[69]

EGFR INHIBITORS

EGF and its receptor (EGFR) have been well characterized. It has been shown to have altered expression and acts to increase proliferation and angiogenesis, and decrease apoptosis in a variety of cancers including lung, colon, head and neck, and pancreatic.[70] Mechanism for tumorigenesis include (1) ligand-independent tyrosine kinase activation of EGFR, usually the result of a constitutively active receptor mutant; (2) overexpression of ligand; and (3) overexpression of EGFR resulting from increased transcriptional, posttranscriptional mechanisms, or gene amplification.[71] Targeting EGFR with novel inhibitors, such as erlotinib or gefitinib, has resulted in modest clinical responses.[72] However, in the case of non–small cell lung cancer, a select population with EGFR tyrosine kinase domain mutations has been shown to have impressive responses.[73] In a variety of tumors, increased EGFR gene copy number has also been associated with response and OS.[74–76] Given the important role of this receptor in tumorigenesis, it has been a target of drug development.

There are two main strategies to target EGFR: monoclonal antibodies (trastuzumab, pertuzumab, and EMD7200) and small molecule TKIs (gefitinib, erlotinib, and lapatinib). These agents have been investigated in a variety of gynecologic malignancies but unlike the case with non–small cell lung cancer, it is unclear who may respond to these agents.

Ovarian Cancer

Both monoclonal antibodies and TKIs have been studied in women with recurrent ovarian cancer with generally disappointing results (**Table 5**).[77–84] It is possible that patients with EGFR amplification, EGFR mutation (rare), overexpression of pHER2, or low expression of HER3 may represent select populations more likely to respond to these drugs. Clinical trials focusing on these select populations are ongoing. Additionally, a new monoclonal antibody MM121, a human monoclonal antibody targeting ErbB3, is being combined with paclitaxel in a phase II trial in women with recurrent ovarian cancer (ClinicalTrials.gov identifier NCT01447706).

Endometrial Cancer

Erlotinib was evaluated in women with chemotherapy-naive, recurrent or metastatic endometrial cancer.[85] One prior line of hormonal therapy was permitted. Erlotinib was given at the standard dose of 150 mg orally a day. Thirty-two patients were assessable for response. There were 4 patients (12.5%) with confirmed PR lasting 2 to 36 months and 15 patients (47%) who had SD with a median duration of 3.7 months. The treatment was very well tolerated with the only grade 4 toxicity being elevated transaminases. EGFR expression was noted to be positive in 19 patients and negative in 9 patients. Three of the 19 patients with overexpression (16%) had a PR. There were no EGFR mutations identified, and there was no correlation with gene amplification and response. Comparatively, this response rate is similar to single-agent cytotoxic agents and suggests that erlotinib should be developed as an agent in future trials.

Cervical Cancer

Cetuximab has been studied fairly extensively in carcinoma of the cervix. In a GOG study, 35 women with recurrent, measurable, or persistent cervical cancer were treated with cetuximab, 400 mg/m^2 initial dose, followed by 250 mg/m^2 weekly. Nearly 90% of patients had received prior radiation treatment and one or two lines of chemotherapy. Cetuximab was well tolerated with minimal grade 3 toxicities, mainly dermatologic and GI. There were no clinical responses, whereas five patients (14.3%) remained progression free for at least 6 months. All of these patients had squamous cell histology. The median PFS and OS were 1.9 and 6.7 months, respectively.[86] When combining cetuximab with cisplatin in a similar patient population, responses remained limited: 9% in those who had received prior chemotherapy and 16% in those

Table 5
Recent clinical trials evaluating epidermal growth factor receptor inhibitor agents in the management of ovarian cancer

Study	Drug	N	RR (%)	SD (%)	PFS (mo)
Gordon et al[77]	Erlotinib	34	6	44	—
Schilder et al[78]	Gefitinib	27	4	14	2.1
Posadas et al[79]	Gefitinib	24	0	37	—
Wagner et al[80]	Gefitinib + tamoxifen	56	0	28.5	2
Bookman et al[81]	Trastuzumab	41	7.3	39	2
Seiden et al[82]	EMD72000	37	0	21	2
Gordon et al[83]	Pertuzumab	116	4.3	6.8	1.5
Secord et al[84]	Cetuximab + carbplatin	28	32	28	9.4

Abbreviations: RR, response rate; SD, stable disease; PFS, progression free survival.

who had not. When EGFR protein expression was analyzed, nearly all tumors were noted to be positive and there was a trend between the percentage of cells expressing EGFR protein and PFS.[87] Erlotinib has also been evaluated in patients with recurrent or persistent cervical cancer. With no objective responses, only four patients (15%) with SD, and only one patient (4%) progression free at 6 months, this drug was deemed inactive.[88]

Lapatinib is a dual anti-EGFR and anti-HER2/neu TKI that was recently studied in a randomized trial as a single agent versus the multitargeted antivascular agent pazopanib or in combination with pazopanib in women with measurable stage IV persistent or recurrent cervical cancer. The results of this study are described previously in the section on antiangiogenesis. The combination therapy arm was discontinued because of futility and toxicities, and single-agent lapatinib was inferior to pazopanib and had limited activity in this patient population.[50]

Vulvar Cancer

Previous studies, using immunohistochemistry, have demonstrated high levels of EGFR protein expression in vulvar squamous cell carcinomas and have correlated these with advanced stage, lymph node metastases, and survival.[89–91] Additionally, work by our group evaluated approximately 50 vulvar cancers with immunohisto-chemistry, fluorescence in situ hybridization, and mutational analysis. EGFR gene amplification and chromosome 7 high polysomy were observed in 12% and 6% of cases, respectively. Immunohistochemistry of malignant tissue with 3+ staining demonstrated a high sensitivity and specificity for identifying EGFR gene amplifica-tion.[92] Based on this background we initiated a phase II trial evaluating erlotinib in the management of women with squamous cell vulvar carcinoma. A total of 41 women were enrolled. The drug was well tolerated, with the major toxicities including renal failure, electrolyte abnormalities, rash, and diarrhea. An overall clinical benefit rate of 63% was observed with 23% having a PR and 40% SD that lasted a median of 8 weeks. Pretreatment and posttreatment tumor biopsies were evaluated for immuno-histochemistry expression of EGFR, gene amplification, and mutation analysis. All tumors had 2 to 3+ expression of EGFR. Four or nine patients were noted to have EGFR amplification (N = 3) or trisomy (N = 1). All the gene amplifications were noted in the posttreatment biopsies and all four had either a PR (N = 3) or SD (N = 1). There were no activating mutations identified.

PI3K/AKT PATHWAY INHIBITORS

The PI3K family phosphorylates the 3′-hydroxyl group of phosphoinositides. In the normal cell, the PI3K pathway allows cells to adapt to changes in the environment but is also one of the most commonly activated pathways in cancers.[93,94] AKT is a serine-threonine kinase that is directly activated in response to PI3K and is critical to the tumorigenic effect of the PI3K pathway. Activation of AKT directly leads to cancer cell growth, metabolism, and survival. One of the downstream effectors of AKT is mTORC1, which is controlled by a variety of environmental factors. Activation of mTORC1 leads to the increased translation of mRNAs that encode many cell cycle regulators that control cell progression from G1 to S-phase. Dysregulation of the PI3K/AKT pathway can happen by a variety of mechanisms but the two most commonly implicated are activation by receptor tyrosine kinase and somatic mutations of specific components of the signaling pathway, most notably the loss of the PTEN tumor suppressor gene or gain of function mutation in PI3KCA that encodes the catalytic subunit p110α. It is important to understand the multiple components of

PI3K/AKT pathway and the tight link between this pathway and others, such as RAS-Erk. This knowledge will allow the most effective therapeutic approach for new agents in this class and likely determine the clinical benefit from PI3K inhibition. **Table 6** lists selected inhibitors of the PI3K pathway that are in clinical trials.

Endometrial Cancer

Endometrial cancers have been the primary gynecologic malignancy targeted by PI3K/AKT inhibitors. This is not surprising when one considers that loss of PTEN is seen in greater than 50% of endometrial cancers, whereas other PI3K pathway activating mutations are seen in 25% to 30% of endometrial cancers. Although many of the agents listed in **Table 6** are beginning to enter into phase I and II clinical trials, the mTOR inhibitors are furthest along in development. As single agents, temsirolimus, deforolimus, and everolimus have shown limited responses rates between 0% and 14% depending on the amount of prior chemotherapy. Importantly, however, SD was achieved in 30% to 80% with median duration of approximately 4 months **(Table 7)**.[95–97] Across all studies, mTOR inhibitors were well tolerated with the predominate toxicities being fatigue; hematologic; and metabolic (cholesterol, triglycerides, and glucose control). To improve responses with temsirolimus, this agent is being combined with cytotoxic agents, such as carboplatin and paclitaxel; antiangiogenic agents, such as bevacizumab (GOG trial # 229G, ClinicalTrials.gov identifier: NCT00723255); or hormonal therapy, such as megace and tamoxifen (GOG trial #248, ClinicalTrials.gov identifier: NCT00729586).

Table 6
Selected PI3K pathway inhibitors under investigation in phase I/II clinical trials in gynecologic cancers

Inhibitor Type	Company
PI3K inhibitors	
XL-147	Exelixis
BKM 120	Novartis
GDC 0941	Genentech/Piramed/Roche
PX866	Oncothyreon
AKT inhibitors	
MK2206	Merck
GSK 2,141,795	GlaxoSmithKline
GDC-0068	Genentech
Perifosine	Keryx
mTOR inhibitors	
Temsirolimus	Wyeth
Everolimus	Novartis
Deforolimus	ARIAD
Dual PI3K and mTOR inhibitors	
BEZ- 235	Novartis
GDC-0980	Genentech
XL765	Exelixis
GSK 1,059,615	GlaxoSmithKline
PWT33597	Pathway Therapeutics

Table 7
Results of recent clinical trials evaluating mTOR inhibitors in recurrent endometrial cancer

Reference	Drug	Patient Population	Response Rate (%)	Stable Disease Rate (%)
Oza et al[96]	Temsirolimus (CCI-779)	Pretreated, all histologies	7.4	44
Oza et al[96]	Temsirolimus	Chemo-naive, all histologies	26	63
Slomovitz et al[95]	Everolimus (Rad001)	Pretreated, endometrioid only	0	44
Columbo et al[97]	Ridaforolimus (AP23573)	Pretreated, all histologies	7.4	34

FUTURE DIRECTIONS OF TARGETED THERAPIES FOR GYNECOLOGIC CANCERS

Molecular characterization of ovarian cancer, specifically ovarian HGSC, has led to the identification of potential molecular targets for new treatments. The Cancer Genome Atlas Project has investigated the messenger RNA expression, microRNA expression, promoter methylation, and DNA copy number in 489 HGSCs along with the DNA sequences of exons from coding genes[98]; similar efforts are underway in endometrial cancer. In this study, homologous recombination deficiency was found in approximately half of the cancers and that the NOTCH and FOXM1 signaling pathways are aberrant in HGSC. PARP inhibitors and other drugs that target defects in DNA repair are currently underway. Based on these Cancer Genome Atlas Project data, testing inhibitors of the NOTCH and FOXM1 signaling pathways in ovarian HGSC has rationale. In addition, low-level somatic mutations are found in HGSC, so molecular analysis of ovarian cancer samples for mutations in known oncogenes for which targeted therapies exist is warranted, thus increasing the therapeutic options available to patients.[99]

SUMMARY

The discovery of new biologic targeted agents and appropriately matching them to specific gynecologic tumor types either based on histology or the genetic make-up of the cancer is an exciting new chapter in the treatment of gynecologic malignancies. Therapeutic targets of multiple pathways are currently in study, and combinations with chemotherapy as well as combinations of pathway inhibitors are currently in development.

REFERENCES

1. Martin L, Schilder R. Novel approaches in advancing the treatment of epithelial ovarian cancer: the role of angiogenesis inhibition. J Clin Oncol 2007;25:2894–901.
2. Zhang L, Yang N, Garcia JR, et al. Generation of a syngeneic mouse model to study the effects of vascular endothelial growth factor in ovarian carcinoma. Am J Pathol 2002;161:2295–309.
3. Cooper BC, Ritchie JM, Broghammer CL, et al. Preoperative serum vascular endothelial growth factor levels: significance in ovarian cancer. Clin Cancer Res 2002;8:3193–7.

4. Hefler LA, Zeillinger R, Grimm C, et al. Preoperative serum vascular endothelial growth factor as a prognostic parameter in ovarian cancer. Gynecol Oncol 2006;103:512–7.
5. Burger RA, Sill MW, Monk BJ, et al. Phase II trial of bevacizumab in persistent or recurrent epithelial ovarian cancer or primary peritoneal cancer: a Gynecologic Oncology Group study. J Clin Oncol 2007;25:5165–71.
6. Cannistra SA, Matulonis UA, Penson RT, et al. Phase II study of bevacizumab in patients with platinum-resistant ovarian cancer or peritoneal serous cancer. J Clin Oncol 2007;5:5180–6.
7. Randall LM, Monk BJ. Bevacizumab toxicities and their management in ovarian cancer. Gynecol Oncol 2010;117:497–504.
8. Tew WP, Colombo N, Ray-Coquard I, et al. VEGF-Trap for patients with recurrent platinum-resistant epithelial ovarian cancer: preliminary results of a randomized, multicenter phase II study [abstract 5508]. In: Proceedings of the 2007 American Society of Clinical Oncology meeting.
9. Matulonis UA, Berlin S, Ivy P, et al. Cediranib, an oral inhibitor of vascular endothelial growth factor receptor kinases, is an active drug in recurrent epithelial ovarian, fallopian tube, and peritoneal cancer. J Clin Oncol 2009;27:5601–6.
10. Matei D, Sill MW, Lankes HA, et al. Activity of sorafenib in recurrent ovarian cancer and primary peritoneal carcinomatosis: a Gynecologic Oncology Group Trial. J Clin Oncol 2011;29:69–75.
11. Biagi JJ, Oza AM, Chalchal HI, et al. A phase II study of sunitinib in patients with recurrent epithelial ovarian and primary peritoneal carcinoma: an NCIC Clinical Trials Group study. Ann Oncol 2011;22:335–40.
12. Friedlander M, Hancock KC, Rischin D, et al. A phase II, open-label study evaluating pazopanib in patients with recurrent ovarian cancer. Gynecol Oncol 2010;119:32–7.
13. Matulonis U, Tew WP, Matei D, et al. A phase II study of ENMD2076 in platinum-resistant ovarian cancer [abstract 5021]. In: Proceedings of the 2011 American Society of Clinical Oncology meeting.
14. Vergote I, Sella A, Bedell C, et al. Phase II study of XL184 in a cohort of ovarian cancer patients with measurable soft tissue disease [abstract 407]. Proceedings of the 22nd EORTC-NCI-AACR Symposium on Molecular Targets and Cancer Therapeutics conference. 2010.
15. Ledermann JA, Hackshaw A, Kaye S, et al. Randomized phase II placebo-controlled trial of maintenance therapy using the oral triple angiokinase inhibitor BIBF 1120 after chemotherapy for relapsed ovarian cancer. J Clin Oncol 2011;29:3798–804.
16. Matulonis UA. Bevacizumab and its use in epithelial ovarian cancer. Future Oncol 2011;7:365–79.
17. Burger RA. Overview of anti-angiogenic agents in development for ovarian cancer. Gynecol Oncol 2011;121:230–8.
18. Garcia AA, Hirte H, Fleming G, et al. Phase II clinical trial of bevacizumab and low-dose metronomic oral cyclophosphamide in recurrent ovarian cancer: a trial of the California, Chicago, and Princess Margaret Hospital phase II consortia. J Clin Oncol 2008;26:76–82.
19. Penson RT, Dizon DS, Cannistra SA, et al. Phase II study of carboplatin, paclitaxel, and bevacizumab with maintenance bevacizumab as first-line chemotherapy for advanced mullerian tumors. J Clin Oncol 2010;28:154–9.
20. Rose PG, Drake R, Braly PS, et al. Preliminary results of a phase II study of oxaliplatin, docetaxel, and bevacizumab as first-line therapy of advanced cancer of

the ovary, peritoneum, and fallopian tube [abstract 5546]. In: Proceedings of the 2009 American Society of Clinical Oncology meeting.

21. Tillmanns TD, Lowe MP, Schwartzberg LS, et al. A phase II study of bevacizumab with nab-paclitaxel in patients with recurrent, platinum-resistant primary epithelial ovarian or primary peritoneal carcinoma [abstract 5009]. In: Proceedings of the 2010 American Society of Clinical Oncology meeting.

22. Raja FA, Griffin CL, Qian W, et al. Initial toxicity assessment of ICON6: a randomised trial of cediranib plus chemotherapy in platinum-sensitive relapsed ovarian cancer. Br J Cancer 2011;105:884–9.

23. Coleman RL, Duska LR, Ramirez PT, et al. Phase 1–2 study of docetaxel plus aflibercept in patients with recurrent ovarian, primary peritoneal, or fallopian tube cancer. Lancet Oncol 2011;12(12):1109–17.

24. Karlan BY, Oza AM, Hansen VL, et al. Randomized, double-blind, placebo-controlled phase II study of AMG 386 combined with weekly paclitaxel in patients with recurrent ovarian carcinoma [abstract 5000]. In: Proceedings of the 2010 American Society of Clinical Oncology meeting.

25. NCT00390611. Paclitaxel and carboplatin with or without sorafenib in the first-line treatment of patients with ovarian cancer. Available at: http://www.clinicaltrials.gov/ct2/show/NCT00390611. Accessed November 15, 2011.

26. Burger RA, Brady MF, Bookman MA, et al. Phase III trial of bevacizumab (BEV) in the primary treatment of advanced epithelial ovarian cancer (EOC), primary peritoneal cancer (PPC), or fallopian tube cancer (FTC): a Gynecologic Oncology Group study [abstract LBA1]. In: Proceedings of the 2010 American Society of Clinical Oncology meeting.

27. Perren T, Swart AM, Pfisterer J, et al. ICON7: a phase III randomised Gynaecologic Cancer Intergroup trial of concurrent bevacizumab and chemotherapy followed by maintenance bevacizumab, versus chemotherapy alone in women with newly diagnosed epithelial ovarian cancer, primary peritoneal cancer or fallopian tube cancer [abstract LBA4]. In: Proceedings of the 2010 European Society of Medical Oncology meeting.

28. Kristensen GB, Perren T, Qian W, et al. Result of interim analysis of overall survival in the GCIG ICON7 phase III randomized trial of bevacizumab in women with newly diagnosed ovarian cancer [abstract LBA 5006]. In: Proceedings of the 2011 American Society of Clinical Oncology meeting.

29. NCT01015118. BIBF 1120 or placebo in combination with paclitaxel and carboplatin in first line treatment of ovarian cancer. Available at: http://www.clinicaltrials.gov/ct2/show/NCT01015118. Accessed November 15, 2011.

30. NCT00866697. Efficacy and safety of pazopanib monotherapy after first line chemotherapy in ovarian, fallopian tube, or primary peritoneal cancer. Available at: http://www.clinicaltrials.gov/ct2/show/NCT00866697. Accessed November 15, 2011.

31. NCT00951496. Bevacizumab and intravenous or intraperitoneal chemotherapy in treating patients with stage II, stage III, or stage IV ovarian epithelial cancer, fallopian tube cancer, or primary peritoneal cancer. Available at: http://www.clinicaltrials.gov/ct2/show/NCT00951496. Accessed November 15, 2011.

32. NCT01167712. Paclitaxel and carboplatin with or without bevacizumab in treating patients with stage III or stage IV ovarian epithelial cancer, primary peritoneal cancer, or fallopian tube cancer. Available at: http://www.clinicaltrials.gov/ct2/show/NCT01167712. Accessed November 15, 2011.

33. Aghajanian C, Finkler NJ, Rutherford T, et al. OCEANS: a randomized, double-blinded, placebo-controlled phase III trial of chemotherapy with or without bevacizumab in patients with platinum-sensitive recurrent epithelial ovarian, primary

peritoneal, or fallopian tube cancer [abstract LBA 5007]. In: Proceedings of the 2011 American Society of Clinical Oncology meeting.

34. NCT00565851. Carboplatin and paclitaxel with or without bevacizumab after surgery in treating patients with recurrent ovarian epithelial cancer, primary peritoneal cavity cancer, or fallopian tube cancer. Available at: http://www.clinicaltrials.gov/ct2/show/NCT00565851. Accessed November 15, 2011.

35. NCT00544973. An RCT of concurrent and maintenance cediranib in women with platinum-sensitive relapsed ovarian cancer (ICON6). Available at: http://www.clinicaltrials.gov/ct2/show/NCT00544973. Accessed November 15, 2011.

36. NCT01204749. TRINOVA-1: a study of AMG386 or placebo, in combination with weekly paclitaxel chemotherapy, as treatment for ovarian cancer, primary peritoneal cancer and fallopian tube cancer. Available at: http://www.clinicaltrials.gov/ct2/show/NCT01204749. Accessed November 15, 2011.

37. Kamat AA, Merritt WM, Coffey D, et al. Clinical and biological significance of vascular endothelial growth factor in endometrial cancer. Clin Cancer Res 2007;13:7487–95.

38. Aghajanian C, Sill MW, Darcy KM, et al. Phase II trial of bevacizumab in recurrent or persistent endometrial cancer: a Gynecologic Oncology Group study. J Clin Oncol 2011;29:2259–65.

39. Correa R, Mackay H, Hirte HW, et al. A phase II study of sunitinib in recurrent or metastatic endometrial carcinoma: a trial of the Princess Margaret Hospital, The University of Chicago, and California Cancer Phase II Consortia [abstract 5038]. In: Proceedings of the 2010 American Society of Clinical Oncology meeting.

40. Nimeiri HS, Oza AM, Morgan RJ, et al. A phase II study of sorafenib in advanced uterine carcinoma/carcinosarcoma: a trial of the Chicago, PMH, and California Phase II Consortia. Gynecol Oncol 2010;117:37–40.

41. McMeekin DS, Sill MW, Benbrook D, et al. A phase II trial of thalidomide in patients with refractory endometrial cancer and correlation with angiogenesis biomarkers: a Gynecologic Oncology Group study. Gynecol Oncol 2007;105:508–16.

42. Cheng WF, Chen CA, Lee CN, et al. Vascular endothelial growth factor and prognosis of cervical carcinoma. Obstet Gynecol 2000;96:721–6.

43. Cooper R, Logue J, Davidson S, et al. Vascular endothelial growth factor (VEGF) expression is a prognostic factor for radiotherapy outcome in advanced carcinoma of the cervix. Br J Cancer 2000;83:620–5.

44. Guidi AJ, Abu-Jawdeh G, Berse B, et al. Vascular permeability factor (vascular endothelial growth factor) expression and angiogenesis in cervical neoplasia. J Natl Cancer Inst 1995;87:1237–45.

45. Toussaint-Smith E, Donner DB, Roman A. Expression of human papillomavirus type 16 E6 and E7 oncoproteins in primary foreskin keratinocytes is sufficient to alter the expression of angiogenic factors. Oncogene 2004;23:2988–95.

46. López-Ocejo O, Viloria-Petit A, Bequet-Romero M, et al. Oncogenes and tumor angiogenesis: the HPV-16 E6 oncoprotein activates the vascular endothelial growth factor (VEGF) gene promoter in a p53 independent manner. Oncogene 2000;19:4611–20.

47. Monk BJ, Sill MW, Burger RA, et al. Phase II study of bevacizumab in the treatment of persistent or recurrent squamous cell carcinoma of the cervix: a Gynecologic Oncology Group. J Clin Oncol 2009;27:1069–74.

48. NCT00803062. Paclitaxel and cisplatin or topotecan with or without bevacizumab in treating patients with stage IVB, recurrent, or persistent cervical cancer. Available at: http://www.clinicaltrials.gov/ct2/show/NCT00803062. Accessed November 15, 2011.

49. Mackay HJ, Tinker A, Winquist E, et al. A phase II study of sunitinib in patients with locally advanced or metastatic cervical carcinoma: NCIC CTG Trial IND.184. Gynecol Oncol 2009;116:163–7.

50. Monk BJ, Mas Lopez L, Zarba JJ, et al. Phase II, open-label study of pazopanib or lapatinib monotherapy compared with pazopanib plus lapatinib combination therapy in patients with advanced and recurrent cervical cancer. J Clin Oncol 2010;28:3562–9.

51. Iglehart JD, Silver DP. Synthetic lethality: a new direction in cancer-drug development. N Engl J Med 2009;361:189–91.

52. Hennessy B, Timms KM, Carey MS, et al. Somatic mutations in BRCA1 and BRCA2 could expand the number of patients that benefit from poly (ADP Ribose) polymerase inhibitors in ovarian cancer. J Clin Oncol 2010;28:3570–6.

53. Fong PC, Boss DS, Yap TA, et al. Inhibition of poly (ADP-ribose) polymerase in tumors from BRCA-carriers. N Engl J Med 2009;361:123–34.

54. Audeh MW, Carmichael J, Penson RT, et al. Oral poly(ADP-ribose) polymerase inhibitor olaparib in patients with BRCA1 or BRCA2 mutations and recurrent ovarian cancer: a proof-of-concept trial. Lancet 2010;376:245–51.

55. Gelmon KA, Tischkowitz M, Mackay H, et al. Olaparib in patients with high grade serous or poorly differentiated ovarian carcinoma or triple negative breast cancer: a phase 2, multicenter, open-label, non-randomized study. Lancet Oncol 2011;12:852–61.

56. Kaye SB, Lubinski J, Matulonis U, et al. A phase II, open-label, randomized, multi-center study to compare the efficacy and safety of olaparib, a poly(ADP-ribose) polymerase (PARP) inhibitor, and pegylated liposomal doxorubicin (PLD) in patients with BRCA1 or BRCA2 mutations and recurrent ovarian cancer. J Clin Oncol, in press.

57. Ledermann JA, Harter P, Gourley C, et al. Phase II randomized placebo-controlled study of olaparib (AZD2281) in patients with platinum-sensitive relapsed serous ovarian cancer [abstract 5003]. In: Proceedings of the 2011 American Society of Clinical Oncology meeting.

58. Plummer R. Perspective on the pipeline of drugs being developed with modulation of DNA damage as a target. Clin Cancer Res 2010;16:4527–31.

59. Bhattacharya R, Kwon J, Ali B, et al. Role of hedgehog signaling in ovarian cancer. Clin Cancer Res 2008;14(23):7659–66.

60. Kaye S, Fehrenbacher L, Holloway R, et al. A phase 2, randomized, placebo-controlled study of hedgehog pathway inhibitor GDC-0449 as maintenance therapy in patients with ovarian cancer in 2nd and 3rd complete remission. Late breaking [abstract 25]. In: Proceedings of the 2010 European Society of Medical Oncology.

61. Elnakat H, Ratnam M. Role of folate receptor genes in reproduction and related cancers. Front Biosci 2006;11:506–19.

62. Ebel W, Routhier EL, Foley B, et al. Preclinical evaluation of MORAb-003, a humanized monoclonal antibody antagonizing folate recetor-alpha. Cancer Immun 2007;7:6–13.

63. Armstrong DK, Bicher R, Coleman RL, et al. Exploratory phase II efficacy study of MORAb-003, a monoclonal antibody against folate receptor alpha in platinum sensitive ovarian cancer in first relapse [abstract 5500]. In: Proceedings of the 2008 American Society of Clinical Oncology meeting.

64. Naumann RW, Coleman RL, Burger RA, et al. PRECEDENT: a randomized phase II trial comparing EC145 and pegylated liposomal doxorubicin (PLD) in combination, versus PLD alone in subjects with platinum-resistant ovarian cancer [abstract #5045]. In: Proceedings of the 2011 American Society of Clinical Oncology meeting.

65. Miller DS, Blessing JA, Krasner CN, et al. Phase II evaluating pemetrexed in the treatment of recurrent or persistent platinum-resistant ovarian cancer or primary peritoneal carcinoma: a Gynecologic Oncology Group study. J Clin Oncol 2009;27:2686–91.

66. Matulonis UA, Horowitz NS, Campos SM, et al. Phase II study of carboplatin and pemetrexed for the treatment of platinum-sensitive ovarian cancer. J Clin Oncol 2008;26:5761–6.

67. Miller DS, Blessing JA, Drake RD, et al. A phase II evaluation of pemetrexed (Alimta, LY231514, IND#40061) in the treatment of recurrent or persistent endometrial cancer: a phase II study of the Gynecologic Oncology Group. Gynecol Oncol 2009;115:443–6.

68. Miller DS, Blessing JA, Bodurka DC, et al. Evaluation of pemetrexed (Alimta, LY231514) as second line chemotherapy in persistent or recurrent carcinoma of the cervix: a phase II study of the Gynecologic Oncology Group. Gynecol Oncol 2008;110:65–70.

69. Lorusso D, Ferrandina G, Pignata S, et al. Evaluation of pemetrexed (Alimta, LY231514) as second line chemotherapy in persistent or recurrent carcinoma of the cervix: the CERVIX 1 study of the MITO (Multicentre Italian Trials in Ovarian Cancer and Gynecologic Malignancies) Group. Ann Oncol 2010;21(1):61–6.

70. Ciardiello F, Tortora G. EGFR antagonists in cancer treatment. N Engl J Med 2008; 358:1160–74.

71. Grandal MV, Madshus IH. Epidermal growth factor receptor and cancer: control of oncogenic signaling by endocytosis. J Cell Mol Med 2008;12:1527–34.

72. Baselga J, Arteaga CL. Critical update and emerging trends in epidermal growth factor receptor targeting in cancer. J Clin Oncol 2005;23:2445–59.

73. Janne PA, Engelman JA, Johnson BE. Epidermal growth factor receptor mutations in non small cell lung cancer: implications for treatment and tumor biology. J Clin Oncol 2005;23:3227–34.

74. Hirsch FR, Herbst RS, Olsen C, et al. Increased EGFR gene copy number detected by fluorescent in situ hybridization predicts outcome in non small cell lung cancer patients treated with cetuximab and chemotherapy. J Clin Oncol 2008;26:3351–7.

75. Moroni M, Veronese S, Benvenuti S, et al. Gene copy number for epidermal growth factor receptor (EGFR) and clinical response to antiEGFR treatment in colorectal cancer: a cohort study. Lancet Oncol 2005;6:279–86.

76. Chung CH, Ely K, McGazvran L, et al. Increased epidermal growth factor receptor gene copy number is associated with poor prognosis in head and neck squamous cell carcinomas. J Clin Oncol 2006;24:4170–6.

77. Gordon AN, Finkler N, Edward RP, et al. Efficacy and safety of eroltinib HCL, and epidermal growth factor receptor (HER1/EGFR) tyrosine kinase inhibitor in patients with advanced ovarian cancer: results of a phase II multicenter study. Int J Gynecol Cancer 2005;15:785–92.

78. Schilder RJ, Sill MW, Chen X, et al. Phase II study of gefitinib in patients with relapsed or persistent ovarian cancer or primary peritoneal carcinoma and evaluation of epidermal growth factor receptor mutations and immunohistochemical expression: a Gynecologic Oncology Group study. Clin Cancer Res 2005;11:5539–48.

79. Posadas EM, Liel MS, Kwitkowski V, et al. A phase II and pharmocodynamic study of gefitinib in patients with refractory or recurrent epithelial ovarian cancer. Cancer 2007;109:1323–30.

80. Wagner U, du bois A, Pfisterer J, et al. Gefitinib in combination with tamoxifen in patients with ovarian cancer refractory or resistant to platinum-taxane based

therapy: a phase II trial of the AGO Ovarian Cancer Study Group (AGO-OVAR 2.6). Gynecol Oncol 2007;105:132–7.

81. Bookman MA, Darcy KM, Clarke-Pearson D, et al. Evaluation of monoclonal humanized anti-HER2 antibody, trastuzumab, in patients with recurrent or refractory ovarian or primary peritoneal carcinoma with overexpression of HER2: a phase II trial of the Gynecologic Oncology group. J Clin Oncol 2003;21:283–90.

82. Seiden MV, Burris HA, Matulonis U, et al. A phase II trial of EMD72000 (matuzumab), humanized anti EGFR monoclonal antibody, in patients with platinum-resistant ovarian and primary peritoneal malignancies. Gynecol Oncol 2007; 104:727–31.

83. Gordon MS, Matei D, Aghajanian C, et al. Clinical activity of pertuzumab (rhuMAB 2C4), a HER dimerization inhibitor in advanced ovarian cancer: potential predictive relationship with tumor HER2 activation status. J Clin Oncol 2006;24(26): 4324–32.

84. Secord AA, Blessing JA, Armstrong DK, et al. Phase II trial of cetuximab and carboplatin in relapsed platinum-sensitive ovarian cancer and evaluation of epidermal growth factor receptor expression: a Gynecologic Oncology Group trial. Gynecol Oncol 2008;108:493–9.

85. Oza AM, Eisenhauer EA, Elit L, et al. Phase II study of erlotinib in recurrent or metastatic endometrial cancer: NCIC IND-148. J Clin Oncol 2008;26:4319–25.

86. Santin AD, Sill MW, McMeekin DS, et al. Phase II trial of cetuximab in the treatment of persistent or recurrent squamous or non-squamous cell carcinoma of the cervix: a Gynecologic Oncology Group study. Gynecol Oncol 2011;122: 495–500.

87. Farley J, Sill MW, Birrer M, et al. Phase II study of cisplatin plus cetuximab in advanced, recurrent, and previously treated cancers of the cervix and evaluation of epidermal growth factor receptor immunohistochemical expression; a Gynecologic Oncology Group study. Gynecol Oncol 2011;121:303–8.

88. Schilder RJ, Sill MW, Lee YC, et al. A phase II trial of erlotinib in recurrent squamous cell carcinoma of the cervix: a Gynecologic Oncology Group study. Int J Gynecol Cancer 2009;19:929–33.

89. Johnson GA, Mannel R, Khalifa M, et al. Epidermal growth factor receptor in vulvar malignancies and its relationship to metastasis and patient survival. Gynecol Oncol 1997;65:425–9.

90. Oonk MH, de Bock GH, van der Veen DJ, et al. EGFR expression is associated with groin node metastases in vulvar cancer but does not improve their prediction. Gynecol Oncol 2007;104:109–13.

91. Berchuck A, Rodriguez G, Kamel A, et al. Expression of epidermal growth factor receptor and HER-2/new in normal and neoplastic cervix, vulva, and vagina. Obstet Gynecol 1990;76:381–7.

92. Growdon WB, Boisvert SL, Akhavanfard S, et al. Decreased survival in EGFR gene amplified vulvar carcinoma. Gynecol Oncol 2008;111:289–97.

93. Emerling BM, Akcakanat A. Targeting PI3K/mTOR signaling in cancer. AACR Meeting Report. Cancer Res 2011. [Epub ahead of print].

94. Engelman JA. Targeting PI3K signaling in cancer: opportunities, challenges, and limitations. Nat Rev Cancer 2009;9:550–62.

95. Slomovitz BM, Lu KH, Johnston T, et al. Target of rapamycin inhibitor, everolimus, in patients with recurrent endometrial carcinoma. Cancer 2010;116:5415–9.

96. Oza AM, Elit L, Tsao MS, et al. Phase II study of temsirolimus in women with recurrent or metastatic endometrial cancer: a trial of the NCIC Clinical Trials Group. J Clin Oncol 2011;29:3278–385.

97. Colombo N, McMeekin S, Schwartz P, et al. A phase II trial of the mTOR inhibitor AP23573 as a single agent in advanced endometrial cancer [abstract 5516]. In: Proceedings of the 2007 American Society of Clinical Oncology meeting.

98. Cancer Genome Atlas Research Network. Integrated genomic analyses of ovarian carcinoma. Nature 2011;474:609–15.

99. Matulonis UA, Hirsch M, Palescandolo E, et al. High throughput interrogation of somatic mutations in high grade serous cancer of the ovary. PLoS One 2011; 6(9):e24433.

Advances in the Use of Radiation for Gynecologic Cancers

Akila N. Viswanathan, MD, MPH

KEYWORDS

• Gynecologic cancer • Cervical cancer • Vulvar cancer
• Radiation • Endometrial cancer

Radiation is an important component in the curative management of malignancies of the gynecologic tract, in particular cervical, vulvar, vaginal, and endometrial cancers.[1] Although ovarian cancer has historically shown significant clinical response to radiation, the toxicity rates with the requisite radiation to the whole abdomen, coupled with improvements in chemotherapy and the integration of paclitaxel-based regimens, have limited the role of radiation in ovarian cancer in the United States to patients with recurrent disease.[2] The development and integration of highly refined radiologic imaging has resulted in more precise tumor targeting, thereby reducing dose to normal tissues while escalating the dose to the target. In addition, the integration of concurrent chemotherapy as a radiation sensitizer has significantly improved survival rates in gynecologic cancers and is one of the most important shifts in cancer management in the past century.

CERVICAL CANCER

The successful treatment of cervical cancer with radiation began approximately 100 years ago, demonstrating a long record of success in the postoperative setting and for patients with inoperable disease. Careful assessment of the extent of disease via a manual examination, including rectovaginal palpation of the parametrial and uterosacral ligaments, is required for International Federation of Gynecology and Obstetrics (FIGO) staging. In the United States, radiologic imaging, such as magnetic resonance imaging (MRI) and positron emission tomography (PET) scans, at diagnosis may provide additional information about the extent of disease spread. Patients with MRI evidence of parametrial or vaginal involvement receive radiation, whereas those with cervical cancers smaller than 4 cm with no adjacent parametrial or vaginal invasion may be candidates for a radical hysterectomy. PET scan evidence of nodal involvement similarly is related to prognosis.[3]

Department of Radiation Oncology, Brigham and Women's Hospital, 75 Francis Street, ASB 1, L2, Boston, MA 02115, USA
E-mail address: aviswanathan@lroc.harvard.edu

Hematol Oncol Clin N Am 26 (2012) 157–168
doi:10.1016/j.hoc.2011.11.004
0889-8588/12/$ – see front matter © 2012 Elsevier Inc. All rights reserved.
hemonc.theclinics.com

Postoperative Radiation for Cervical Cancer

Patients with early-stage (FIGO IA–IB1) cervical cancer with no evident nodal spread on PET imaging may undergo a radical hysterectomy with bilateral complete lymphadenectomy. One randomized trial of 469 patients compared outcomes for patients with stages IB-IIA cervical cancer treated with either external beam radiation therapy (EBRT) or with a radical hysterectomy.[4] Due to adverse features, 54% of the stage IB1 and 84% of the stage IB2 postoperative patients required adjuvant radiation. Although overall survival was 83% for both arms, there was a significant difference in toxicity (28% vs 12%; $P = .0004$), favoring the radiation arm. The primary toxicity was an increase in small-bowel obstruction in patients who had a lymphadenectomy. Therefore, the combination of a radical hysterectomy and postoperative radiation places patients at a higher risk of complications than single-modality therapy. To date, no randomized trial has compared concurrent chemotherapy with radiation to radical hysterectomy for early-stage disease. Younger patients are more likely to choose surgery to preserve ovarian function.

Postoperatively, prognostic factors may categorize cases into high-risk, intermediate-risk, or low-risk disease. Low-risk disease, with tumors less than 4 cm at diagnosis and no other adverse features, does not require adjuvant radiation. Intermediate-risk cervical cancers have lymphovascular invasion (LVI), deep stromal invasion, large tumor size, or a combination of these. Intermediate-risk patients benefit from postoperative EBRT.[5] After a follow-up of approximately 10 years, a 46% reduction in the risk of recurrence was seen in patients who received postoperative radiation. There was a 30% improvement in overall survival with the use of radiation ($P = .07$) but also an increase in grades 3 and 4 toxicity by 4.5%.[5] Whether concurrent chemotherapy with radiation may be of benefit to postoperative cervical cancer patients with intermediate risk factors is the focus of a randomized trial currently accruing patients.

High-risk features in the postoperative setting include positive lymph nodes, positive margins at the resection edge, and parametrial spread. A randomized trial demonstrated a 10% overall survival advantage with the use of platinum-based concurrent chemoradiation in patients with high-risk disease and this remains the standard of care.[6] A currently accruing randomized trial is assessing the efficacy of carboplatin and paclitaxel chemotherapy after concurrent chemoradiation in this population.

Patients treated with radiation postoperatively may receive EBRT with a 3-D conformal, CT-planned, 4-field approach, sparing small bowel as much as possible with patients simulated in the prone position on a belly board.[7] Alternatively, they may be treated with intensity-modulated radiation (IMRT). As a highly conformal novel technique using multiple (5 or more) beams and dynamic integration of blocking IMRT creates a region of dose covering the target that may spare adjacent normal tissues more than 3-D conformal radiation. Issues with IMRT in the postoperative setting include a potential for a higher integral dose, longer daily treatments, and an increase in complexity requiring more stringent quality assurance measures. Most centers in the United States prescribe female pelvic EBRT 1.8 Gy per day for 25 fractions to a total dose of 45 Gy. The use of vaginal brachytherapy (BT) after EBRT is dependent on the cumulative EBRT dose and the presence of high-risk features, such as LVI or nodal involvement.

Locally Advanced Disease

Patients with inoperable cervical cancer (stages IB2–IVA) are treated curatively with a combination of EBRT and intrauterine BT. BT is a highly specialized and conformal method of escalating radiation dose directly in the center of the tumor. The use of BT in addition to EBRT reduces the pelvic relapse rate and improves local control as well as survival.[8,9]

For the past 10 years, concurrent chemotherapy with radiation has been recommended for all locally advanced cases. In 1999, the National Cancer Institute in the United States released a nationwide clinical alert to all physicians that, due to a significant survival advantage seen with concurrent platinum-based chemotherapy during radiation, this approach would be the new standard of care for cervical cancer patients with FIGO stages IB through IVA. Only one of the reported trials was negative; this not only was the smallest of the studies but also had a high proportion of patients with early-stage disease (**Table 1**). A meta-analysis demonstrated a 12% increase in overall survival with the use of concurrent chemotherapy administered as a radiation sensitizer.[10]

Cisplatin is both cytotoxic and supra-additive with radiation; it inhibits the repair of sublethal and potentially lethal radiation injury by altering DNA repair and enhancing apoptosis. Although the most successful randomized studies combined 5-fluorouracil (5-FU) with cisplatin, the necessity of 5-FU has come into question.[6,11] One trial with 5-FU alone as a radiosensitizer was closed after a high number of recurrences were seen. Most recently, a randomized trial adding weekly gemcitabine to cisplatin during radiation, then adding 4 cycles of cisplatin and gemcitabine after radiation, showed a significant improvement in overall survival and progression-free survival at 3 years (74% vs 65%) compared with weekly cisplatin alone.[12] Similar studies using weekly cisplatin alone but adding outback chemotherapy will be conducted in the near future. In the United States, the most accepted regimen remains weekly cisplatin (40 mg/m^2) on average for 5–6 doses with external beam radiation.

To optimally deliver radiation, all treatment must be completed within 56 days from initiation.[13] Patients should be carefully evaluated by a radiation oncologist, with a clinical examination, detailed history, and assessment of laboratory studies, including complete blood cell count and creatinine test to assess renal function. Patients with hydronephrosis, as seen on CT imaging, may require ureteral stenting by a urologist before simulation. For patients who have negative para-aortic nodes after either imaging or surgical staging evaluation, simulation of the pelvic region may include either anteroposterior-posteroanterior or a 4-field approach, including anterior, posterior, and 2 lateral fields, with blocking to protect the adjacent small bowel, skin, and bone marrow. For women with an intact cervix, IMRT has a high risk of missing the target, given the movement of the cervix, bladder, and bowel; caution is required with IMRT, given the large (≥2 cm) margins necessary around the cervix and uterus.[14,15] For patients with positive para-aortic nodes, extended-field IMRT may assist in reducing the dose of radiation to the small bowel and kidneys.

Image-Guided Brachytherapy for Cervical Cancer

BT is an ideal modality for dose-escalating radiation directly to the center of the tumor. In contrast to EBRT, the BT applicator moves with the organ, delivers low doses of radiation to surrounding normal tissues (given the rapid dose fall-off of the radioactive sources) and may be repositioned based on tumor regression during treatment. The integration of 3-D imaging in radiation treatment planning during the 1990s resulted in early feasibility studies incorporating MRI[16] and CT[17,18] to aid with insertion and BT treatment planning (**Fig. 1**). A survey of physicians in the United States indicated that more than 50% are using CT imaging after BT insertion.[19] In Europe, a larger proportion has incorporated MRI after applicator insertion.[20] Institutional data indicate that imaging with MRI during BT and planning using 3-D–based contours[21,22] may result in a survival benefit compared with the plain-film-radiograph–based planning

Table 1
Randomized trials of chemoradiation for cervical cancer

			Phase III RCTs of Chemoradiation Therapy for Cervical Cancer				
Trial	Stage	No. of Patients	Arms	F/U	OS	DFS	LRF
GOG 85/SWOG 8695[48]	IIB–	368	RT + HU (C)	8.7 y	43%	47%	30%
	IVA		RT + CIS + FU	8.7 y	65% (P = .018)	57% (P = .033)	25% (P = NR)
RTOG 90-01[11]	IB2–	386	RT (C)	6.6 y	41%	36%	35%
	IVA		RT + CIS + FU	8 y	67% (P<.001)	61% (P<.001)	18% (P<.001)
GOG 120[49]	IIB–	526	RT + HU (C)	8.8 y	34%	26%	34%
	IVA		RT + CIS	10 y	53% (P<.001)	46% (P<.001)	22%
			RT + CIS + FU + HU		53% (P<.001)	43% (P<.001)	(P = .014)
							21%
							(P = .009)
GOG 123[50]	IB2	369	RT + H (C)	3 y	74%	63%	21%
			RT + CIS + H	3 y	83% (P = .008)	79% (P<.001)	9% (P = NR)
GOG 109/SWOG 8797[6]	IA2–	243	H + RT (C)	3.5 y	71%	63%	17%
	IIA		H + RT + CIS + FU	4 y	81% (P = .007)	80% (P = .003)	5.5% (P = NR)
NCIC[51]	IB–	253	RT (C)	6.8 y	58%	62%	33%
	IVA		RT + CIS	5 y	62% (P = .42)	64% (P = .33)	27% (P = NR)

Abbreviations: F/U, follow-up given as median; (C), control; CIS, cisplatin; DFS, disease-free survival; FU, fluorouracil; H, hysterectomy; HU, hydroxyurea; LRF, locoregional failure; NR, not reported; OS, overall survival; RCT, randomized controlled trial; RT, radiation therapy.

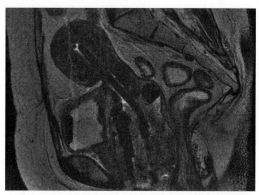

Fig. 1. MRI-guided tandem and ring placement providing anatomic detail of the cervix and normal tissues.

and point dosimetry traditionally used for cervical cancer BT.[23] Future work incorporating MRI and PET imaging into cervical cancer BT may result in optimizing dose while concomitantly reducing the dose to the adjacent normal tissue.[1]

ENDOMETRIAL CANCER

Endometrial cancer has a high survival rate compared with other gynecologic malignancies, due to its early presentation and ease of detection. Most patients with endometrial cancer present with stage I disease. When medically feasible, primary treatment consists of surgical staging, involving total abdominal hysterectomy, bilateral salpingo-oophorectomy, peritoneal washings for cytology, and consideration of pelvic and para-arotic lymph node sampling or dissection. The decision of whether to administer adjuvant radiation and/or chemotherapy is based on pathologic and surgical findings. Staging is based on surgical findings but does not account for all known prognostic factors for recurrence.

Prognostic factors for recurrence in multiple retrospective and prospective studies have included age, tumor grade, depth of myometrial invasion, and evidence of extrauterine disease.[24] Tumor size is also known to be a prognostic factor; women with tumors 2 cm or smaller have a 4% risk of positive lymph nodes compared with 15% for those with tumors larger than 2 cm.[25] LVI may independently increase the risk for recurrence and death from endometrial cancer.[26]

After surgery, patients may be categorized into low risk, intermediate risk, or high risk based on pathologic features. Low-risk patients have grade 1 or 2 disease confined to the uterus, with no or minimal myometrial invasion, no LVI, and a risk of lymph node involvement of less than 5%.[27] The Gynecologic Oncology Group (GOG) 99 study showed that patients in this low-risk group who did not receive radiation had a 1.8% risk of isolated initial local recurrence at 4 years. Therefore, the benefit of any adjuvant therapy is small and no treatment is recommended.[24]

Four randomized trials (the Aalders and colleagues Norwegian Trial, GOG 99, Postoperative Radiation Therapy in Endometrial Carcinoma [PORTEC], and ASTEC studies) have evaluated the role of EBRT compared with no adjuvant therapy in the low end of intermediate risk population (**Table 2**). The first of these trials was published in 1980.[28] Aalders and colleagues randomized 540 clinical stage IA patients between 1968 and 1974 after total hysterectomy and bilateral salpingo-oophorectomy to intravaginal radium to 60 Gy to the vaginal surface with or without EBRT to 40 Gy with the

Table 2
Randomized clinical trials in early-stage endometrial cancer

Study	No. of Patients	Inclusion Criteria	Method of Staging	Arms of Study	Overall Survival	5-Year Recurrence Rate
Aalders et al,[28] 1980	540	Stage I (clinical)	Clinical	VBT + EBRT vs VBT alone	89% vs 91%; NS	2% vs 7%; P<.01
PORTEC-1 2000[30]	714	Stage IB (G2/G3); Stage IC (G1/G2)	Surgical, LND not required	EBRT vs none	81% vs 85%; P = .31	4% vs 14%; P<.001
GOG 99 2004[24]	392	Stage IB–IIB (occult)	Surgical, LND required	EBRT vs none (no VBT)	92% vs 86%; P = .56	3% vs 12%; P = .007 at 2 years
ASTEC/EN5 2009[34]	906	Stage IA–IIA	Surgical, LND not required	EBRT vs none (50% VBT)	84% vs 84%; P = .77	3% vs 6%; P = .02
PORTEC-2 2010[33]	427	>60 years of age; stage IC G1/G2; stage IB G3; any age stage IIA G3	Surgical, LND exclusion criteria	EBRT vs VBT	84% vs 80%; P = .57	5% vs 2%; P = .17

Abbreviations: EBRT, external beam radiation therapy; G, grade; LND, lymph node dissection; NS, not significant; VBT, vaginal brachytherapy.

midline block after 20 Gy. Patients who received radiation had a 5-year local-regional recurrence rate of 1.9% compared with 6.9% for those who did not (P<.01). There was no survival difference between the two groups. On subset analysis, patients with greater than 50% myometrial invasion and grade 3 disease had an increased mortality rate even if they received adjuvant therapy. LVI was associated with a significantly higher mortality rate (26.7% vs 9.1%; P<.01). The investigators recommended post-operative pelvic irradiation and vaginal cuff BT for patients with high-risk features.

The results of PORTEC-1 were published in 2000. A total of 715 patients with stage I papillary serous or clear cell carcinoma and either grade 1 disease and greater than 50% myometrial invasion, grade 2 disease with any amount of myometrial invasion, or grade 3 disease with less than 50% myometrial invasion were randomized to received pelvic irradiation or no radiation.[29] Patients who had a hysterectomy were not permitted to have lymph node dissection; however, suspicious lymph nodes were removed. Irradiated patients received 46 Gy with EBRT. Local-regional recurrence rates at 5 years were 4% in the radiation group and 14% in the control group (P<.01). With an updated median follow-up time of 13.3 years, the 15-year rates were 6% for EBRT and 15.5% for no treatment.[30] Overall survival was not different (81% vs 85%; P = .31). There were more grade 1 complications in the radiation group, 25% versus 6%, although there were only 6 grade 3 complications and 1 grade 4 complication in the radiation group, for an overall actuarial grade 3+ complication rate after radiation of 2% to 3%. The PORTEC group separately reported results on patients with greater than 50% myometrial invasion with grade 3 disease, because this group was required to have EBRT, given the high risk of pelvic nodal involvement. There was a 15% risk of distant metastases, indicating a role for chemotherapy in this group with stage I uterine cancer.[31]

Subsequently, the PORTEC-2 trial randomized patients with the same criteria as PORTEC-1 to vaginal BT versus EBRT. It showed a significantly higher rate of diarrhea, with a decrement in quality of life, with the EBRT.[32] The overall rate of nodal relapse was 3.5% in those who did not receive pelvic irradiation.[33] After central pathology review, however, there was a substantial shift from grade 2 to grade 1 disease and 14% of enrolled patients would not have been eligible for inclusion in the trial. This indicates that central pathology review is critical for any randomized trial given the heterogeneity of pathology reporting.

GOG 99, published in 2004, randomized patients between 1987 and 1995 after a complete lymphadenectomy and hysterectomy. Patients received 50.4 Gy EBRT versus no adjuvant therapy.[24] There was a 2-year significant reduction in recurrences, 12% in the observation group versus 3% in the radiation group; however, this did not translate into a significant 5-year survival difference (92% vs 86%). Patients were categorized by age (<50, 50–70, and >70), and the following were considered risk factors: grade 2 or 3 disease, invasion to the outer third of the myometrial wall, and LVI. The high-intermediate risk group was defined as patients older than 70 years of age with 1 risk factor, or 50 to 70 years of age with 2 risk factors, or any age with all 3 risk factors. The 2-year cumulative incidence of recurrence in the high-intermediate risk group was 26% in the observation group and 6% in the radiation group.

The ASTEC trial similarly randomized 505 patients to EBRT versus no further therapy. Vaginal BT was optional and was administered to approximately 50% of women enrolled in the trial. No overall survival benefit was seen with the addition of pelvic irradiation although it significantly reduced the risk of local recurrence.[34]

High-risk patients are those with positive pelvic or para-aortic nodes, cervical involvement, or extrauterine spread to the fallopian tubes, ovaries, or serosal surface of the uterus. High-risk patients are candidates for a combination of EBRT, BT, and chemotherapy, although the exact regimen, sequencing, and use of chemotherapy agents are the topics of much debate.

Two randomized trials compared pelvic irradiation to cyclophosphamide and Adriamycin chemotherapy in patients with stages IC3 to III endometrial carcinoma; neither study showed a difference in progression-free survival or overall survival.[35,36] The GOG 122 trial randomized patients with stage III or IV (<2 cm residual disease) to either whole-abdominal radiation therapy (WART) or Adriamycin-cisplatin therapy (AP) for 8 cycles.[37] After adjusting for stage, a significant progression-free survival and overall survival benefit was noted favoring chemotherapy. A high pelvic failure rate, however, was seen in both arms: 18% for AP versus 13% for WART. Abdominal and distant recurrences accounted for 32% of failures in the AP arm and 38% of recurrences after WART. Three trials have asked whether chemoradiation is better than radiation, and to date none has shown an advantage in overall survival,[38,39] although one demonstrated a progression-free survival advantage for chemoradiation.[40] Based on the results of these studies, ongoing trials are comparing the role of chemoradiation therapy versus chemotherapy alone and chemoradiation therapy versus radiation therapy alone. A phase II study demonstrated the feasibility of concurrent chemoradiation therapy followed by chemotherapy for stages IC through IVA uterine cancer.[41] One phase II trial currently accruing patients through the Radiation Therapy Oncology Group (RTOG) will assess toxicities with the addition of bevacizumab to concurrent radiation with cisplatin, followed by 4 cycles of carboplatin and paclitaxel chemotherapy.

The optimal sequencing of chemotherapy and EBRT for patients at high risk is not known. The GOG published a randomized trial of pelvic radiation followed by cisplatin and Adriamycin with or without paclitaxel, showing the feasibility of this approach.[42] In a retrospective series of 109 patients treated at multiple institutions, with approximately 50% having endometrioid histology, the analysis was adjusted for multiple factors, including age, grade, histology, stage, and surgical extent. The results showed that patients treated with a sandwich approach of radiation between chemotherapy had a progression-free survival advantage compared with either radiation first or chemotherapy first.[43] Whether the results may be biased based on the large percentage of non-endometrioid histology, the large number of adjustment variables relative to the number of recurrences, or the heterogeneity of the different treatment regimens is unclear.

The institutional approach pursued at Brigham and Women's Hospital is that patients with endometrioid adenocarcinoma grade 1 disease with no or less than 50% myometrial invasion receive no adjuvant therapy. Patients who have a complete lymphadenectomy with stage I disease and either grade 2 disease or grade 1 disease with greater than 50% myometrial invasion receive vaginal BT alone. Exceptions to this include patients with aggressive histologies, such as papillary serous or clear cell adenocarcinoma, or the presence of LVI. Any patient with grade 3 disease with myometrial invasion who has not had a lymphadenectomy receives EBRT and BT. After a radical hysterectomy, patients with stage II disease may require radiation. Women with stage II cancers who have not had a lymphadenectomy, women have not had a radical hysterectomy, or those with a large, bulky cervix receive pelvic irradiation. In general, patients with stage III through IVA endometrioid adenocarcinoma and those with aggressive histologies, such as papillary serous and clear cell adenocarcinoma with any stage, receive a combination of chemotherapy and EBRT and BT.

VULVAR CANCER

Vulvar carcinoma is an uncommon and aggressive disease, affecting approximately 2% of women with gynecologic cancer. Radiation may be used to improve local control and plays a role in postoperative treatment for patients with either close (<8 mm fixed) or positive margins at the vulvar primary specimen[44] or for patients with positive nodes.[45] The doses of radiation vary based on the extent of disease and whether any residual disease is present. Close margins of the primary vulvar specimen require a dose of more than 56 Gy to the vulvar region. For the inguinal region, patients with nodal spread but no extracapsular extension receive more than 50 Gy. Patients with extracapsular extension may receive more than 60 Gy whereas those with gross residual disease require 65 Gy or more.

Cisplatin-based chemotherapy concurrent with radiation is recommended, similar to the approach used in cervical cancer, although older patients should be assessed carefully, because they may not tolerate chemotherapy.[46] Concurrent chemotherapy is given to many postoperative patients able to tolerate it, although comorbidities and age may prohibit administration. Patients with unresectable disease at diagnosis may receive chemoradiation in an attempt to render the tumor operable. Those with tumors deemed unresectable may receive a combination of EBRT and BT to try to escalate the radiation dose to a curative limit of approximately 70 Gy. Recent advances in the use of IMRT may spare the femoral heads, but extreme caution must be used because undercoverage of the inguinal nodes and oversparing of the vulvar skin may occur.[47]

SUMMARY

Radiation plays an integral role in the management of gynecologic cancers. The specific regimen must be carefully coordinated based on the details of a patient's personal history and pathologic findings. An integrated multidisciplinary approach that merges pathology, radiology, medical oncology, gynecologic oncology, and radiation oncology results in a greater understanding and, ideally, better outcomes for women suffering from gynecologic cancer.

REFERENCES

1. Viswanathan AN, Kirisits C, Erickson B, et al. Gynecologic radiation therapy: novel approaches to image-guidance and management. Berlin: Springer; 2011.
2. Rubin SC, Sabbatini P, Viswanathan AN. Ovarian cancer. In: Pazdur R, Wagman LD, Camphausen KA, et al, editors. Cancer management: a multidisciplinary approach. 11th edition. CMP Medica; 2011.
3. Kidd EA, Siegel BA, Dehdashti F, et al. Lymph node staging by positron emission tomography in cervical cancer: relationship to prognosis. J Clin Oncol 2010;28: 2108–13.
4. Landoni F, Maneo A, Colombo A, et al. Randomised study of radical surgery versus radiotherapy for stage Ib–IIa cervical cancer. Lancet 1997;350:535–40.
5. Sedlis A, Bundy BN, Rotman MZ, et al. A randomized trial of pelvic radiation therapy versus no further therapy in selected patients with stage IB carcinoma of the cervix after radical hysterectomy and pelvic lymphadenectomy: a Gynecologic Group Study. Gynecol Oncol 1999;73:177–83.
6. Peters WA III, Liu PY, Barrett RJ, et al. Concurrent chemotherapy and pelvic radiation therapy compared with pelvic radiation therapy alone as adjuvant therapy after radical surgery in high-risk early stage cancer of the cervix. J Clin Oncol 2000;18:1606–13.
7. Pinkawa M, Gagel B, Demirel C, et al. Dose-volume histogram evaluation of prone and supine patient position in external beam radiotherapy for cervical and endometrial cancer. Radiother Oncol 2003;69:99–105.

8. Lanciano RM, Won M, Coia LR, et al. Pretreatment and treatment factors associated with improved outcome in squamous cell carcinoma of the uterine cervix: a final report of the 1973 and 1978 patterns of care studies. Int J Radiat Oncol Biol Phys 1991;20:667–76.

9. Montana GS, Hanlon AL, Brickner TJ, et al. Carcinoma of the cervix: patterns of care studies: review of 1978, 1983, and 1988-1989 surveys. Int J Radiat Oncol Biol Phys 1995;32:1481–6.

10. Goodman HM, Buttlar CA, Niloff JM, et al. Adenocarcioma of the uterine cervix: prognostic factors and patterns of recurrence. Gynecol Oncol 1989;33:241–7.

11. Eifel PJ, Winter K, Morris M, et al. Pelvic irradiation with concurrent chemotherapy versus pelvic and para-aortic irradiation for high risk cervical cancer: an update of Radiation Therapy Oncology Group Trial (RTOG) 90-01. J Clin Oncol 2004;22:872–80.

12. Duenas-Gonzalez A, Zarba JJ, Patel F, et al. Phase III, open-label, randomized study comparing concurrent gemcitabine plus cisplatin and radiation followed by adjuvant gemcitabine and cisplatin versus concurrent cisplatin and radiation in patients with stage IIB to IVA carcinoma of the cervix. J Clin Oncol 2011;29:1678–85.

13. Lanciano RM, Pajak TF, Martz K, et al. The influence of treatment time on outcome for squamous cell cancer of the uterine cervix treated with radiation: a Patterns-of-Care Study. Int J Radiat Oncol Biol Phys 1993;25:391–8.

14. Lim K, Small W Jr, Portelance L, et al. Consensus guidelines for delineation of clinical target volume for intensity-modulated pelvic radiotherapy for the definitive treatment of cervix cancer. Int J Radiat Oncol Biol Phys 2011;79:348–55.

15. Beadle BM, Jhingran A, Salehpour M, et al. Cervix regression and motion during the course of external beam chemoradiation for cervical cancer. Int J Radiat Oncol Biol Phys 2009;73:235–41.

16. Viswanathan AN, Racine ML, Cormack R. Final results of a prospective study of MR-Based interstitial brachytherapy. Brachytherapy 2008;7:148.

17. Eisbruch A, Johnston CM, Martel MK, et al. Customized gynecologic interstitial implants: CT-based planning, dose evaluation, and optimization aided by laparotomy. Int J Radiat Oncol Biol Phys 1998;40:1087–93.

18. Erickson B, Albano K, Gillin M. CT-guided interstitial implantation of gynecologic malignancies. Int J Radiat Oncol Biol Phys 1996;36:699–709.

19. Viswanathan AN, Erickson BA. Three-dimensional imaging in gynecologic brachytherapy: a survey of the American Brachytherapy Society. Int J Radiat Oncol Biol Phys 2010;76:104–9.

20. Viswanathan AN, Creutzberg CL, Craighead P, et al. International Brachytherapy Practice Patterns: A Survey of the Gynecologic Cancer Intergroup (GCIG). Int J Radiat Oncol Biol Phys 2010. [Epub ahead of print].

21. Haie-Meder C, Potter R, Van Limbergen E. Recommendations from Gynaecological (GYN) GEC-ESTRO Working Group (I): concepts and terms in 3D image based 3D treatment planning in cervix cancer brachytherapy with emphasis on MRI assessment of GTV and CTV. Radiother Oncol 2005;74:235–45.

22. Potter R, Haie-Meder C, Van Limbergen E, et al. Recommendations from gynaecological (GYN) GEC ESTRO working group (II): concepts and terms in 3D image-based treatment planning in cervix cancer brachytherapy-3D dose volume parameters and aspects of 3D image-based anatomy, radiation physics, radiobiology. Radiother Oncol 2006;78:67–77.

23. Potter R, Georg P, Dimopoulos JC, et al. Clinical outcome of protocol based image (MRI) guided adaptive brachytherapy combined with 3D conformal

radiotherapy with or without chemotherapy in patients with locally advanced cervical cancer. Radiother Oncol 2011;100:116–23.

24. Keys HM, Roberts JA, Brunetto VL, et al. A phase III trial of surgery with or without adjunctive external pelvic radiation therapy in intermediate risk endometrial adenocarcinoma: a Gynecologic Oncology Group study. Gynecol Oncol 2004; 92:744–51.

25. Schink J, Lurain J, Wallemark C, et al. Tumor size in endometrial cancer: a prognostic factor for lymph node metastasis. Obstet Gynecol 1987;70:216–9.

26. Briet JM, Hollema H, Reesink N, et al. Lymphvascular space involvement: an independent prognostic factor in endometrial cancer. Gynecol Oncol 2005;96: 799–804.

27. Creasman W, Morrow C, Bundy B, et al. Surgical pathologic spread patterns of endometrial cancer. A Gynecologic Oncology Group Study. Cancer 1987;60:2035–41.

28. Aalders J, Abeler V, Kolstad P, et al. Postoperative external irradiation and prognostic parameters in Stage I endometrial carcinoma. Obstet Gynecol 1980;56: 419–27.

29. Creutzberg CL, van Putten WL, Koper PC, et al. Treatment morbidity in patients with endometrial cancer: results from a multicenter randomized trial. Lancet 2000;355:1404–11.

30. Creutzberg CL, Nout RA, Lybeert ML, et al. Fifteen-Year Radiotherapy Outcomes of the Randomized PORTEC-1 Trial for Endometrial Carcinoma. Int J Radiat Oncol Biol Phys 2011;81(4):e631–8.

31. Creutzberg CL, van Putten WL, Warlam-Rodenhuis CC, et al. Outcome of high-risk stage IC, grade 3, compared with stage I endometrial carcinoma patients: the Postoperative Radiation Therapy in Endometrial Carcinoma Trial. J Clin Oncol 2004;22:1234–41.

32. Nout RA, Putter H, Jurgenliemk-Schulz IM, et al. Quality of life after pelvic radiotherapy or vaginal brachytherapy for endometrial cancer: first results of the randomized PORTEC-2 trial. J Clin Oncol 2009;27:3547–56.

33. Nout RA, Smit VT, Putter H, et al. Vaginal brachytherapy versus pelvic external beam radiotherapy for patients with endometrial cancer of high-intermediate risk (PORTEC-2): an open-label, non-inferiority, randomised trial. Lancet 2010; 375:816–23.

34. Blake P, Swart AM, Orton J, et al. Adjuvant external beam radiotherapy in the treatment of endometrial cancer (MRC ASTEC and NCIC CTG EN.5 randomised trials): pooled trial results, systematic review, and meta-analysis. Lancet 2009; 373:137–46.

35. Susumu N, Sagae S, Udagawa Y, et al. Randomized phase III trial of pelvic radiotherapy versus cisplatin-based combined chemotherapy in patients with intermediate- and high-risk endometrial cancer: a Japanese Gynecologic Oncology Group study. Gynecol Oncol 2008;108:226–33.

36. Maggi R, Lissoni A, Spina F, et al. Adjuvant chemotherapy vs radiotherapy in high-risk endometrial carcinoma: results of a randomised trial. Br J Cancer 2006;95:266–71.

37. Randall ME, Filiaci VL, Muss H, et al. Randomized phase III trial of whole-abdominal irradiation versus doxorubicin and cisplatin chemotherapy in advanced endometrial carcinoma: a Gynecologic Oncology Group Study. J Clin Oncol 2006;24:36–44.

38. Kuoppala T, Maenpaa J, Tomas E, et al. Surgically staged high-risk endometrial cancer: randomized study of adjuvant radiotherapy alone vs. sequential chemoradiotherapy. Gynecol Oncol 2008;110:190–5.

39. Morrow CP, Bundy BN, Homesley HD, et al. Doxorubicin as an adjuvant following surgery and radiation therapy in patients with high-risk endometrial carcinoma, stage I and occult stage II: a Gynecologic Oncology Group Study. Gynecol Oncol 1990;36:166–71.

40. Hogberg T, Signorelli M, de Oliveira CF, et al. Sequential adjuvant chemotherapy and radiotherapy in endometrial cancer–results from two randomised studies. Eur J Cancer 2010;46:2422–31.

41. Greven K, Winter K, Underhill K, et al. Final analysis of RTOG 9708: adjuvant postoperative irradiation combined with cisplatin/paclitaxel chemotherapy following surgery for patients with high-risk endometrial cancer. Gynecol Oncol 2006;103:155–9.

42. Homesley HD, Filiaci V, Gibbons SK, et al. A randomized phase III trial in advanced endometrial carcinoma of surgery and volume directed radiation followed by cisplatin and doxorubicin with or without paclitaxel: a Gynecologic Oncology Group study. Gynecol Oncol 2009;112:543–52.

43. Secord AA, Havrilesky LJ, O'Malley DM, et al. A multicenter evaluation of sequential multimodality therapy and clinical outcome for the treatment of advanced endometrial cancer. Gynecol Oncol 2009;114:442–7.

44. Heaps JM, Fu YS, Montz FJ, et al. Surgical-pathologic variables predictive of local recurrence in squamous cell carcinoma of the vulva. Gynecol Oncol 1990;38:309–14.

45. Kunos C, Simpkins F, Gibbons H, et al. Radiation therapy compared with pelvic node resection for node-positive vulvar cancer: a randomized controlled trial. Obstet Gynecol 2009;114:537–46.

46. Mak RH, Halasz LM, Tanaka CK, et al. Outcomes after radiation therapy with concurrent weekly platinum-based chemotherapy or every-3-4-week 5-fluorouracil-containing regimens for squamous cell carcinoma of the vulva. Gynecol Oncol 2011;120:101–7.

47. Beriwal S, Coon D, Heron DE, et al. Preoperative intensity-modulated radiotherapy and chemotherapy for locally advanced vulvar carcinoma. Gynecol Oncol 2008;109:291–5.

48. Whitney CW, Sause W, Bundy BN, et al. A randomized comparison of fluorouracil plus cisplatin versus hydroxyurea as an adjunct to radiation therapy in stages IIB-IVA carcinoma of the cervix with negative para-aortic lymph nodes. J Clin Oncol 1999;17:1339–48.

49. Rose PG, Bundy BN, Watkins EB, et al. Concurrent cisplatin-based chemoradiation improves progression free and overall survival in advanced cervical cancer: results of a randomized Gynecologic Oncology Group Study. N Engl J Med 1999; 340:1144–53.

50. Keys HM, Bundy BM, Stehman FB, et al. Cisplatin, radiation and adjuvant hysterectomy compared with radiation and adjuvant hysterectomy for bulky stage IB cervical carcinoma. N Engl J Med 1999;340:1154–61.

51. Pearcey R, Brundage M, Drouin P, et al. Phase III trial comparing radical radiotherapy with and without cisplatin chemotherapy in patients with advanced squamous cell cancer of the cervix. J Clin Oncol 2002;20:966–72.

Contemporary Quality of Life Issues Affecting Gynecologic Cancer Survivors

Jeanne Carter, PhD[a,b], Richard Penson, MD, MRCP[c],
Richard Barakat, MD[a], Lari Wenzel, PhD[d,*]

KEYWORDS

• Quality of life • Sexual function • Chemotherapy toxicities

Gynecologic cancers account for approximately 11% of the newly diagnosed cancers in women in the United States and 18% in the world.[1] The most common gynecologic malignancies occur in the uterus and endometrium (53%), ovary (25%), and cervix (14%).[2] Cervical cancer is most prevalent in premenopausal women, during their childbearing years, whereas uterine and ovarian cancers tend to present in the peri-menopausal or menopausal period. Vaginal and vulvar cancers and malignancies arising from gestation, or gestational trophoblastic neoplasms, occur to a lesser extent. Regardless of cancer origin or age of onset, the disease and its treatment can produce short- and long-term sequelae (ie, sexual dysfunction, infertility, or lymphedema) that adversely affect quality of life (QOL). This article outlines the primary contemporary issues or concerns that may affect QOL and offers strategies to offset or mitigate QOL disruption. These contemporary issues are identified within the domains of sexual functioning, reproductive issues, lymphedema, and the contribution of health-related QOL (HRQOL) in influential gynecologic cancer clinical trials.

[a] Gynecology Service, Department of Surgery, Memorial Sloan-Kettering Cancer Center, New York, NY 10065, USA
[b] Psychiatry and Behavioral Sciences, Memorial Sloan-Kettering Cancer Center, New York, NY 10065, USA
[c] Medical Gynecologic Oncology, Department of Medicine, Harvard Medical School, Massachusetts General Hospital, Boston, MA 02114, USA
[d] Department of Medicine and Public Health, University of California Irvine, 839 Health Sciences Court, Sprague Hall, Suite 212, Irvine, CA 92697, USA
* Corresponding author.
E-mail address: lwenzel@uci.edu

Hematol Oncol Clin N Am 26 (2012) 169–194
doi:10.1016/j.hoc.2011.11.001
0889-8588/12/$ – see front matter © 2012 Elsevier Inc. All rights reserved.

CANCER, TREATMENT, AND SEXUALITY

Gynecologic cancer and its treatment directly affect the sexual and reproductive organs. Surgical staging is the standard of care in treating most gynecologic malignancies and may involve the removal of the uterus and ovaries. Any cancer treatment that impairs (or removes) the ovaries can negatively affect vaginal health because of hormonal deprivation, resulting in abrupt, intense, and prolonged symptoms, including hot flashes, vaginal dryness, dyspareunia, and an overall decrease in QOL.[3–7] Premenopausal and perimenopausal women diagnosed with gynecologic cancer are at high risk for ovarian failure (or surgical menopause) and sexual dysfunction,[6] leading to emotional distress, possible disruption of social and intimate relationships, and in some cases treatment-induced infertility.[8–10] Women diagnosed after menopause who have been using estrogen replacement are often advised to stop taking the hormone (especially with uterine cancer), triggering an abrupt and severe exacerbation of menopausal symptoms.[11,12] Vaginal atrophy can be severe for those treated with surgical removal of the ovaries, pelvic radiation, or chemotherapy.[6]

Other factors, such as age and relationships, can impact the sexual function of gynecologic cancer patients and survivors. Reported rates of sexual activity range from 10% to 50% in older ovarian cancer patients[13,14] compared with 77% to 81% in younger patients.[15,16] Many women are not sexually active because of the physical health of their partner[17] or quality of their relationship.[18] Misperceptions among couples, such as female cancer survivors reporting greater vaginal changes and dryness than their partner, highlight the need for relationship communication, especially for those experiencing pain.[18]

Sexual morbidity is associated with poor psychologic adjustment and QOL in women treated for gynecologic cancer[19–21] in the immediate posttreatment period[16,22,23] and in long-term survival.[24,25] Dyspareunia, vaginal dryness, and loss of desire are the most common sexual difficulties after cancer treatment.[6,8,13,26,27] Women experiencing persistent, bothersome menopausal symptoms (ie, vaginal dryness) are at higher risk for distress and depression.[16] Vasomotor symptoms can also be sexually disruptive by interfering with sleep and energy,[28,29] and therefore require early assessment and management. Vaginal atrophy is associated with vaginal dryness, tightness, itching, burning, and pain during sexual activity or gynecologic examinations. It can also increase risk of vaginal and urinary tract infections. To alleviate these symptoms, it is important to improve lubrication, moisture, and the pH of the vagina.

Simple solutions to improve vaginal health include vaginal moisturizers and lubricants. Vaginal moisturizers are nonhormonal, over-the-counter products intended to be used several times a week consistently for overall vaginal health and comfort, regardless of sexual activity. Vaginal moisturizers hydrate the vaginal mucosa; improve the balance of intracellular fluids in the vaginal epithelium for up to 2 to 3 days (or two times per week); and restore a premenopausal vaginal pH in postmenopausal women. Women with a history of cancer often need to administer vaginal moisturizers up to three to five times per week because of the abrupt estrogen deprivation associated with cancer treatment (ie, ovarian failure or removal). For best absorption and benefit, vaginal moisturizers should be applied at bedtime and used regularly.

Vaginal lubricants, made in liquid or gel form, minimize dryness and pain during sexual activity. Water- or silicone-based lubricants are recommended, and when used properly can prevent irritation and mucosal tears, which can lead to postcoital pain or infection.[30] Treating vaginal dryness and pain (dyspareunia) often leads to improvement in sexual response, such as better desire, subjective arousal, and ability to reach orgasm. The literature shows psychoeducational interventions promote sexual function, satisfaction, and well-being.[31]

Surgery and Sexuality

Type and radicality of surgery is often linked to extent of sexual dysfunction.[32] Treatment of vulvar intraepithelial neoplasia or vulvar cancer can range from local vulvar excision to radical vulvectomy, and in some cases, resection may involve the clitoral area. Older age and extensive vulvar excisions are associated with poorer sexual function and QOL.[32] Decreased lubrication, shortened vaginal length, lack of sensation, and dyspareunia are associated with radical hysterectomy[33–35]; however, nerve-sparing approaches have led to improved QOL and reduction of bladder, sexual, and intestinal sequelae, without compromising surgical outcome.[36] Pelvic exenteration is one of the most radical, but potentially curative, treatment strategies for advanced or recurrent gynecologic malignancy. The procedure is an en bloc resection of the pelvic organs (ie, uterus, cervix, vagina, ovaries, lower urinary tract, and rectosigmoid colon) first described by Brunschwig in 1948. This procedure requires a motivated patient, with a good support network to assist in the recovery period.[37] Provision of information and presurgical preparation for potential changes to a woman's body (ie, sexual function and ostomy care) are crucial for postoperative adjustment.[37,38] Technologic improvements in imaging have allowed for better selection of patients (no distant metastases) most likely to benefit from this extensive surgical procedure.[39] The best candidates are those who are younger and have recurrent cervical cancer and pathologically negative surgical margins.[39]

Radiation and Sexuality

Studies show external-beam radiation therapy (EBRT) is associated with bowel side effects (eg, diarrhea and fecal leakage), which limit patient activities and QOL.[40,41] Pelvic radiation to the vagina, especially at high doses, can cause agglutination, ulceration, or stenosis.[33,42] Vaginal lubrication is often decreased because of loss of small blood vessels and direct damage to the vaginal mucosa.[43] Vaginal depth and elasticity can be compromised by radiation therapy,[44,45] adversely affecting sexual function.[33,46] Inflammation to mucosal surfaces of the vagina can contribute to dyspareunia. Chronic fibrotic changes to the pelvis may worsen vaginal atrophy over time, creating chronic difficulties up to 5 years or more posttreatment,[47] although sexual activity or vaginal dilator therapy can help.[48]

High-dose intravaginal radiation therapy (HDIVRT) has recently shown decreased morbidity compared with EBRT.[49–52] The Postoperative Radiation Therapy in Endometrial Carcinoma (PORTEC) study showed that HDIVRT was effective in vaginal disease control, with fewer toxicities and better QOL than EBRT.[41,53] Other studies comparing EBRT with HDIVRT have reported excellent recurrence-free and overall survival rates.[54] These findings suggest that early stage endometrial cancer patients can avoid the high morbidity associated with EBRT by receiving HDIVRT.[52] The PORTEC-2 Trial did confirm, however, that HDIVRT patients experience vaginal toxicities (dryness, tightening, and shortened vagina) and dyspareunia. The paucity of data regarding the influence of these side effects on sexual function, survivorship, and QOL was noted by the authors. This area of research warrants further investigation because IVRT is gaining favor as a treatment modality.

Informational Needs and Communication

Recent survey studies have assessed cancer patients' satisfaction and awareness of available sexual health resources and intervention strategies. Sexuality is important to cancer patients, but less than half (45%) receive information on the potential impact of cancer treatment on sexual function.[55] Preliminary survey results demonstrate that female cancer survivors (gynecologic and breast) are not satisfied with current sexual health resources and are not communicating concerns with their medical team. In this cohort, over two-thirds (77%) expressed comfort mentioning sexual health issues with their medical team, but less than one-third (32%) discussed the topic. Sixty-five percent indicated a preference to receive written educational material followed by a discussion with their medical team. Even though 72% thought it would be helpful to speak with a sexual health expert, only 10% had done so.[56]

Because of a lack of time and overcrowded schedules, many physicians prefer to focus on physical assessment and "combating the disease" rather than intimacy, sexuality, or other issues of QOL and survivorship.[57,58] Furthermore, many healthcare providers do not have the training or resources to discuss, assess, or provide treatment plans for sexual problems.[59–61] In the setting of open communication, women can often gain insight, reduce concerns, and have their experience normalized, in addition to having health promotion strategies (eg, vaginal moisturizers) suggested and reinforced.[62] Some patients may be unaware that cancer can have latent effects or significantly influence sexuality and vaginal health, which is especially problematic in women with gynecologic cancer; as a result, sexual concerns are seldom addressed.[30,63]

Female patients with cancer have indicated that treatment toxicities, prognosis, and long-term effects are among the most important topics to discuss during follow-up,[64] and they welcome the opportunity to discuss sexual function, side effects, and symptoms.[63] However, physicians cite a lack of time as an impediment to exploring QOL issues.[65] Checklists or brief surveys may be an excellent method to screen for vaginal dryness, discomfort, and other survivorship concerns (ie, lymphedema).[66–68] These methods are ideal because of the minimal amount of materials and personnel needed, and allow for an opportunity to elicit concerns in a time-efficient manner within the clinical setting to provide information or triage for referrals.

Assessment of Sexual Function

For evidence-based research, validated empiric measures are needed. Although many sexual function measures have been developed,[69] the contemporary measures of sexual health have focused on the use of the Female Sexual Function Index (FSFI), both in long and short forms, and recently the Patient-Reported Outcomes Measurement Information System (PROMIS). Sexual dysfunction and symptoms in cancer survivors may differ from those experienced by women in the general population. Although the FSFI has strong psychometric qualities, it has not been validated in cancer cohorts. Recent data suggest the FSFI is a reliable, valid measure of sexual functioning for cancer populations,[70] but scoring issues must be addressed to avoid reporting artificially low FSFI scores and estimates of female sexual dysfunction prevalence. Short versions of the FSFI have also been developed in the general population (FSFI-6 SF [Italy]) and tested in the oncology setting (FSFI CA-6)[71] to facilitate screening for sexual dysfunction in busy clinical practices. An abridged FSFI-6 short form (SF) of the full FSFI-19 was recently validated in female outpatients reporting sexual dysfunction.[72] However, when the psychometrics of the FSFI-6 SF was investigated in a sample of cancer survivors, a different six-item set was found to perform better. The revised items' contents measured sexual functioning more reliably in this cohort, particularly in the domains of lubrication and satisfaction, perhaps reflecting differences in the nature of dysfunction between cancer survivors and outpatients in reproductive medicine clinics. The FSFI CA-6 SF was also examined using the Item

Response Theory models to identify the one item on each of the six FSFI domains that had the most optimal measurement properties. The results are very promising, with internal consistency reliability of 0.86 and Pearson correlation of 0.97 with the full FSFI.[71]

The recent development of the PROMIS Network (http://www.nihpromis.org/) has offered a system of highly reliable, valid, flexible, precise, and responsive assessment tools to measure patient-reported health status. The objective of the PROMIS-Sexual Function tool continues this work by providing a flexible and psychometrically robust measure of sexual function within oncology. To date, development procedures have included review of the sexual function measure literature, focus group methodology, and development of a conceptual model for PROMIS sexual function measures for cancer patients.[69,73,74] Future steps for the PROMIS sexual function measure include large-scale item testing, psychometric evaluation, validation, and translation.[74] Brief assessment tools are essential to reduce patient burden and allow for assessment of this important domain within future clinical trials.

REPRODUCTIVE ISSUES

Cancer-related infertility can cause persistent feelings of sadness and grief lasting well into survivorship.[8,75] Premature menopause or loss of reproductive function is not only associated with poorer emotional functioning but also greater risk for sexual difficulties.[76] The relationship between infertility and long-term QOL in female cancer survivors shows that reproductive concerns are of great importance[77,78] and centrally linked to psychosocial outcomes.[10] Even women who undergo fertility-preserving surgery experience distress and reproductive concerns postoperatively over time.[79]

Fertility-preserving surgery is an option for a select group of young gynecologic cancer patients.[80–82] Cervical cancer is one of the most common cancers in women less than age 40,[1] who are still in their childbearing years. Over the past two decades, radical trachelectomy, which allows for the preservation of the uterus, has been established as a feasible alternative in the management of cervical cancer for those desiring future fertility.[83–85] An estimated 48% of women diagnosed with early stage cervical cancer in their reproductive years would meet the criteria for radical trachelectomy.[86] The recurrence rate is less than 5% and the death rate is less than 2%,[82] comparable with those of radical hysterectomy. Most pregnancies ($\sim$75%) after radical trachelectomy reach the third trimester and are delivered at term (37+ weeks). These women, however, often have reproductive concerns and anxiety.[67] A recent large series noted a 15% infertility rate in these patients with the need for reproductive assistance. Forty percent of the infertility was caused by neocervical stenosis.[82] Other issues include dyspareunia and lymphedema.[16,85] Women may not spontaneously offer information about these issues unless specifically queried because they may not consider perceived mild or intermittent issues worthy of discussion with their doctor.[87] It may be useful and time efficient to use a checklist or symptom diaries to review potential survivorship concerns.[68]

Young women diagnosed with endometrial cancer in their childbearing years may be eligible for conservative management with hormonal therapy. This option can be used in the treatment of complex atypical hyperplasia (precancerous condition) and low-risk endometrial cancer (ie, grade 1 histology with no myometrial invasion).[88–92] Complex atypical hyperplasia of the endometrium is often treated with hysterectomy because of the high risk (29%) of progression to endometrial cancer[93] and the 25% to 42% risk of having unidentified endometrial cancer within the specimen.[94] Women should only be considered for conservative management after careful evaluation, including a dilatation and curettage and radiologic imaging.[80,95] Patients should be counseled on the limited data with a conservative approach, risk of disease progression both during and after progestin therapy, duration of treatment, the 5% risk of ovarian metastasis,[96] and the 10% to 29% risk of synchronous ovarian malignancy.[96–99] Patients undergoing conservative nonsurgical treatment for early endometrial cancer should have regular follow-up, with endometrial sampling every 3 to 6 months.[80] Some experts advocate definitive surgical treatment on completion of childbearing or tumor recurrence.[96,100–102]

Ovarian cancer is less common in premenopausal women; yet, some women, including those with a diagnosis of malignant germ cell tumors, sex cord tumors, tumors of low malignant potential, or stage IA invasive ovarian cancer, may be appropriate for fertility-sparing treatment.[80,95,103–107] One of the largest series on the experience of treating young women with fertility-sparing surgery for the treatment of malignant germ cell tumors showed 81% undergoing unilateral salpingo-oophorectomy and staging, with a 90% to 100% survival rate.[104] Adult granulosa cell tumors of the ovary tend to exhibit disease unilaterally, yet 2% to 8% of these tumors may present bilaterally in the ovary.[107,108] It is reasonable, but controversial, to consider removal of the other ovary and completion hysterectomy in women treated conservatively after childbearing has been completed. In women diagnosed with borderline tumors with a strong desire to preserve fertility, conservative management is not an unreasonable option if the tumor is confined to one ovary and treated with unilateral salpingo-oophorectomy plus complete surgical staging.[109,110] Stage I epithelial ovarian cancer can be managed conservatively in some cases if the cancer is confined to the ovary. However, preservation of the uterus and contralateral ovary needs to be conducted in the setting of a comprehensive surgical staging procedure, with in-depth counseling about the risk of recurrence and possible adjuvant therapy. Patients treated conservatively for stage I ovarian cancer should also be closely followed with CA-125 monitoring every 3 months and transvaginal ultrasound for a minimum of 2 years. Definitive surgery may be advised after childbearing is complete.

Reproductive Options

Reproductive assistance consisting of cryopreservation of gametes (oocyte or sperm) or embryos[111–113] can be a viable option for biologic offspring when there are concerns about premature menopause and infertility. Nevertheless, this option requires a functional uterus on treatment completion or may require the assistance of another individual or third party for family-building options. Techniques include egg (oocyte) donation; sperm donation; embryo donation; and in vitro fertilization with or without a gestational carrier (surrogacy). Adoption is another alternative, although the literature notes that some adoption agencies may be reluctant to consider cancer survivors as potential parents[114] because of concerns about recurrence or late health risks after cancer treatment.[115,116] Despite the risk of cancer-related infertility, many women report unmet informational needs about reproductive health either before or during treatment.[63,78] Delivery of adequate information and proper preparation has been noted to reduce anxiety and distress and enhance coping and QOL.[87]

SURGICAL TREATMENT AND RISK OF LYMPHEDEMA OF THE LOWER EXTREMITY

The incidence of lymphedema of the lower extremity (LLE) after treatment for gynecologic cancer, and its risk factors, are not well known.[117,118] Retrospective studies indicate nodal sampling as a factor in LLE development.[119] A recent trial reported statistically significant early and late postoperative complications in women who underwent lymphadenectomy (N = 81; P = .001) compared with those who did not. Lymphedema and lymphocysts were the main difference in noted morbidity between the groups.[120] Shorter length of hospitalization has significantly differed between women undergoing and not undergoing lymphadenectomy (6 vs 5 days, respectively),[120] although it is unclear if this finding translates into a quicker recovery by surgical type. Resumption of activities was a significant finding in the evaluation of other surgical studies (LAP2)[23,121] and could be an important consideration in future cost and QOL analyses.

There are no prospective data empirically assessing LLE to determine the implications of lymph node factors (number of lymph nodes removed). Formal assessment in future study designs is crucial because it may be vastly underrecognized. Patient-reported outcomes (PROs) should be included to determine the potential impact of adverse effects on activities and QOL. Infection is also a contributing factor and may be a concern when conducting nodal dissection as part of the staging process. Carlson and colleagues[122] showed that vulvar infection and inguinal wound breakdown were prevalent in women undergoing lymphadenectomy.

Lymphedema has been identified as a chronic, disruptive, and disfiguring condition, and requires long-term management. Although not life threatening, this late effect of cancer treatment is gaining more attention as patients live longer because of improved survival outcomes. Research on the psychomorbidity of upper-extremity lymphedema allows clinicians to extrapolate information about the potential difficulties faced by women with LLE. Nevertheless, there are no empiric data to fully comprehend psychosocial, functional, or QOL issues experienced by gynecologic cancer survivors coping with lymphedema. Many cancer survivors struggle with changes to their body long after treatment has been completed. Thus, the psychomorbidity of LLE on a patient's QOL can be significant.[123] Lymphedema can be socially embarrassing or undermine confidence in appearance or body image. A small retrospective study with vulvar cancer survivors showed LLE decreased QOL through loss of work, decreased socialization, and poor self-esteem and body image.[124] Recurrent infections have also been highlighted as a negative compounding result of this condition.[125] Some patients associated lymphedema with a sign of recurrence or progression of disease, causing heightened anxiety and fear. The chronic nature of this condition also serves as a constant reminder of one's cancer history. The significance of the current research on the psychological and QOL data is directly related to the study design and methods in which these domains were measured. Many studies did not include lymphedema-specific measures when assessing emotional, social, and QOL impact of this condition.[126] It is also difficult to fully comprehend the prevalence or extent of burden in those living with this condition without accurate incidence data. This lack of clarity stresses the importance of prospectively studying QOL variables in conjunction with lymphedema and disease-specific measurements.[127]

New Surgical Techniques

Over the past several decades, minimally invasive surgical procedures, including laparscopically assisted and robotically assisted approaches, have been increasingly used. Minimally invasive surgical techniques can decrease patient morbidity for women undergoing surgical staging for gynecologic cancer[128] by reducing blood loss, complications, postoperative pain, and length of hospitalization compared with laparotomy.[129] The Gynecologic Oncology Group (GOG) conducted a national cooperative trial (LAP2) comparing laparoscopy with laparotomy for comprehensive surgical staging of uterine cancer. Laparoscopic surgical staging was found to be a feasible and safe alternative to laparotomy and demonstrated shorter hospitalization (2 days less), less pain, and fewer moderate-to-severe postoperative adverse events.[121] In addition, patients undergoing laparoscopic surgical staging had higher QOL, better physical functioning, positive body image, less pain and interference with QOL, and a faster recovery (resumption of activities and return to work) than those receiving laparotomy over the 6-week postoperative period.[23]

Robotically assisted surgical procedures use computer-assisted technology to provide improved dexterity and precision of instruments, with three-dimensional imaging. Compared with laparoscopy, robotic-assisted procedures are fairly new; however, the use of the da Vinci surgical system has quickly become an integral part of gynecologic oncology.[130] Robotically assisted techniques have been used in the treatment of early stage endometrial and cervical cancers.[128,131] A recent retrospective study showed that the robotically assisted hysterectomy in patients with endometrial cancer had a higher lymph node yield ($P<.0001$), decreased hospital stay ($P<.0001$) and estimated blood loss ($P<.001$), and lower postoperative complication rate (5.9%) compared with laparotomy (29.7%; $P<.0001$). A recent cost comparison of robotic, laparoscopic, and open hysterectomy for treatment of endometrial cancer found laparoscopic surgery to be the least expensive, but robotic surgery was associated with a shorter recovery time.[132] Robotically assisted hysterectomy may be preferable to laparoscopic hysterectomy,[131] but prospective studies evaluating long-term outcomes with robotically assisted procedures are lacking.

The sentinel lymph node (SLN) concept was initially introduced for the treatment of melanoma, which revolutionized the field, and has now been examined in other diseases.[133] Sentinel lymph node biopsy (SLNB) is a technique that provides accurate information about the status of lymph nodes without subjecting patients to comprehensive lymphadenectomy. This surgical innovation has been associated with a significant reduction in morbidity in the short (ie, infection) and the long term (ie, LLE).[134] Studies have confirmed that objectively measured lymphedema rates after SLNB[123,135–138] are significantly decreased compared with axillary lymph node dissection, with lymphedema rates of approximately 3% with SLNB versus approximately 20% with axillary lymph node dissection at 6 months' follow-up,[139–141] without compromise to outcome. Specifically for gynecologic cancers, surgical treatment of vulvar cancer requires inguinal lymph node dissection (unilateral or bilateral) to assess regional metastasis; as a result, the risk of postoperative complications and wound breakdown are particularly high for these women.[142,143] SLNB may be a reasonable option for a select group of these patients. Recent studies have shown its value in early stage cervical cancer,[144] and treatment algorithms have been suggested.[145] Research with patients with endometrial cancer has suggested that the extent of nodal sampling is a factor in the development of symptomatic lymphedema,[119] although the extent (ie, number of lymph nodes removed) is debatable,[146] and SLNB may help solve the debate. Overall, SLNB is an innovative technique with the potential to improve QOL by minimizing morbidity; however, before implementing this as standard of care outside of the cancer center setting, larger validation studies are needed to establish safety and accuracy of this concept in gynecologic oncology.

HRQOL AND PROS IN CLINICAL TRIALS

QOL data can accurately describe a population, predict outcomes, guide clinical decisions, screen for disease or dysfunction, and inform the allocation of resources.[147] Although potentially illuminating the meaning of the experience of illness, it also opens the appreciation of the complexity of medical issues, and reflects disease- and treatment-related symptoms, physical performance, patient satisfaction, control of disease,[148] fears and hopelessness,[149] expectations,[150] social and cultural context, and personal values.[151] Given the chronic and often incurable nature of many gynecologic malignancies, the toxicity or tolerability of a specific therapy can be as important as its efficacy, and HRQOL measurement can provide information about the impact of the disease and its treatment to aid clinicians in selecting antineoplastic and supportive care therapy. PROs are data collected directly from the patient, and the field has evolved to recognize HRQOL and symptom-specific measures and outcomes that influence trial development and care.

HRQOL in Clinical Trials

Approximately 10% of all cancer clinical trials include HRQOL as one of the main end points.[152,153] Vital data that quantify the impact of treatment on HRQOL have been provided in recent upfront (first line) ovarian cancer clinical trials. To date, five completed phase III studies in the upfront treatment of ovarian cancer have included validated HRQOL outcome measures, and in every instance HRQOL was helpful in determining the best regimen.

For example, the Canadian European Intergroup trial OV.10 established the benefit of paclitaxel in treating ovarian carcinoma.[154] One hundred fifty-two of the patients accrued in Canada completed the European Organization for Research and Treatment of Cancer Quality of Life Questionnaire C30 and a trial-specific checklist. Compliance was excellent (81%–93%), and although there was a deterioration in HRQOL domains immediately after chemotherapy (Day 8 of cycle 1), in both arms there was an improvement in global HRQOL during treatment and follow-up. Although there was greater neurologic and muscle toxicity for paclitaxel, this did not adversely affect HRQOL.

The Arbeitsgemeinschaft Gynaekologische Onkologie trial established the benefit of carboplatin.[155] Previous data had confirmed that carboplatin and cisplatin resulted in equivalent survival. However, this study showed that the carboplatin/paclitaxel arm was associated with superior HRQOL (physical, role, and cognitive) in functioning and better outcomes in three symptom scales (carboplatin/paclitaxel associated with less nausea and vomiting [$P<.001$]; less appetite loss [$P<.001$]; and less fatigue [$P = .033$]), with better overall HRQOL ($P = .012$).

The SCOTROC trial validated the role of docetaxel where HRQOL was a primary end point.[156] The SCOTROC study compared carboplatin/docetaxel with carboplatin/paclitaxel as first-line chemotherapy for stage IC to IV ovarian cancer and demonstrated a clear advantage for docetaxel in terms of less neurotoxicity.[156] SCOTROC demonstrated that meaningful HRQOL differences between treatment regimens can be reported by patients using validated instruments.[157]

However, in recurrent and resistant disease where combinations do not provide a survival advantage over single-agent palliative chemotherapy in women with relapsed ovarian cancer, the EORTC's QLQ-30 did not detect between-arm HRQOL differences, although excessive toxicity was observed.[158] Some of these toxicities are "paper" (laboratory) toxicities (with potential consequences), such as thrombocytopenia, and therefore not assessed by PROs.

Although some investigators remind us that it is impossible to measure a "sunbeam with a ruler,"[159] the systematic development of validated instruments (questionnaires) has allowed important randomized clinical trials to report HRQOL.[160,161] The present challenge is to translate what has been learned from clinical trials into clinical practice.[162] Ovarian cancer has provided an opportunity to develop and validate new tools, such as the abdominal discomfort module[163] and neurotoxicity subscale,[164] both piloted in protocol GOG-172 (IV vs IP chemotherapy). This has contributed to lowering the dose and changing the schedule of drugs in clinical practice and in the new study (GOG-252).

Cardinal Symptoms and Concerns During the Gynecologic Cancer Disease Trajectory

Multiple factors influence HRQOL: demographic, physical, psychological, social, sexual, and spiritual.[165,166] Prominent among the toxicities and symptoms that can diminish HRQOL in patients with gynecologic cancer are pain, bowel and bladder problems, emotional distress, neuropathy, alopecia, nausea and vomiting, anemia, and fatigue.[167] In ovarian cancer, for example, there are clearly defined seasons in the disease trajectory of gynecologic tumors when the goals are cure (initial therapy); remission (for potentially platinum-sensitive disease); durable palliation (of relatively resistant disease); and the relief of suffering (palliative care). Initial presentation of ovarian cancer is associated with nonspecific symptoms, but may be more commonly associated with pelvic or abdominal pain, increased abdominal size or bloating, and difficulty eating or feeling full.[168] Different phases of the disease have unique symptom issues, and the field is starting to evaluate subtle influences on HRQOL, such as disrupted sleep.[169] Some data suggest that patients may be most compromised in functional well-being, and this is harder to elucidate and harder still to help.[170]

PALLIATIVE CHEMOTHERAPY: HRQOL IMPLICATIONS

Many currently used first- and second-line chemotherapeutic agents can induce significant toxicities, and potentially diminish HRQOL.[171,172] The treatment of recurrent ovarian cancer has defined the popular paradigm of continual single-agent palliative chemotherapy despite little evidence for a survival advantage for this approach[173] and powerful, randomized controlled data that suggest premature initiation of chemotherapy is associated with poorer HRQOL.[174] Eventually, all women develop chemotherapy-resistant tumors, and response rates are poor, with a median 2-year survival of only 20% for those with platinum-resistant ovarian cancer.[175] Women with recurrent ovarian cancer experience an average of 12 concurrent symptoms, and these symptoms directly influence HRQOL, some related to the disease and some directly related to the treatment.[176] The most common side effects of chemotherapy include hair loss and peripheral neuropathy, one obvious and one hidden, but both constant reminders of being a cancer patient.[177] The most important symptoms identified in surveying 455 physicians and nurses at 17 National Comprehensive Cancer Network institutions were fatigue, pain, nausea, weight loss, fear, and HRQOL.[178] This has been further revised to reduce the 30 items to 18 in the NFOSI-18 symptom index, assessing 51 women with advanced ovarian cancer and 10 gynecologic oncologists.[179]

With respect to ovarian cancer, the suggestion that there may be a survival advantage for a subgroup of patients on maintenance therapy mandates that there is a better appreciation of impact of treatment on QOL.[180–182] For patients with advanced disease, the worth of palliative chemotherapy can be anecdotally clear, but is supported only by a limited evidence base. Doyle and colleagues[183] examined the value of palliative chemotherapy in 27 women with refractory and recurrent ovarian cancer, only 26% of whom had a documented tumor response and in whom overall median survival was subsequently only 11 months. Sixty-five percent of women expected that chemotherapy would make them live longer, and 42% expected that it would cure them. After two cycles of chemotherapy, HRQOL improvements were seen in global and emotional functioning using the EORTC QLQ C-30. These improvements lasted a median of 2 and 3 months, respectively. The diminishing returns of benefit with later lines of chemotherapy, however, mandate carefully weighing the merits of every intervention. More recently, large randomized ovarian cancer trials incorporating HRQOL endpoints have been reported.[156,184] However, the sample size and power to detect differences is important. For example, ICON IV reported no significant difference in HRQOL despite survival differences between platinum treatment and carboplatin in combination with paclitaxel in patients with platinum-sensitive recurrent disease, reinforcing that the better control of disease often translates into better HRQOL and can compensate for treatment-related morbidity.[184]

Chemotherapy Toxicity: Neurotoxicity

Platinum compounds, the mainstay of treatment for most gynecologic malignancies,[185] are associated with cumulative myelosuppression neurotoxicity; nephrotoxicity; and severe noncumulative toxicities, including anemia and nausea and vomiting.[172,186] Neurotoxicity, anemia, and nausea and vomiting all have well-known adverse effects on HRQOL. Paclitaxel in combination with a platinum compound is now considered the standard of care as first-line chemotherapy for advanced ovarian cancer.[171,177] However, paclitaxel has a number of toxicities (eg, granulocytopenia, anemia, and thrombocytopenia) that overlap those of the platins, and the coadministration of paclitaxel and a platinum compound can potentially increase the frequency or severity of shared toxicities. Additionally, paclitaxel itself is associated with peripheral neuropathy, which can add to the disease burden.[187] In a study of multimodal therapy, radiation therapy in combination with cisplatin alone, cisplatin plus fluorouracil and hydroxyurea, or hydroxyurea alone was assessed in women with locally advanced cervical cancer.[188] Both cisplatin groups achieved gains in overall survival and progression-free survival; however, patients who received radiation therapy plus the three-drug regimen experienced more leukopenia and other hematologic effects of grade 3 and grade 4 toxicity than did patients in the other two groups ($P<.001$).

Administration of glutamine or the antidepressant venlafaxine may be helpful in cases of paclitaxel-induced neuropathy, and amifostine may provide protection from cisplatin-induced neuropathy[189,190]; however, there is no drug to reliably prevent or cure chemotherapy-induced neuropathy.[191] Therapeutic interventions for neurotoxicity remain controversial, with vitamin B_6 possibly reducing the efficacy of alkylator chemotherapy. Nonpharmacologic approaches to treatment of chemotherapy-induced neuropathy are based on patient education about potential neuropathic side effects; impact of these side effects on performance of daily activities (eg, buttoning clothes, walking, sensing control pedals while driving, or checking water temperature); and related safety issues.

Chemotherapy Toxicity: Intraperitoneal Therapy

Ovarian cancer tends to be chemosensitive and confines itself to the surface of the peritoneal cavity for much of its natural history. These features have made it an obvious target for intraperitoneal (IP) chemotherapy. At least eight well-conducted randomized trials in nearly 2000 women receiving primary treatment for ovarian cancer showed women were less likely to die if they received an IP component to the chemotherapy (hazard ratio [HR] = 0.79; 95% confidence interval [CI], 0.70–0.90), and the disease-free interval (HR = 0.79; 95% CI, 0.69–0.90) was also significantly prolonged.[192,193] There was greater serious toxicity with regard to gastrointestinal effects, pain, and fever but less ototoxicity with the IP than intravenous route.[193]

Wenzel and colleagues[194] reported the first analysis of the HRQOL results of the widely cited phase III study of IV paclitaxel and cisplatin versus IV paclitaxel, IP cisplatin, and IP paclitaxel in optimal stage III epithelial ovarian cancer (GOG-172) using the FACT-O, GOG-NTX, and FACT-GOG Abdominal Discomfort measures. HRQOL was assessed before randomization (baseline); before cycle 4; and 3 to 6 weeks and 12 months posttreatment. Patients receiving IP therapy reported significantly worse HRQOL and abdominal pain before cycle 4 (P<.0001) and worse HRQOL 3 to 6 weeks posttreatment (P = .0035). Neurotoxicity was significantly worse both 3 to 6 weeks after completing chemotherapy (P = .0004) and 1 year later (P = .0018). However, there were no significant HRQOL or abdominal discomfort differences between arms 1 year posttreatment. Clinicians are aware of this trade-off and the magnitude of the impact of using this route for chemotherapy. This clearly contributes to the continued reluctance to accept IP therapy as a standard of care, but drives the next phase of studies designed to find more acceptable, less toxic therapeutic combinations.

Chemotherapy Toxicity: Combination Therapy

In the palliation of recurrent metastatic solid tumors, a popular paradigm is the sequential use of single-agent therapy to minimize toxicity.[173,195] In contrast, when tumors are chemosensitive, combination platinum-based therapy is the standard in almost all gynecologic malignancies. In only two diseases is a triplet of chemotherapy the standard of care: germ cell tumors and endometrial cancer. The Cochrane meta-analysis of less chemotherapy compared with combination in advanced endometrial cancer included more than 1000 patients.[192] Progression-free survival was significantly improved, but there was only a trend toward improved survival (HR = 0.90; 95% CI, 0.80–1.03). As expected, toxicity was generally higher with the combination chemotherapy regimens. Only one trial, GOG-177, showed a significant survival benefit from the addition of paclitaxel to combination chemotherapy, again with the expense of increased toxicity.[196] Paclitaxel, adriamycin, and cisplatin with granulocyte colony-stimulating factor produced less grade 4 neutropenia (36% vs 50%) but more grade 3 peripheral neuropathy (12% vs 1%), for an absolute improvement in 12-month overall survival of 58% for paclitaxel, adriamycin, and cisplatin versus 50% for adriamycin and cisplatin.

In cervical cancer, HRQOL has been assessed using FACT-Cx, consisting of the Functional Assessment of Cancer Therapy (FACT-G) plus a cervix cancer-specific subscale, the Brief Pain Inventory-Short Form, and a neurotoxicity subscale.[197] Scores were stable over time and considerably lower than the general population norms. The addition of paclitaxel to cisplatin produced a significantly higher response rate and progression-free survival, with no overall survival advantage. Despite greater myelosuppression with combination chemotherapy, there was no significant impact on the overall HRQOL score, but HRQOL and PROs have supported this as the standard of care.

Chemotherapy Toxicity: Integration of Novel Biologics

The recent attempt to add chemotherapy agents in a rational fashion in the treatment of advanced ovarian cancer (GOG-182/ICON-V) has not substantially impacted the cure rate for the disease.[198] With the addition of gemcitabine to carboplatin and paclitaxel, there was considerable excess grade 3 and 4 toxicity. However, just as the era of increasing benefit to chemotherapy draws asymptotically to a ceiling, the hope of benefit from novel biologics has dawned, adding complex HRQOL measurement questions.[199] The term "novel biologic" is potentially misleading in that many cytotoxics are targeted to specific biologic functions, but the term is taken to mean agents that are designed, rather than discovered, and target biologic pathways important in the development of cancer. Many affect fundamental mechanisms of cellular life in which fatigue may be a prominent side effect, and therefore a major focus of future PRO research.[200]

BOWEL OBSTRUCTION

Bowel obstruction frequently occurs late in the course of gynecologic malignancies, usually from disease progression but occasionally from treatment complications. Palliative surgery in the last year of life has a mortality rate as high as 30%, and may lead to serious complications and colostomy. Nonsurgical choices can achieve effective palliation for bowel obstruction. Percutaneous endoscopic gastric tube placement is highly effective, with one informative series reporting 86 (91%) of 94 patients with advanced ovarian cancer achieving symptomatic relief (no nausea and vomiting) within a week.[201] Total parenteral nutrition may prolong life, at the cost of edema, thrombosis, infections, and medicalizing the dying process, and chemotherapy is typically ineffective in restoring bowel function in heavily pretreated patients with recurrent disease.[202] Octreotide, a synthetic somatostatin analog, reduces secretions and may improve obstruction, and new long-acting release preparation is convenient, although expensive.[203] Stenting may provide effective palliation in gastric outlet or colon obstruction, but is often painful, and stents can migrate or cause bleeding, reobstruction, or perforation.[204]

HRQOL, UTILITY, AND COST EFFECTIVENESS

The science behind the evaluation of outcomes rarely translates into simple formulae; such that 1 year of life at a quality of "x" must be as desirable as 6 months of life at a quality of "2x." In anticipation, patient-centered exploration of gambles and tradeoffs can inform decisions, and in retrospect, calibrate cost-effectiveness. New measurement initiatives, such as the PROMIS, will make it easier to compare patients' HRQOL.[205]

To be approved, new drugs must significantly impact survival or patients' QOL. PROs have become an important outcome measure of the use of new medical interventions.[206] Quality-adjusted survival is an increasingly recognized measure for evaluating interventions across health care, combined with growing awareness of the cost effectiveness of anticancer interventions. Therefore, additional analyses will be conducted to evaluate comparative effectiveness, cost-effectiveness, and use across clinical trials.[207] Resource use and cost for cancer patients will likely be an increasing focus of study.[183,208–210]

CONNECTION AND CARE

The impulse to "not just stand there, but to do something" is a powerful driver in oncology, and yet insight, awareness, and offering one's presence may do more than chemotherapy.[153] Compassionate attention may halve the amount of analgesia needed.[211] Keeping equanimity in stressful and distressing situations also affords the opportunity to fully evaluate and critically review. Counterintuitive observations are often reported: the decline in QOL over time for newly diagnosed patients, although it seems to improve for those with recurrent disease,[212] especially when considering abandoning palliative chemotherapy.[213] Integrating PROs of HRQOL with feedback to oncologists seems to improve disclosure and discussion of symptoms, but many potentially serious issues seem to remain unaddressed.[214] These delicate and demanding tasks need greater priority, training, protected time, and an empowering human connection.

Gynecologic cancer demands complex multimodality care. There is a Hippocratic responsibility to the commission to cure, and also need the Aesculepian commitment to care. To live life fully is the goal.[215] Recent advances have improved and challenged HRQOL. Evaluating and addressing treatment, survivorship, and HRQOL issues is an important part of the entire package of modern medical care.

REFERENCES

1. Jemal A, Siegel R, Xu JQ, et al. Cancer statistics, 2010. CA Cancer J Clin 2010; 60(5):277–300.
2. Siegel R, Ward E, Brawley O, et al. The impact of eliminating socioeconomic and racial disparities on premature cancer deaths. CA Cancer J Clin 2011;61(4): 212–36.
3. Harris PF, Remington PL, Trentham-Dietz A, et al. Prevalence and treatment of menopausal symptoms among breast cancer survivors. J Pain Symptom Manage 2002;23(6):501–9.
4. Crandall C, Petersen L, Ganz PA, et al. Association of breast cancer and its therapy with menopause-related symptoms. Menopause 2004;11(5):519–30.
5. Gupta P, Sturdee DW, Palin SL, et al. Menopausal symptoms in women treated for breast cancer: the prevalence and severity of symptoms and their perceived effects on quality of life. Climacteric 2006;9(1):49–58.
6. Schover LR. Premature ovarian failure and its consequences: vasomotor symptoms, sexuality, and fertility. J Clin Oncol 2008;26(5):753–8.
7. Ganz PA, Greendale GA, Petersen L, et al. Breast cancer in younger women: reproductive and late health effects of treatment. J Clin Oncol 2003;21(22): 4184–93.
8. Carter J, Rowland K, Chi D, et al. Gynecologic cancer treatment and the impact of cancer-related infertility. Gynecol Oncol 2005;97(1):90–5.
9. Wenzel L, Cella D. Quality of life issues in gynecologic cancer. In: Hoskins WJ, Perez CA, Young RC, et al, editors. Principles and practices of gynecologic oncology. 4th edition. Philadelphia: Lippincott, Williams & Wilkins; 2005. p. 1333–42.
10. Wenzel L, Dogan-Ates A, Habbal R, et al. Defining and measuring reproductive concerns of female cancer survivors. J Natl Cancer Inst Monogr 2005;(34):94–8.
11. Greendale GA, Petersen L, Zibecchi L, et al. Factors related to sexual function in postmenopausal women with a history of breast cancer. Menopause 2001;8(2): 111–9.
12. Haskell SG, Bean-Mayberry B, Gordon K. Discontinuing postmenopausal hormone therapy: an observational study of tapering versus quitting cold turkey: is there a difference in recurrence of menopausal symptoms? Menopause 2009; 16(3):494–9.
13. Matulonis UA, Kornblith A, Lee H, et al. Long-term adjustment of early-stage ovarian cancer survivors. Int J Gynecol Cancer 2008;18(6):1183–93.
14. Carmack Taylor CL, Basen-Engquist K, Shinn EH, et al. Predictors of sexual functioning in ovarian cancer patients. J Clin Oncol 2004;22(5):881–9.
15. Greenwald HP, McCorkle R. Sexuality and sexual function in long-term survivors of cervical cancer. J Womens Health 2008;17(6):955–63.
16. Carter J, Sonoda Y, Baser RE, et al. A 2-year prospective study assessing the emotional, sexual, and quality of life concerns of women undergoing radical

trachelectomy versus radical hysterectomy for treatment of early-stage cervical cancer. Gynecol Oncol 2010;119(2):358–65.

17. Greimel ER, Winter R, Kapp KS, et al. Quality of life and sexual functioning after cervical cancer treatment: a long-term follow-up study. Psychooncology 2009; 18(5):476–82.

18. Stafford L, Judd F. Partners of long-term gynaecologic cancer survivors: psychiatric morbidity, psychosexual outcomes and supportive care needs. Gynecol Oncol 2010;118(3):268–73.

19. Likes WM, Stegbauer C, Tillmanns T, et al. Pilot study of sexual function and quality of life after excision for vulvar intraepithelial neoplasia. J Reprod Med 2007;52(1):23–7.

20. Carpenter KM, Fowler JM, Maxwell GL, et al. Social support among gynecologic cancer survivors. Ann Behav Med 2010;39(1):79–90.

21. Levin AO, Carpenter KM, Fowler JM, et al. Sexual morbidity associated with poorer psychological adjustment among gynecological cancer survivors. Int J Gynecol Cancer 2010;20(3):461–70.

22. Le T, Menard C, Samant R, et al. Longitudinal assessments of quality of life in endometrial cancer patients: effect of surgical approach and adjuvant radiotherapy. Int J Radiat Oncol Biol Phys 2009;75(3):795–802.

23. Kornblith AB, Huang HQ, Walker JL, et al. Quality of life of patients with endometrial cancer undergoing laparoscopic international federation of gynecology and obstetrics staging compared with laparotomy: a gynecologic oncology group study. J Clin Oncol 2009;27(32):5337–42.

24. Lindau ST, Gavrilova N, Anderson D. Sexual morbidity in very long term survivors of vaginal and cervical cancer: a comparison to national norms. Gynecol Oncol 2007;106(2):413–8.

25. Canada AL, Schover LR. The psychosocial impact of interrupted childbearing in long-term female cancer survivors. Psychooncology 2010. [Epub ahead of print].

26. Cella D, Fallowfield LJ. Recognition and management of treatment-related side effects for breast cancer patients receiving adjuvant endocrine therapy. Breast Cancer Res Treat 2008;107(2):167–80.

27. Ganz PA, Rowland JH, Desmond K, et al. Life after breast cancer: understanding women's health-related quality of life and sexual functioning. J Clin Oncol 1998;16(2):501–14.

28. Joffe H, Soares CN, Thurston RC, et al. Depression is associated with worse objectively and subjectively measured sleep, but not more frequent awakenings, in women with vasomotor symptoms. Menopause 2009;16(4):671–9.

29. Williams RE, Levine KB, Kalilani L, et al. Menopause-specific questionnaire assessment in US population-based study shows negative impact on health-related quality of life. Maturitas 2009;62(2):153–9.

30. Carter J, Goldfrank D, Schover LR. Simple strategies for vaginal health promotion in cancer survivors. J Sex Med 2011;8(2):549–59.

31. Brotto LA, Heiman JR, Goff B, et al. A psychoeducational intervention for sexual dysfunction in women with gynecologic cancer. Arch Sex Behav 2008;37(2): 317–29.

32. Likes WM, Stegbauer C, Tillmanns T, et al. Correlates of sexual function following vulvar excision. Gynecol Oncol 2007;105(3):600–3.

33. Bergmark K, Avall-Lundqvist E, Dickman PW, et al. Vaginal changes and sexuality in women with a history of cervical cancer. N Engl J Med 1999;340(18): 1383–9.

34. Jensen PT, Groenvold M, Klee MC, et al. Early-stage cervical carcinoma, radical hysterectomy, and sexual function: a longitudinal study. Cancer 2004;100(1): 97–106.

35. Pieterse QD, Maas CP, ter Kuile MM, et al. An observational longitudinal study to evaluate miction, defecation, and sexual function after radical hysterectomy with pelvic lymphadenectomy for early-stage cervical cancer. Int J Gynecol Cancer 2006;16(3):1119–29.

36. Ditto A, Martinelli F, Borreani C, et al. Quality of life and sexual, bladder, and intestinal dysfunctions after class III nerve-sparing and class II radical hysterectomies a questionnaire-based study. Int J Gynecol Cancer 2009;19(5): 953–7.

37. Carter J, Chi DS, Abu-Rustum N, et al. Brief report: total pelvic exenteration: a retrospective clinical needs assessment. Psychooncology 2004;13(2):125–31.

38. Maggioni A, Roviglione G, Landoni F, et al. Pelvic exenteration: ten-year experience at the European Institute of Oncology in Milan. Gynecol Oncol 2009; 114(1):64–8.

39. Benn T, Brooks RA, Zhang Q, et al. Pelvic exenteration in gynecologic oncology: a single institution study over 20 years. Gynecol Oncol 2011;122(1):14–8.

40. Creutzberg CL, van Putten WL, Koper PC, et al. The morbidity of treatment for patients with stage I endometrial cancer: results from a randomized trial. Int J Radiat Oncol Biol Phys 2001;51(5):1246–55.

41. Nout RA, Putter H, Jurgenliemk-Schulz IM, et al. Quality of life after pelvic radiotherapy or vaginal brachytherapy for endometrial cancer: first results of the randomized PORTEC-2 trial. J Clin Oncol 2009;27(21):3547–56.

42. Saibishkumar EP, Patel FD, Sharma SC. Evaluation of late toxicities of patients with carcinoma of the cervix treated with radical radiotherapy: an audit from India. Clin Oncol (R Coll Radiol) 2006;18(1):30–7.

43. Vistad I, Cvancarova M, Fossa SD, et al. Postradiotherapy morbidity in long-term survivors after locally advanced cervical cancer: how well do physicians' assessments agree with those of their patients? Int J Radiat Oncol Biol Phys 2008;71(5):1335–42.

44. Flay LD, Matthews JH. The effects of radiotherapy and surgery on the sexual function of women treated for cervical-cancer. Int J Radiat Oncol Biol Phys 1995;31(2):399–404.

45. Bruner DW, Lanciano R, Keegan M, et al. Vaginal stenosis and sexual function following intracavitary radiation for the treatment of cervical and endometrial carcinoma. Int J Radiat Oncol Biol Phys 1993;27(4):825–30.

46. Jensen PT, Groenvold M, Klee MC, et al. Longitudinal study of sexual function and vaginal changes after radiotherapy for cervical cancer. Int J Radiat Oncol Biol Phys 2003;56(4):937–49.

47. Frumovitz M, Sun CC, Schover LR, et al. Quality of life and sexual functioning in cervical cancer survivors. J Clin Oncol 2005;23(30):7428–36.

48. Keys HM, Roberts JA, Brunetto VL, et al. A phase III trial of surgery with or without adjunctive external pelvic radiation therapy in intermediate risk endometrial adenocarcinoma: a Gynecologic Oncology Group study. Gynecol Oncol 2004;92(3):744–51.

49. Alektiar KM, Venkatraman E, Chi DS, et al. Intravaginal brachytherapy alone for intermediate-risk endometrial cancer. Int J Radiat Oncol Biol Phys 2005;62(1): 111–7.

50. Petereit DG, Tannehill SP, Grosen EA, et al. Outpatient vaginal cuff brachytherapy for endometrial cancer. Int J Gynecol Cancer 1999;9(6):456–62.

51. Anderson JM, Stea B, Hallum AV, et al. High-dose-rate postoperative vaginal cuff irradiation alone for stage IB and IC endometrial cancer. Int J Radiat Oncol Biol Phys 2000;46(2):417–25.

52. MacLeod C, Fowler A, Duval P, et al. High-dose-rate brachytherapy alone post-hysterectomy for endometrial cancer. Int J Radiat Oncol Biol Phys 1998;42(5): 1033–9.

53. Nout RA, Smit VT, Putter H, et al. Vaginal brachytherapy versus pelvic external beam radiotherapy for patients with endometrial cancer of high-intermediate risk (PORTEC-2): an open-label, non-inferiority, randomised trial. Lancet 2010; 375(9717):816–23.

54. Kumar VJ, Nin CY, Kuei LY, et al. Survival and disease relapse in surgical stage I endometrioid adenocarcinoma of the uterus after adjuvant vaginal vault brachytherapy. Int J Gynecol Cancer 2010;20(4):564–9.

55. Flynn KE, Smith MA, Davis MK. From physician to consumer: the effectiveness of strategies to manage health care utilization. Med Care Res Rev 2002;59(4): 455–81.

56. Stabile C, Barakat R, Abu-Rustum N, et al. Preliminary data-a survey of female cancer patients' preference for sexual health interventions. J Sex Med 2011;8: 65–6.

57. Rogers M, Todd C. Information exchange in oncology outpatient clinics: source, valence and uncertainty. Psychooncology 2002;11(4):336–45.

58. Hordern AJ, Street AF. Communicating about patient sexuality and intimacy after cancer: mismatched expectations and unmet needs. Med J Aust 2007; 186(5):224–7.

59. Berman L, Berman J, Felder S, et al. Seeking help for sexual function complaints: what gynecologists need to know about the female patient's experience. Fertil Steril 2003;79(3):572–6.

60. Shifren JL, Johannes CB, Monz BU, et al. Help-seeking behavior of women with self-reported distressing sexual problems. J Womens Health 2009;18(4):461–8.

61. Wiggins DL, Wood R, Granai CO, et al. Sex, intimacy, and the gynecologic oncologist: survey results of the New England Association of Gynecologic Oncologists (NEAGO). J Psychosoc Oncol 2007;25(4):61–70.

62. Zachariae R, Pedersen CG, Jensen AB, et al. Association of perceived physician communication style with patient satisfaction, distress, cancer-related self-efficacy, and perceived control over the disease. Br J Cancer 2003;88(5): 658–65.

63. Stead ML, Brown JM, Fallowfield L, et al. Lack of communication between healthcare professionals and women with ovarian cancer about sexual issues. Br J Cancer 2003;88(5):666–71.

64. de Bock GH, Bonnema J, Zwaan RE, et al. Patient's needs and preferences in routine follow-up after treatment for breast cancer. Br J Cancer 2004;90(6): 1144–50.

65. Rogausch A, Sigle J, Seibert A, et al. Feasibility and acceptance of electronic quality of life assessment in general practice: an implementation study. Health Qual Life Outcomes 2009;7:51.

66. Detmar SB, Muller MJ, Schornagel JH, et al. Health-related quality-of-life assessments and patient-physician communication: a randomized controlled trial. JAMA 2002;288(23):3027–34.

67. Carter J, Sonoda Y, Chi DS, et al. Radical trachelectomy for cervical cancer: postoperative physical and emotional adjustment concerns. Gynecol Oncol 2008;111(1):151–7.

68. Carter J, Raviv L, Sonoda Y, et al. Recovery issues of fertility-preserving surgery in patients with early-stage cervical cancer and a model for survivorship the physician checklist. Int J Gynecol Cancer 2011;21(1):106–16.

69. Jeffery DD, Tzeng JP, Keefe FJ, et al. Initial report of the cancer patient-reported outcomes measurement information system (PROMIS) sexual function committee review of sexual function measures and domains used in oncology. Cancer 2009;115(6):1142–53.

70. Baser RE, Carter J, Li Y. Psychometric validation of the female sexual function index (FSFI) in cancer survivors. Cancer Res, in press.

71. Baser RE, Carter J, Li Y. Psychometric evaluation of a 6-item short form of the Female Sexual Function Index (FSFI) in a sample of cancer survivors. London, England: International Society for Quality of Life Research (ISOQOL) Annual Conference. Oct 27–30, 2010.

72. Isidori AM, Pozza C, Esposito K, et al. Development and validation of a 6-item version of the Female Sexual Function Index (FSFI) as a diagnostic tool for female sexual dysfunction. J Sex Med 2010;7(3):1139–46.

73. Flynn KE, Jeffery DD, Keefe FJ, et al. Sexual functioning along the cancer continuum: focus group results from the Patient-Reported Outcomes Measurement Information System (PROMIS (R)). Psychooncology 2011; 20(4):378–86.

74. Flynn KE, Reese JB, Jeffery D, et al. Patient experiences with communication about sex during and after treatment for cancer. Psychooncology 2011. [Epub ahead of print].

75. Carter J. Cancer-related infertility. Gynecol Oncol 2005;99(Suppl. 1):S122–3.

76. Ganz PA, Moinpour CM, Pauler DK, et al. Health status and quality of life in patients with early-stage Hodgkin's disease treated on Southwest Oncology Group study 9133. J Clin Oncol 2003;21(18):3512–9.

77. Duffy CM, Allen SM, Clark MA. Discussions regarding reproductive health for young women with breast cancer undergoing chemotherapy. J Clin Oncol 2005;23(4):766–73.

78. Thewes B, Meiser B, Rickard J, et al. The fertility- and menopause-related information needs of younger women with a diagnosis of breast cancer: a qualitative study. Psychooncology 2003;12(5):500–11.

79. Carter J, Sonoda Y, Abu-Rustum NR. Reproductive concerns of women treated with radical trachelectomy for cervical cancer. Gynecol Oncol 2007;105(1): 13–6.

80. Gershenson DM. Fertility-sparing surgery for malignancies in women. J Natl Cancer Inst Monogr 2005;(34):43–7.

81. Abu-Rustum NR, Sonoda Y, Black D, et al. Fertility-sparing radical abdominal trachelectomy for cervical carcinoma: technique and review of the literature. Gynecol Oncol 2006;103(3):807–13.

82. Plante M, Gregoire J, Renaud MC, et al. The vaginal radical trachelectomy: an update of a series of 125 cases and 106 pregnancies. Gynecol Oncol 2011; 121(2):290–7.

83. Plante M. Vaginal radical trachelectomy: an update. Gynecol Oncol 2008; 111(Suppl. 2):S105–10.

84. Abu-Rustum NR, Neubauer N, Sonoda Y, et al. Surgical and pathologic outcomes of fertility-sparing radical abdominal trachelectomy for FIGO stage IB1 cervical cancer. Gynecol Oncol 2008;111(2):261–4.

85. Lanowska M, Mangler M, Spek A, et al. Radical vaginal trachelectomy (RVT) combined with laparoscopic lymphadenectomy: prospective study of 225

patients with early-stage cervical cancer. Int J Gynecol Cancer 2011;21(8): 1458–64.

86. Sonoda Y, Abu-Rustum NR, Gemignani ML, et al. A fertility-sparing alternative to radical hysterectomy: how many patients may be eligible? Gynecol Oncol 2004; 95(3):534–8.

87. Toubassi D, Himel D, Winton S, et al. The informational needs of newly diagnosed cervical cancer patients who will be receiving combined chemoradiation treatment. J Cancer Educ 2006;21(4):263–8.

88. Benshushan A. Endometrial adenocarcinoma in young patients: evaluation and fertility-preserving treatment. Eur J Obstet Gynecol Reprod Biol 2004;117(2): 132–7.

89. Kim YB, Holschneider CH, Ghosh K, et al. Progestin alone as primary treatment of endometrial carcinoma in premenopausal women. Report of seven cases and review of the literature. Cancer 1997;79(2):320–7.

90. Mazzon I, Corrado G, Morricone D, et al. Reproductive preservation for treatment of stage IA endometrial cancer in a young woman: hysteroscopic resection. Int J Gynecol Cancer 2005;15(5):974–8.

91. Vinker S, Shani A, Open M, et al. Conservative treatment of adenocarcinoma of the endometrium in young patients. Is it appropriate? Eur J Obstet Gynecol Reprod Biol 1999;83(1):63–5.

92. Wang CB, Wang CJ, Huang HJ, et al. Fertility-preserving treatment in young patients with endometrial adenocarcinoma. Cancer 2002;94(8):2192–8.

93. Kurman RJ, Kaminski PF, Norris HJ. The behavior of endometrial hyperplasia. A long-term study of "untreated" hyperplasia in 170 patients. Cancer 1985;56(2): 403–12.

94. Trimble CL, Kauderer J, Zaino R, et al. Concurrent endometrial carcinoma in women with a biopsy diagnosis of atypical endometrial hyperplasia: a Gynecologic Oncology Group study. Cancer 2006;106(4):812–9.

95. Leitao MM Jr, Chi DS. Fertility-sparing options for patients with gynecologic malignancies. Oncologist 2005;10(8):613–22.

96. Duska LR, Garrett A, Rueda BR, et al. Endometrial cancer in women 40 years old or younger. Gynecol Oncol 2001;83(2):388–93.

97. Evans-Metcalf ER, Brooks SE, Reale FR, et al. Profile of women 45 years of age and younger with endometrial cancer. Obstet Gynecol 1998;91(3):349–54.

98. Gitsch G, Hanzal E, Jensen D, et al. Endometrial cancer in premenopausal women 45 years and younger. Obstet Gynecol 1995;85(4):504–8.

99. Walsh C, Holschneider C, Hoang Y, et al. Coexisting ovarian malignancy in young women with endometrial cancer. Obstet Gynecol 2005;106(4): 693–9.

100. Jadoul P, Donnez J. Conservative treatment may be beneficial for young women with atypical endometrial hyperplasia or endometrial adenocarcinoma. Fertil Steril 2003;80(6):1315–24.

101. Lowe MP, Cooper BC, Sood AK, et al. Implementation of assisted reproductive technologies following conservative management of FIGO grade I endometrial adenocarcinoma and/or complex hyperplasia with atypia. Gynecol Oncol 2003;91(3):569–72.

102. Niwa K, Tagami K, Lian Z, et al. Outcome of fertility-preserving treatment in young women with endometrial carcinomas. BJOG 2005;112(3):317–20.

103. Low JJ, Perrin LC, Crandon AJ, et al. Conservative surgery to preserve ovarian function in patients with malignant ovarian germ cell tumors. A review of 74 cases. Cancer 2000;89(2):391–8.

104. Zanetta G, Bonazzi C, Cantu M, et al. Survival and reproductive function after treatment of malignant germ cell ovarian tumors. J Clin Oncol 2001;19(4): 1015–20.
105. Morice P, Camatte S, El Hassan J, et al. Clinical outcomes and fertility after conservative treatment of ovarian borderline tumors. Fertil Steril 2001;75(1): 92–6.
106. Schilder JM, Thompson AM, DePriest PD, et al. Outcome of reproductive age women with stage IA or IC invasive epithelial ovarian cancer treated with fertility-sparing therapy. Gynecol Oncol 2002;87(1):1–7.
107. Brown C, Dharmendra B, Barakat R. Preserving fertility in patients (Pts) with epithelial ovarian cancer (EOC): the role of conservative surgery in the treatment of early stage disease [abstract #36]. Gynecol Oncol 2000;76:240.
108. Savage P, Constenla D, Fisher C, et al. Granulosa cell tumours of the ovary: demographics, survival and the management of advanced disease. Clin Oncol (R Coll Radiol) 1998;10(4):242–5.
109. Rao GG, Skinner EN, Gehrig PA, et al. Fertility-sparing surgery for ovarian low malignant potential tumors. Gynecol Oncol 2005;98(2):263–6.
110. Cadron I, Leunen K, Van Gorp T, et al. Management of borderline ovarian neoplasms. J Clin Oncol 2007;25(20):2928–37.
111. Noyes N, Knopman JM, Long K, et al. Fertility considerations in the management of gynecologic malignancies. Gynecol Oncol 2011;120(3):326–33.
112. Oktay K, Sonmezer M. Fertility issues and options in young women with cancer. Recent Results Cancer Res 2008;178:203–24.
113. Sonmezer M, Oktay K. Fertility preservation in female patients. Hum Reprod Update 2004;10(3):251–66.
114. Rosen A. Third-party reproduction and adoption in cancer patients. J Natl Cancer Inst Monogr 2005;(34):91–3.
115. Alizadeh AA, Eisen MB, Davis RE, et al. Distinct types of diffuse large B-cell lymphoma identified by gene expression profiling. Nature 2000;403(6769): 503–11.
116. Schover LR. Psychosocial aspects of infertility and decisions about reproduction in young cancer survivors: a review. Med Pediatr Oncol 1999;33(1):53–9.
117. Nunns D, Williamson K, Swaney L, et al. The morbidity of surgery and adjuvant radiotherapy in the management of endometrial carcinoma. Int J Gynecol Cancer 2000;10(3):233–8.
118. Fujiwara K, Kigawa J, Hasegawa K, et al. Effect of simple omentoplasty and omentopexy in the prevention of complications after pelvic lymphadenectomy. Int J Gynecol Cancer 2003;13(1):61–6.
119. Abu-Rustum NR, Alektiar K, Iasonos A, et al. The incidence of symptomatic lower-extremity lymphedema following treatment of uterine corpus malignancies: a 12-year experience at Memorial Sloan-Kettering Cancer Center. Gynecol Oncol 2006;103(2):714–8.
120. Panici PB, Basile S, Maneschi F, et al. Systematic pelvic lymphadenectomy vs no lymphadenectomy in early-stage endometrial carcinoma: randomized clinical trial. J Natl Cancer Inst 2008;100(23):1707–16.
121. Walker JL, Piedmonte MR, Spirtos NM, et al. Laparoscopy compared with laparotomy for comprehensive surgical staging of uterine cancer: gynecologic oncology group study LAP2. J Clin Oncol 2009;27(32):5331–6.
122. Carlson JW, Kauderer J, Walker JL, et al. A randomized phase III trial of VH fibrin sealant to reduce lymphedema after inguinal lymph node dissection: a Gynecologic Oncology Group study. Gynecol Oncol 2008;110(1):76–82.

123. Ryan M, Stainton MC, Jaconelli C, et al. The experience of lower limb lymphedema for women after treatment for gynecologic cancer. Oncol Nurs Forum 2003;30(3):417–23.

124. Janda M, Obermair A, Cella D, et al. Vulvar cancer patients' quality of life: a qualitative assessment. Int J Gynecol Cancer 2004;14(5):875–81.

125. Pereira de Godoy JM, Braile DM, de Fatima Godoy M, et al. Quality of life and peripheral lymphedema. Lymphology 2002;35(2):72–5.

126. Cella DF, Wiklund I, Shumaker SA, et al. Integrating health-related quality of life into cross-national clinical trials. Qual Life Res 1993;2(6):433–40.

127. Carter J, Raviv L, Appollo K, et al. A pilot study using the Gynecologic Cancer Lymphedema Questionnaire (GCLQ) as a clinical care tool to identify lower extremity lymphedema in gynecologic cancer survivors. Gynecol Oncol 2010; 117(2):317–23.

128. Boggess JF, Gehrig PA, Cantrell L, et al. A comparative study of 3 surgical methods for hysterectomy with staging for endometrial cancer: robotic assistance, laparoscopy, laparotomy. Am J Obstet Gynecol 2008;199(4):360.e1–9.

129. Mendivil A, Holloway RW, Boggess JF. Emergence of robotic assisted surgery in gynecologic oncology: American perspective. Gynecol Oncol 2009;114(2): S24–31.

130. duPont NC, Chandrasekhar R, Wilding G, et al. Current trends in robot assisted surgery: a survey of gynecologic oncologists. Int J Med Robot 2010;6(4): 468–72.

131. Boggess JF, Gehrig PA, Cantrell L, et al. A case-control study of robot-assisted type III radical hysterectomy with pelvic lymph node dissection compared with open radical hysterectomy. Am J Obstet Gynecol 2008;199(4):357.e1–7.

132. Barnett JC, Judd JP, Wu JM, et al. Cost comparison among robotic, laparoscopic, and open hysterectomy for endometrial cancer. Obstet Gynecol 2010; 116(3):685–93.

133. Gervasoni JE, Sbayi S, Cady B. Role of lymphadenectomy in surgical treatment of solid tumors: an update on the clinical data. Ann Surg Oncol 2007;14(9): 2443–62.

134. Zivanovic O, Khoury-Collado F, Abu-Rustum NR, et al. Sentinel lymph node biopsy in the management of vulvar carcinoma, cervical cancer, and endometrial cancer. Oncologist 2009;14(7):695–705.

135. Badger C, Preston N, Seers K, et al. Physical therapies for reducing and controlling lymphoedema of the limbs. Cochrane Database Syst Rev 2004;4: CD003141.

136. Werngrenelgstrom M, Lidman D. Lymphedema of the lower-extremities after surgery and radiotherapy for cancer of the cervix. Scand J Plast Reconstr Surg Hand Surg 1994;28(4):289–93.

137. Bergmark K, Avall-Lundqvist E, Dickman PW, et al. Lymphedema and bladder-emptying difficulties after radical hysterectomy for early cervical cancer and among population controls. Int J Gynecol Cancer 2006;16(3):1130–9.

138. Gaarenstroom KN, Kenter GG, Trimbos JB, et al. Postoperative complications after vulvectomy and inguinofemoral lymphadenectomy using separate groin incisions. Int J Gynecol Cancer 2003;13(4):522–7.

139. Burak WE, Hollenbeck ST, Zervos EE, et al. Sentinel lymph node biopsy results in less postoperative morbidity compared with axillary lymph node dissection for breast cancer. Am J Surg 2002;183(1):23–7.

140. Petrek JA, Senie RT, Peters M, et al. Lymphedema in a cohort of breast carcinoma survivors 20 years after diagnosis. Cancer 2001;92(6):1368–77.

141. Schrenk P, Rieger R, Shamiyeh A, et al. Morbidity following sentinel lymph node biopsy versus axillary lymph node dissection for patients with breast carcinoma. Cancer 2000;88(3):608–14.
142. Burke TW, Stringer CA, Gershenson DM, et al. Radical wide excision and selective inguinal node dissection for squamous-cell carcinoma of the vulva. Gynecol Oncol 1990;38(3):328–32.
143. Hacker NF, Leuchter RS, Berek JS, et al. Radical vulvectomy and bilateral inguinal lymphadenectomy through separate groin incisions. Obstet Gynecol 1981;58(5):574–9.
144. Roy M, Bouchard-Fortier G, Popa I, et al. Value of sentinel node mapping in cancer of the cervix. Gynecol Oncol 2011;122(2):269–74.
145. Cormier B, Diaz JP, Shih K, et al. Establishing a sentinel lymph node mapping algorithm for the treatment of early cervical cancer. Gynecol Oncol 2011; 122(2):275–80.
146. American College of Obstetricians and Gynecologists. ACOG practice bulletin, clinical management guidelines for obstetrician-gynecologists: management of endometrial cancer. Obstet Gynecol 2005;65(106):413–25.
147. Chapman RH, Berger M, Weinstein MC, et al. When does quality-adjusting life-years matter in cost-effectiveness analysis? Health Econ 2004;13(5): 429–36.
148. Gotay CC, Korn EL, McCabe MS, et al. Quality-of-life assessment in cancer treatment protocols: research issues in protocol development. J Natl Cancer Inst 1992;84(8):575–9.
149. Bodurka-Bevers D, Basen-Engquist K, Carmack CL, et al. Depression, anxiety, and quality of life in patients with epithelial ovarian cancer. Gynecol Oncol 2000; 78(3 Pt 1):302–8.
150. Calman KC. Quality of life in cancer patients: an hypothesis. J Med Ethics 1984; 10(3):124–7.
151. Study protocol for the World Health Organization project to develop a quality of life assessment instrument (WHOQOL). Qual Life Res 1993;2(2):153–9.
152. Bottomley A. The cancer patient and quality of life. Oncologist 2002;7(2): 120–5.
153. Cella D. What do global quality-of-life questions really measure? Insights from Hobday et al and the "do something" rule. J Clin Oncol 2003;21(16):3178–9 [author reply: 3179].
154. Bezjak A, Tu D, Bacon M, et al. Quality of life in ovarian cancer patients: comparison of paclitaxel plus cisplatin, with cyclophosphamide plus cisplatin in a randomized study. J Clin Oncol 2004;22(22):4595–603.
155. Greimel ER, Bjelic-Radisic V, Pfisterer J, et al. Randomized study of the Arbeitsgemeinschaft Gynaekologische Onkologie Ovarian Cancer Study Group comparing quality of life in patients with ovarian cancer treated with cisplatin/paclitaxel versus carboplatin/paclitaxel. J Clin Oncol 2006;24(4):579–86.
156. Vasey PA, Jayson GC, Gordon A, et al. Phase III randomized trial of docetaxel-carboplatin versus paclitaxel-carboplatin as first-line chemotherapy for ovarian carcinoma. J Natl Cancer Inst 2004;96(22):1682–91.
157. Gralla RJ. Silk purse in Atlanta: a commentary on SWOG 9509, an advanced non-small cell lung cancer trial. Oncologist 1999;4(3):188–90.
158. Sehouli J, Stengel D, Oskay-Oezcelik G, et al. Nonplatinum topotecan combinations versus topotecan alone for recurrent ovarian cancer: results of a phase III study of the North-Eastern German Society of Gynecological Oncology Ovarian Cancer Study Group. J Clin Oncol 2008;26(19):3176–82.

159. Lederberg M, Fitchett G. Can you measure a sunbeam with a ruler? Psychoon-cology 1999;8:375–7.
160. Levine MN, Ganz PA. Beyond the development of quality-of-life instruments: where do we go from here? J Clin Oncol 2002;20(9):2215–6.
161. Browman GP. Science, language, intuition, and the many meanings of quality of life. J Clin Oncol 1999;17(6):1651–3.
162. Efficace F, Bottomley A, Osoba D, et al. Beyond the development of health-related quality-of-life (HRQOL) measures: a checklist for evaluating HRQOL outcomes in cancer clinical trials. Does HRQOL evaluation in prostate cancer research inform clinical decision making? J Clin Oncol 2003;21(18):3502–11.
163. Wenzel L, Huang HQ, Cella D, et al. Validation of FACT/GOG-AD subscale for ovarian cancer-related abdominal discomfort: a Gynecologic Oncology Group study. Gynecol Oncol 2008;110(1):60–4.
164. Huang HQ, Brady MF, Cella D, et al. Validation and reduction of FACT/GOG-Ntx subscale for platinum/paclitaxel-induced neurologic symptoms: a gynecologic oncology group study. Int J Gynecol Cancer 2007;17(2):387–93.
165. Ferrell B, Smith SL, Cullinane CA, et al. Psychological well being and quality of life in ovarian cancer survivors. Cancer 2003;98(5):1061–71.
166. Kornblith AB, Thaler HT, Wong G, et al. Quality of life of women with ovarian cancer. Gynecol Oncol 1995;59(2):231–42.
167. Wenzel L, Monk B, Huang H, et al. Clinically meaningful quality-of-life changes in ovarian cancer: results from Gynecologic Oncology Group Clinical Trial 152. Paper presented at Quality of Life III: translating the science of quality-of-life assessment into clinical practice. An example-driven approach for practicing clinicians and clinical researchers. Scottsdale, AZ. November 28, 2011.
168. Goff BA, Mandel LS, Drescher CW, et al. Development of an ovarian cancer symptom index: possibilities for earlier detection. Cancer 2007;109(2):221–7.
169. Sandadi S, Frasure H, Broderick M, et al. The effect of sleep disturbance on quality of life in women with ovarian cancer. Gynecol Oncol 2011;123(2):351–5.
170. von Gruenigen VE, Huang HQ, Gil KM, et al. A comparison of quality-of-life domains and clinical factors in ovarian cancer patients: a Gynecologic Oncology Group study. J Pain Symptom Manage 2010;39(5):839–46.
171. McGuire WP, Hoskins WJ, Brady MF, et al. Cyclophosphamide and cisplatin compared with paclitaxel and cisplatin in patients with stage III and stage IV ovarian cancer. N Engl J Med 1996;334(1):1–6.
172. Armstrong DK. Relapsed ovarian cancer: challenges and management strate-gies for a chronic disease. Oncologist 2002;7(Suppl. 5):20–8.
173. Markman M. Viewing ovarian cancer as a "chronic disease": what exactly does this mean? Gynecol Oncol 2006;100(2):229–30.
174. Rustin GJ, van der Burg ME, Griffin CL, et al. Early versus delayed treatment of relapsed ovarian cancer (MRC OV05/EORTC 55955): a randomised trial. Lancet 2010;376(9747):1155–63.
175. Gordon AN, Tonda M, Sun S, et al. Long-term survival advantage for women treated with pegylated liposomal doxorubicin compared with topotecan in a phase 3 randomized study of recurrent and refractory epithelial ovarian cancer. Gynecol Oncol 2004;95(1):1–8.
176. Donovan HS, Hartenbach EM, Method MW. Patient-provider communication and perceived control for women experiencing multiple symptoms associated with ovarian cancer. Gynecol Oncol 2005;99(2):404–11.
177. Ozols RF, Bundy BN, Greer BE, et al. Phase III trial of carboplatin and paclitaxel compared with cisplatin and paclitaxel in patients with optimally resected stage

III ovarian cancer: a Gynecologic Oncology Group study. J Clin Oncol 2003; 21(17):3194–200.

178. Cella D, Paul D, Yount S, et al. What are the most important symptom targets when treating advanced cancer? A survey of providers in the National Comprehensive Cancer Network (NCCN). Cancer Invest 2003;21(4): 526–35.

179. Jensen SE, Rosenbloom SK, Beaumont JL, et al. A new index of priority symptoms in advanced ovarian cancer. Gynecol Oncol 2011;120(2):214–9.

180. Gelber RD, Goldhirsch A, Cavalli F. Quality-of-life-adjusted evaluation of adjuvant therapies for operable breast cancer. The International Breast Cancer Study Group. Ann Intern Med 1991;114(8):621–8.

181. Hirte H, Vergote IB, Jeffrey JR, et al. A phase III randomized trial of BAY 12-9566 (tanomastat) as maintenance therapy in patients with advanced ovarian cancer responsive to primary surgery and paclitaxel/platinum containing chemotherapy: a National Cancer Institute of Canada Clinical Trials Group study. Gynecol Oncol 2006;102(2):300–8.

182. Markman M. Management of ovarian cancer. An impressive history of improvement in survival and quality of life. Oncology (Williston Park) 2006;20(4):347–54 [discussion: 354, 357–348, 364 passim].

183. Doyle C, Crump M, Pintilie M, et al. Does palliative chemotherapy palliate? Evaluation of expectations, outcomes, and costs in women receiving chemotherapy for advanced ovarian cancer. J Clin Oncol 2001;19(5):1266–74.

184. Parmar MK, Ledermann JA, Colombo N, et al. Paclitaxel plus platinum-based chemotherapy versus conventional platinum-based chemotherapy in women with relapsed ovarian cancer: the ICON4/AGO-OVAR-2.2 trial. Lancet 2003; 361(9375):2099–106.

185. Pignata S, De Placido S, Biamonte R, et al. Residual neurotoxicity in ovarian cancer patients in clinical remission after first-line chemotherapy with carboplatin and paclitaxel: the Multicenter Italian Trial in Ovarian cancer (MITO-4) retrospective study. BMC Cancer 2006;6:5.

186. Dunton CJ. Management of treatment-related toxicity in advanced ovarian cancer. Oncologist 2002;7(Suppl. 5):11–9.

187. Seiden MV. Ovarian cancer. Oncologist 2001;6(4):327–32.

188. Rose PG, Bundy BN, Watkins EB, et al. Concurrent cisplatin-based radiotherapy and chemotherapy for locally advanced cervical cancer. N Engl J Med 1999; 340(15):1144–53.

189. Hilpert F, Stahle A, Tome O, et al. Neuroprotection with amifostine in the first-line treatment of advanced ovarian cancer with carboplatin/paclitaxel-based chemotherapy: a double-blind, placebo-controlled, randomized phase II study from the Arbeitsgemeinschaft Gynakologische Onkologoie (AGO) Ovarian Cancer Study Group. Support Care Cancer 2005;13(10):797–805.

190. Lorusso D, Ferrandina G, Greggi S, et al. Phase III multicenter randomized trial of amifostine as cytoprotectant in first-line chemotherapy in ovarian cancer patients. Ann Oncol 2003;14(7):1086–93.

191. Annas GJ. Informed consent, cancer, and truth in prognosis. N Engl J Med 1994;330(3):223–5.

192. Available at: http://www.cochrane.org/. Accessed October 4, 2011.

193. Armstrong DK, Bundy B, Wenzel L, et al. Intraperitoneal cisplatin and paclitaxel in ovarian cancer. N Engl J Med 2006;354(1):34–43.

194. Wenzel LB, Huang HQ, Armstrong DK, et al. Health-related quality of life during and after intraperitoneal versus intravenous chemotherapy for optimally

debulked ovarian cancer: a Gynecologic Oncology Group study. J Clin Oncol 2007;25(4):437–43.

195. Markman M. Challenging ovarian cancer: how can we improve quantity and quality of life? MedGenMed 2002;4(4):10.

196. Fleming GF, Brunetto VL, Cella D, et al. Phase III trial of doxorubicin plus cisplatin with or without paclitaxel plus filgrastim in advanced endometrial carcinoma: a Gynecologic Oncology Group study. J Clin Oncol 2004;22(11): 2159–66.

197. McQuellon RP, Thaler HT, Cella D, et al. Quality of life (QOL) outcomes from a randomized trial of cisplatin versus cisplatin plus paclitaxel in advanced cervical cancer: a Gynecologic Oncology Group study. Gynecol Oncol 2006; 101(2):296–304.

198. Bookman MA, Brady MF, McGuire WP, et al. Evaluation of new platinum-based treatment regimens in advanced-stage ovarian cancer: a Phase III Trial of the Gynecologic Cancer Intergroup. J Clin Oncol 2009;27(9):1419–25.

199. Atkins M. Presented at Journal of Clinical Oncology, ASCO Annual Meeting Proceedings. vol. 24, Plenary discussion; 2006.

200. Donnelly CM, Blaney JM, Lowe-Strong A, et al. A randomised controlled trial testing the feasibility and efficacy of a physical activity behavioural change intervention in managing fatigue with gynaecological cancer survivors. Gynecol Oncol 2011;122(3):618–24.

201. Pothuri B, Montemarano M, Gerardi M, et al. Percutaneous endoscopic gastrostomy tube placement in patients with malignant bowel obstruction due to ovarian carcinoma. Gynecol Oncol 2005;96(2):330–4.

202. Abu-Rustum NR, Barakat RR, Venkatraman E, et al. Chemotherapy and total parenteral nutrition for advanced ovarian cancer with bowel obstruction. Gynecol Oncol 1997;64(3):493–5.

203. Matulonis UA, Seiden MV, Roche M, et al. Long-acting octreotide for the treatment and symptomatic relief of bowel obstruction in advanced ovarian cancer. J Pain Symptom Manage 2005;30(6):563–9.

204. Baron TH. Expandable metal stents for the treatment of cancerous obstruction of the gastrointestinal tract. N Engl J Med 2001;344(22):1681–7.

205. Fries JF, Bruce B, Cella D. The promise of PROMIS: using item response theory to improve assessment of patient-reported outcomes. Clin Exp Rheumatol 2005; 23(Suppl. 39):S53–7.

206. Tannock IF, Osoba D, Stockler MR, et al. Chemotherapy with mitoxantrone plus prednisone or prednisone alone for symptomatic hormone-resistant prostate cancer: a Canadian randomized trial with palliative end points. J Clin Oncol 1996;14(6):1756–64.

207. Dobrez D, Cella D, Pickard AS, et al. Estimation of patient preference-based utility weights from the functional assessment of cancer therapy: general. Value Health 2007;10(4):266–72.

208. Cohn DE, Kim KH, Resnick KE, et al. At what cost does a potential survival advantage of bevacizumab make sense for the primary treatment of ovarian cancer? A cost-effectiveness analysis. J Clin Oncol 2011;29(10): 1247–51.

209. Doyle C, Stockler M, Pintilie M, et al. Resource implications of palliative chemotherapy for ovarian cancer. J Clin Oncol 1997;15(3):1000–7.

210. Lewin SN, Buttin BM, Powell MA, et al. Resource utilization for ovarian cancer patients at the end of life: how much is too much? Gynecol Oncol 2005;99(2): 261–6.

211. Lang EV, Benotsch EG, Fick LJ, et al. Adjunctive non-pharmacological analgesia for invasive medical procedures: a randomised trial. Lancet 2000; 355(9214):1486–90.

212. Lakusta CM, Atkinson MJ, Robinson JW, et al. Quality of life in ovarian cancer patients receiving chemotherapy. Gynecol Oncol 2001;81(3):490–5.

213. von Gruenigen VE, Daly BJ. Treating ovarian cancer patients at the end of life: when should we stop? Gynecol Oncol 2005;99(2):255–6.

214. Takeuchi EE, Keding A, Awad N, et al. Impact of patient-reported outcomes in oncology: a longitudinal analysis of patient-physician communication. J Clin Oncol 2011;29(21):2910–7.

215. Kass LR. L'Chaim and its limits: why not immortality? First Things 2001;(113): 17–24.

Index

Note: Page numbers of article titles are in **boldface** type.

A

Abdominal radical trachelectomy, for cervical cancer, 69–70
Adenocarcinoma, vulvar, pathology of, 47–48
Age, epidemiology of ovarian and endometrial cancer, 3–6
Antiangiogenesis therapies, for gynecologic cancers, 133–141
    cervical, 140–141
    endometrial, 140
    ovarian, 133–140

B

Basal cell carcinoma, vulvar, pathology of, 47
Biologic agents. *See* Targeted therapies.
Borderline tumors, ovarian, 97
Bowel obstruction, in gynecologic cancer survivors, 181
BRCA genes, in hereditary breast and ovarian cancer syndrome, 13–18
Breast cancer, hereditary breast and ovarian cancer syndrome, 13–18
    identifying women at risk for, 15–17
    pathology of BRCA-associated, 14
    prognosis and novel therapies, 15
    risk-reducing salpingo-oophorectomy, 17–18
    surveillance, 17

C

Cervical cancer, advances in use of radiation for, 157–161
    new biologic agents for targeted therapy, **133–156**
    precancers, global perspective on, **31–44**
        epidemiology, 32–33
        HPV epidemiology and molecular biology, 33
        HPV infection, immune surveillance, and development of neoplasia, 33–34
        HPV vaccination, 39–40
        limitations of screening worldwide, 38–39
        management of screening abnormalities, 36
        screening and diagnosis, 34–36
        screening in developing settings, 37–38
        treatment options, 36–37
    surgical management of, **63–78**
        fertility-sparing radical surgery, 67–70
        minimally invasive alternatives to radical hysterectomy, 66–67
        pelvic exenteration, 72–74

Hematol Oncol Clin N Am 26 (2012) 195–204
doi:10.1016/S0889-8588(11)00172-9
hemonc.theclinics.com
0889-8588/12/$ – see front matter © 2012 Elsevier Inc. All rights reserved.